Orthopaedics in Infancy and Childhood

Orthopaedics in Infancy and Childhood

Second edition

G. C. Lloyd-Roberts MChir(Cantab.), FRCS
Formerly Consultant Orthopaedic Surgeon, Hospitals for Sick Children, Great Ormond Street
and St George's Hospital, London

J. A. Fixsen, MCh, FRCS
Consultant Orthopaedic Surgeon, Hospitals for Sick Children, Great Ormond Street, London

Butterworth–Heinemann
London   Boston   Singapore   Sydney   Toronto   Wellington

First published 1972
Second edition 1990

© Butterworth–Heinemann Ltd, 1990

British Library Cataloguing in Publication Data
Lloyd-Roberts, G. C. (George Charles) 1918–1986
    Orthopaedics in infancy and childhood. –
2nd ed.
    1. Children. Orthopaedics
I. Title.   II. Fixsen, John A.
617.3
ISBN 750610301

Library of Congress Cataloging-in-Publication Data
Lloyd-Roberts, G. C. (George Charles)
    Orthopaedics in infancy and childhood. – 2nd ed./G.C. Lloyd
-Roberts and J.A. Fixsen
        p. cm.
    Includes bibliographical references.
    ISBN 750610301 :
    1. Pediatric orthopedics.   I. Fixsen, John A.   II. Title.
    [DNLM: 1. Orthopedics–in infancy & childhood.   WS 270 L7930]
RD732.3.C48L56   1989
617.3–dc20
DNLM/DLC
for Library of Congress   89-71251
                                                                CIP

Composition by Genesis Typesetting, Laser Quay, Rochester, Kent
Printed in Great Britain at the University Press, Cambridge

Preface to the Second Edition

The first edition of this book was published in 1971. Its author, the late G. C. Lloyd-Roberts died in January 1986 before the second edition came to fruition. George, as we all knew him, was not very enthusiastic about the production of a second edition. Hence it has been much delayed, despite the undoubted popularity of the first edition. He enlisted my help in general and that of my two colleagues, Peter Webb for the chapter on spinal disorders, and Andrew Jackson for the chapter on the knee. I in my turn have asked many of my colleagues for help and advise, in particular Dr Jon Pritchard for the chapter on bone tumours, the treatment of which has changed so much in the past 15 years.

The aim of the book remains the same. To provide a short concise informative guide to children's orthopaedics for both paediatricians and orthopaedic surgeons, particularly those in training. We have resisted as much as possible an increase in length as the book was never intended to be an exhaustive tome. I have tried to retain as much as possible of George Lloyd-Roberts' distinctive and incisive style, although some of the more anecdotal material, particularly that which was out of date, had to be discarded. I have also retained many of the original references as these remind us that more recent writing often simply repeats or embroiders what has been written earlier.

I must thank Mr Lloyd-Roberts' secretary, Maria Phelan for hours of work on the manuscript and much encouragement. Gillian Clarke has done a marvellous job on editing the material without which I do not think I should ever have finished the task. Finally the Medical Illustration Department at the Hospital for Sick Children have worked extremely hard on the illustrations as the majority of the original ones had been lost and had to be found and re-printed or new ones substituted. I hope that the second edition, which has taken so long to produce, will be considered a worthy successor to the first.

J. A. FIXSEN

Preface to the First Edition

This book was originally intended as a guide to orthopaedic surgery for paediatricians but it has developed rather differently and in its final form will, I hope, be of value to both orthopaedic surgeons and paediatricians. I hope in particular that orthopaedic surgeons in vocational training programmes will gain help and guidance from this book during the time that they are acquiring their experience in orthopaedic surgery of childhood.

If conditions of interest to either specialty are omitted it is because I have not seen them during the last 15 years at The Hospital for Sick Children and elsewhere, or because they do not normally declare themselves before the age of 12 years.

The author of a textbook must accept the possibility that his mind will be henceforward irremediably closed to unfamiliar notions and extraneous influences. Be that as it may, the execution of the task somewhat resembles the judicial variety which when imminent 'clarifies the mind wonderfully'.

My colleagues and friends have helped me considerably with their advice, especially in the areas less familiar to an orthopaedic surgeon. I am specially grateful to those mentioned below and to others, who have both recently and over the years illustrated the darker areas of my uncertainty.

I am indebted to Dr Edward Allen (radiology), Dr Colin Berry (morbid anatomy), Dr Cedric Carter (genetics), Professor Barbara Clayton and Dr Reginald Nassim (metabolic disease), Mr Herbert Eckstein (myelomeningocele), Professor Roger Hardisty (haematology) and Dr John Wilson and Mr Kenneth Till (neurology and neurosurgery) for their generous guidance.

My grateful thanks are also due to me secretary, Miss Maureen Laird, for her forebearance, and to Mr Roger Hoare, who kindly read the manuscript in its final form, for his suggestions.

Lastly, I must acknowledge the contribution of my family. Their dissatisfaction with my preoccupation with this enterprise has hastened its conclusion.

London

G. C. LLOYD-ROBERTS

Acknowledgements

I am very indebted to my colleagues here at Great Ormond Street for their help in producing the second edition of this book. In particular Dr J. Pritchard, Mr P. Webb, Mr A. Jackson and Dr N. Cavanagh, who have all contributed chapters or parts of chapters to the new edition. Also Dr M. Dillon who has given me valuable advice on some sections.

Most of all I must thank my long-suffering secretaries Miss J. Wilson and Miss M. Johnston who have spent hours of time typing the manuscript.

The Medical Illustration Department at the Hospital for Sick Children and the Institute of Child Health have helped enormously in the production of illustrations.

Lastly Miss Gillian Clarke who took on the most difficult task of putting together the new and old manuscripts and without whom I doubt if this second edition would ever have seen the light of day.

Contents

1

The child as an orthopaedic patient

Maturity implies a state of relative physical, emotional, environmental and intellectual stability, whereas in the immature child these factors are always changing. Because appreciation of this apparent truism is fundamental to the successful management of sick children, some of the more important aspects warrant brief discussion.

General development

Without a knowledge of the performance to be expected of a child of a certain age, disability assessment becomes impossible. When a patient is vaguely concerned about delay in motor development and the complaint is valid, the cause may be environmental, emotional, or intellectual, rather than neurological or within the locomotor system. No symptom or sign noted by the parents should ever be dismissed as fanciful.

The difficulty is to establish the significance of the complaint when no abnormal physical signs have been found. An experienced physiotherapist, observing the child at play or in the gymnasium, will frequently be able to confirm or deny that the child's performance falls short of his expected potential. Confirming that a problem exists is vital to the diagnosis of the cause.

Growth

Growth may be either the surgeon's enemy or his ally. It is helpful when correcting a malaligned fracture. It is troublesome when, as a tree growing away from a prevailing wind, increasing deformity develops in response to abnormal pressure such as unbalanced muscle action in patients with myelomeningocele or cerebral palsy. Correction of such deforming forces influencing the growth plates is one of the most important aspects of children's orthopaedics. The growth plates are also sensitive to local disturbances in development, and respond either by inhibition, as in the congenital limb dysplasias (congenital short femur) or by acceleration (congenital arteriovenous communications). Inborn errors, such as achondroplasia, metabolic disorders or endocrine disturbances, produce conspicuous effects. Although less dramatic, the effects of poor nutrition or prolonged ill-health are of great importance.

Adaptability in relation to non-progressive disorders

An adult suffering from hemiplegia secondary to a head injury, having adapted himself to the changed circumstances, develops a relatively static pattern of deformity and function. Not so the baby with cerebral palsy, for here we can expect improvement in function throughout growth, as a quotient of age and experience in relation to the degree of mental and physical damage initially present. This of course assumes a reasonably stable environment and the prevention of disabling secondary deformity or emotional stress. It is important to realize that this improvement is inevitable when considering the effects of 'systems' of treatment.

This adaptability is also well demonstrated in the less complex conditions which are solely mechanical in their presentation. Congenital amputation of the hand is compatible with full function, in contrast to the problems of the adult amputee. Absence of the thumb stimulates the index finger to adopt many of the properties of the thumb, notably the ability to pinch.

Many such examples may be quoted which benefit the child, but sometimes we meet an adaptation which produces a secondary disability. For example, a fixed congenital lumbar scoliosis causes pelvic obliquity and, thus, apparent lengthening of the leg on the side inclined downwards. Not only is the other leg thereby apparently shortened but also it must function and develop in adduction – an unstable position favouring dislocation of the hip. Increase in the apparent shortening may be followed by adaptive leg equalization, in which fixed flexion of the hip and knee on the longer side are added to the original deformity.

Healing and repair

Children recover rapidly from injury or operation – deep and superficial healing are accelerated and wound sepsis is seen much less frequently than in adults. The emotional wound, too, is usually deeper and less readily healed in the parent than in the child, a feature which seems sometimes to be overlooked by those solicitous for the welfare of children in hospital.

The anxiety of both is mitigated if postoperative immobilization excludes both movement of the painful area and prevents the child and mother from seeing the effects of surgery. For both these reasons, plaster of Paris should be used freely in young children. Furthermore, children should be returned to their homes at the earliest moment. For example, there is generally no need to retain a child for more than 3 or 4 days after major hip surgery, if pain and anxiety are relieved by an occlusive plaster.

Although usually fortunate, retrograde amnesia is on occasion a disadvantage, for it demands that injuries receive more prolonged protection than may seem necessary. Thus when a child breaks his tibia it is unwise to remove protection at the stage in healing which would be appropriate in an adult. The child will have already forgotten the fracture, and is likely to be playing football in a few days.

Education

The hospital school developed during the days when skeletal tuberculosis was common. However, because of changing patterns of disease and the general improvement in social conditions, very few children with orthopaedic ailments need now remain in hospital for long periods, and so formal inpatient education is seldom necessary except as occupational therapy.

Nevertheless, we should remember that education implies more than the direct instruction which can be provided in hospital. We must always try to divide the time necessary for treatment into the shortest possible in hospital and the longest at home. Thus the child is not long denied the educational benefits of growing up in a normal environment, with the support, if necessary, of the home tuition service. We must constantly ask ourselves whether the benefit that our patient is likely to gain as an adult, as a result of prolonged inpatient treatment, justifies exposure to the manifest disadvantages. Fortunately, modern orthopaedic practice in conditions such as Perthes' disease, scoliosis and tuberculosis has greatly reduced the time spent in hospital by these patients.

Lastly, we must be alert to the dangers of recommending education in a physically handicapped school, when the physical disability will not prevent the patient from competing on equal terms with his contemporaries when he is grown up. In recent years there has been an encouraging tendency to integrate the physically handicapped into normal schools but the ideal is by no means always possible or available.

The parents

Parents are always an influence in the treatment of children, commonly for the better but unfortunately not always so. Apparent lack of cooperation, obstruction or even antagonism, although not uncommon, are in fact seldom deliberate. Unfortunately, however, whatever their causes or motives these attitudes react adversely on the child. We must therefore try to understand the difficulties and so establish a stable working relationship during the time that we are involved together in the common problem.

The causes of misunderstanding are of course numerous, but most obey a set pattern, the commonest of which are given below.

Anxiety

The parents' understandable anxiety dominates their powers of reasoning and comprehension, so, however carefully the situation is explained to them, they are at best no nearer to an understanding, or at worst leave with new fears based on partially digested statements.

Conflicting statements

These arise more commonly when the child is admitted and another member of the department, medical or nursing, suggests that a line of treatment other than that outlined in the outpatients department will be followed.

Nervousness

This is added to by unfamiliar surroundings, inhibiting their questions or stimulating them to ask the same questions so often, and of so many people, that conflict inevitably arises.

Parental disharmony

The effect is seen at its worst in the mutual child of a separated couple, when both adopt the role of responsible parent.

Uncertainty about the future

This concerns both the sick child and the risk to further children. 'Will he ever walk?' is the commonest unexpressed worry, arising very often when there is no prospect of his doing otherwise. A genetic counselling service should be available at least on a regional basis. Unless the diagnosis is clear and the surgeon well informed on the subject, it is best to ask for expert advice rather than give, however unwittingly, inaccurate information. This subject is discussed further in Chapter 16.

Further reading

Blockey, N. J. (1976) *Children's Orthopaedics – Practical Problems*. London, Boston: Butterworths

Fraser-Roberts, J. A. and Pembury, M. E. (1985) *Introduction to Medical Genetics*, 6th edn. Oxford: Oxford University Press

Harris, N. (1983) *Postgraduate Textbook of Clinical Orthopaedics*. Bristol, London, Boston: Wright P. S. G.

Hensinger, R. N. (1986) *Standards in Pediatric Orthopedics*. New York: Raven Press

Lovell, W. W. and Winter, R. B. (1986) *Pediatric Orthopedics*, 2nd edn. Philadelphia, London: J. B. Lippincott

Sharrard, W. J. W. (1979) *Paediatric Orthopaedics and Fractures*, 2nd edn. Oxford, London: Blackwell Scientific

Tachdjian, M. O. (1987) *Pediatric Orthopedics*, 2nd edn. Philadelphia, London, Toronto: W. B. Saunders

Williams, P. F. (1982) *Orthopaedic Management in Childhood*. Oxford, London: Blackwell Scientific

2

Generalized disorders of the skeleton

In this chapter we have drawn freely from Rubin's monograph (1964), in which the various generalized disorders are described in detail, both in their florid and variant forms as well as in relation to their causes as far as these are known. The reader is also referred to Wynne-Davies and Fairbank (1976) – being a revised edition of Fairbank's original work (1963) which was based on his experience at The Hospitals for Sick Children, London and Wynne-Davies *et al.* (1985). We will concentrate on the typical clinical features, with special reference to associated conditions of importance and, where appropriate, discuss treatment.

Diseases of the epiphysis

Dysplasia epiphysealis hemimelica (Trevor's disease)

Osteochondromas develop eccentrically in the epiphysis; most commonly at the ankle (Figure 2.1), knee and hip, being confined characteristically to one side of the body and epiphysis. The patient presents with a hard swelling close to a joint, with possibly some loss of movement and deformity due to its eccentric position. At first delayed calcification in the transparent chondroma may obscure the diagnosis. In a puzzling hip joint, progressive subluxation, stiffness and deformity of obscure origin was found at operation to be due to this.

Treatment involves surgical remodelling of the epiphysis by excision of the osteocartilaginous overgrowth. There seems little tendency to recurrence.

Spondyloepiphyseal dysplasia (SED) (osteochondrodystrophy)

In this group of diseases epiphyseal growth is disordered and the vertebrae are flattened. There are two distinct entities. The mild

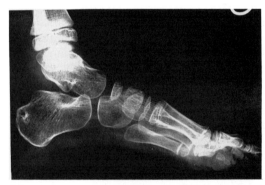

(a)

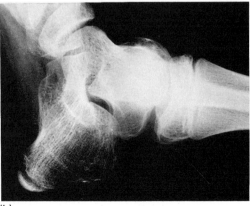

(b)

Figure 2.1 Trevor's disease (dysplasia epiphysealis hemimelica). (a) An osteochondroma is seen on the convex surface of the talus within the ankle joint. (b) This illustrates the destructive effect on the joint

X-linked form, spondyloepiphyseal dysplasia tarda, and the more severe dominantly inherited congenita form. The patients are of short stature with dysplastic joints, the hips, shoulders and knees being particularly affected. In the congenital form there is gross retardation of ossification of the femoral head with severe coxa vara. In the milder form, osteoarthritis is a problem in early adult life. In the severe form, problems will develop at the hips, in the spine from atlantoaxial instability and in the eye with myopia, retinal detachment and glaucoma.

The condition should be distinguished from Morquio's disease (mucopolysaccharidosis type IV) in which keratin sulphate is present in the urine.

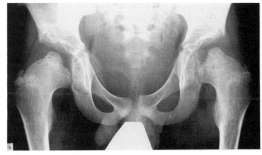

(a)

Multiple epiphyseal dysplasia (MED)

Multiple epiphyseal dysplasia (dysplasia epiphysealis multiplex) is a familial disorder of variable severity. There is some stunting of growth and the joint symptoms often progress later to degenerative arthritis. Apart from shortening, the child is likely to present with hip or knee problems (Figure 2.2 a, b and c). The appearances of the hips may be wrongly interpreted as showing bilateral Perthes' disease. Whenever Perthes' disease is suspected bilaterally, it is prudent to take further radiographs of wrist and ankle, where the typical lateral wedging of the epiphyses is most commonly found. X-rays of the knees show flattening and irregularity of the epiphyses, and other joints should be X-rayed to confirm the diagnosis. Treatment in childhood is usually unnecessary, but occasionally the hips require relief from weight bearing during painful episodes (Maudsley, 1955).

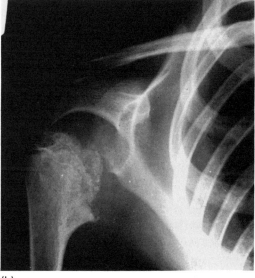

(b)

Chondrodysplasia punctata (Conradi's disease)

This is probably a mixed group showing stippling of the epiphyses and extraepiphyseal calcification in infancy. There is a severe rhizomelic form associated with very short limbs, bilateral cataracts and psychomotor retardation. Death occurs in the perinatal period or first year of life. The milder Conradi Hunermann form shows less limb shortening and has a much better prognosis.

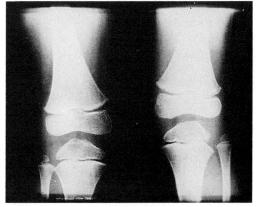

(c)

Figure 2.2 Multiple epiphysealis dysplasia (MED). (a) The hips show flattening and deformity of the femoral heads. Note corresponding acetabular changes. (b) Similar changes at the shoulder joint. (c) The knees, showing characteristic widening of the intercondylar notch

Diastrophic dwarfism

These crooked (diastrophic) dwarfs resemble achondroplasic dwarfs very closely, both clinically and radiologically, but the distinction is of great importance. Diastrophic dwarfism is transmitted as an autosomal recessive. Achondroplasia is an autosomal dominant, so most individuals with the disorder do not reproduce and therefore most cases arise in the population as a result of new mutations.

Although the radiographs are virtually identical except for the skull which is normal in diastrophic dwarfs, the clinical features are quite distinct. Unlike achondroplasiacs, diastrophic dwarfs have multiple peripheral deformities. Club feet, deformities of the hands, dislocated hips (Figure 2.3), scoliosis, deformities of the knees and elbow, and cleft palate are all common.

Furthermore the ears resemble those of a well tested pugilist – the familiar 'cauliflower ear' of that profession. Treatment is difficult, for the deformities are resistant as in arthrogryposis, but respond similarly to aggressive surgery (Wilson, Chrispin and Carter, 1969).

Diseases of the epiphyseal (growth) plate

Achondroplasia

Achondroplasic dwarfs are the commonest type – the familiar circus clown and strong man. Great strength and shortness combine to disqualify them from weight-lifting contests. The trunk is large in proportion to the limbs, and the head, (which is sometimes hydrocephalic) to the face, which is remarkable for frontal bosses and saddle nose. The trident fingers are of near-equal length. Lumbar lordosis and waddling gait may simulate hip dislocation. The narrow pelvic outlet, once a means of selective culling, is now circumvented by caesarean section. In spite of this, the neonatal mortality remains high due to hydrocephalus. Severe bow-leggedness may be an added handicap and requires corrective osteotomy. The neural canal is markedly narrow in the lumbar region making these patients peculiarly prone to compression by a prolapsed intravertebral disc in this region. Such compression demands operation.

Metaphyseal chondrodysplasia

This is an ill-defined group characterized by a failure of growth plate cartilage to remain in ordered columns. There are three main types: type Jansen; type Schmid, which is considerably less severe; and type McKusick, otherwise known as cartilage hair hypoplasia. They show varying degrees of short stature associated with bowing of the long bones which may be mistaken for rickets or dyschondroplasia.

Arachnodactyly (Marfan's syndrome)

Arachnodactyly is associated with multiple abnormalities in various systems. As the name implies, long, thin fingers and toes are prominent features, but these and other

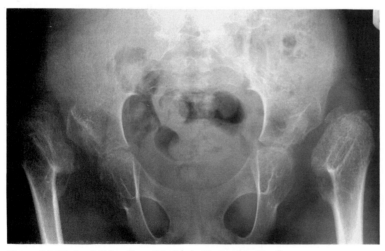

Figure 2.3 Bilateral dislocation of the hip in diastrophic dwarfism

skeletal abnormalities develop late and are not likely to be recognized in early childhood. In contrast, palatal defect, dislocation of the lens, deafness, congenital heart disease (notably aortic aneurysm) and polycystic kidney and lung may present earlier, thus disclosing the diagnosis.

The skeletal features, apart from the hands and feet, comprise scoliosis and joint laxity in an adolescent of uncommon slightness and height for his age. Radiographs show the bones to be long and thin, but otherwise normal. Although usually mild and of late onset, the scoliosis may progress to a degree for which spinal fusion is necessary. Joint laxity may be severe, predisposing to habitual joint dislocation of the patella in particular. The long, thin feet with poor ligamentous support roll into pronation and are frequently sufficiently painful to demand surgical stabilization. Joint laxity is of particular interest in Marfan's disease, for it is of the severe degree seen in osteogenesis imperfecta and both share a tendency to deafness and blue sclera. The suspensory ligament laxity does not, however, seem to cause dislocation of the lens in osteogenesis imperfecta.

Dyschondroplasia (Ollier's disease)

In dyschondroplasia (Figure 2.4 a and b) there is a failure of orderly ossification of the cartilaginous columns of the growth plate, so arrest occurs in the form of translucent metaphyseal chondromas. The process takes time, so it is unlikely to be present in the very young and, although predominantly unilateral, this is not absolute. The clinical features are predictable – widening of the metaphysis, shortening and a liability to fracture. Sometimes, especially when the hands and feet are involved, angiomatous malformations develop in the overlying skin (Maffucci's syndrome).

Treatment may be needed when tumours become massive and unsightly, or interfere with function. Sometimes inequality of leg length requires leg lenthening. Rarely, abnormality in the sphenoid causes cranial nerve disturbance and pituitary dysfunction.

Gargoylism (Hunter-Hurler syndrome, mucopolysaccharidosis I)

Although still classified among the general diseases of the skeleton, gargoylism is metabolic in origin, being a glycoprotein storage disease. The deposits are derived from abnormal mucopolysaccharides which are deposited in excess in the tissues and excreted in the urine. The abnormal urinary constituent is detected by toluidine blue, which becomes purple.

Normal at birth, these children gradually coarsen in appearance and later become obviously dwarfed and defective. The coarse skin and features are both a characteristic and hideous combination – swollen eyelids, lips and tongue, flat nose with flared nostrils, and corneal opacity. The swollen belly topped by umbilical hernia accommodates the liver and spleen, enlarged by cells overloaded and swollen by the abnormal mucopolysaccharide. Similarly, the lymph glands are frequently enlarged. Joints stiffen, especially the hands and spine. Radiologically, the appearances are superficially similar to spondyloepiphyseal dysplasia except that the spinal wedging is confined to the upper lumbar segments where there is an acute angular kyphosis.

Life is fortunately short and within its span no temptation is offered to the surgeon.

Ellis–Van Creveld syndrome (chondroectodermal dysplasia)

The significance of the Ellis–Van Creveld syndrome, which is largely confined to the distal parts of the limbs, is that its recognition should focus attention on the cardiovascular system, which is often affected.

The forearms and lower legs are short in comparison with their proximal segments. Polydactyly and finger and toe deformities (Figure 2.5) with aplastic nails and teeth suggest the diagnosis. Radiographs demonstrate metacarpal and metatarsal confusion, with duplication and cross-unions. Knock knees are common and seem due to maldevelopment of the lateral side of the upper tibial epiphysis. This may require surgical correction, as may the feet in the interests of shoe-fitting, and the hands for polydactyly.

Diseases of the metaphysis

Hypophosphatasia

In hypophosphatasia there is either a failure to produce, or excessive destruction of, alkaline phosphatase, and this is demonstrable in the

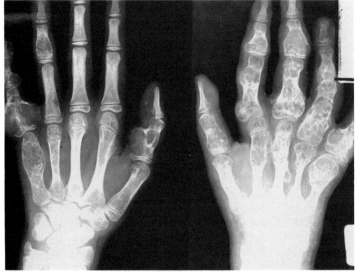

(a)

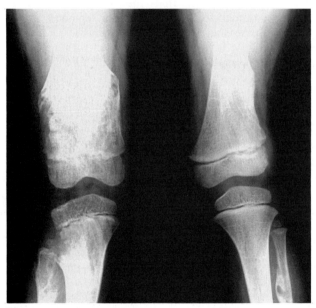

(b)

Figure 2.4 Dyschondroplasia (Ollier's disease, multiple enchondromatosis). (a) Multiple enchondromas in the hands, causing considerable deformity. (b) Knees of same patient, also showing deformity

peripheral blood. The familial influence is sometimes shown by a consistently low, although not clinically obtrusive, level in maternal blood. Lack of this enzyme inhibits the deposition of mineral salts in the mature chondroblasts and osteogenic matrix, thus the clinical and radiological features resemble rickets in a most florid form. The error is encouraged by the clinical state of the baby, who is poorly from the start, prone to intestinal upsets and infectious diseases, and deformed as the softened bones bend. Unlike rickets, the

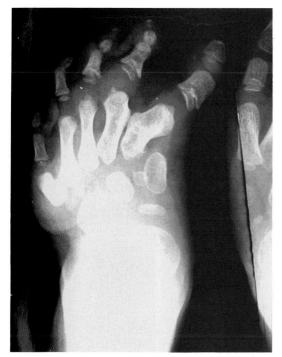

Figure 2.5 Ellis–Van Creveld syndrome (chondroectodermal dysplasia). Note the multiple abnormalities of metatarsals and phalanges with marked hallux varus

condition may be evident at birth or even *in utero* and in these cases the neonatal mortality is high. The survivors, however, frequently improve gradually.

Treatment is largely supportive during the acute early phase, but craniostenosis must be watched for and relieved by surgery to prevent blindness or mental impairment (Schlesinger, Luder and Bodian, 1955).

Osteopetrosis (Albers-Schonberg disease)

Osteopetrosis (Figure 2.6) and osteogenesis imperfecta constitute the two main familial varieties of brittle bone disease. There are two distinct forms of osteopetrosis. The severe variety presents at birth or in early infancy and is of great severity. Death usually occurs in the first decade from obliteration of the marrow cavities and pancytopenia. The less severe or tarda form described by Albers-Schonberg is later in onset and milder in degree.

Recently bone marrow transplants have been used in a few severe cases with dramatic improvement.

Radiographs show homogenous, radio-opaque long bones of normal length and contour except for widening of the metaphysis. Curious bands of translucency are seen in the centre of vertebral bodies and parallel to the iliac crest. Fractures develop from clear-cut partial cracks, reminiscent of stress fractures, later becoming complete and displacing or causing deformity such as coxa vara. More important than fractures are the secondary effects seen in severely affected children. Marrow function is depressed and anaemia develops with its secondary effects – enlargement of the liver, the spleen and the lymph glands. The mortality in this group is high but the less anaemic survive to develop fractures and deformity. Anaemia may recur later, together with hydrocephalus and cranial nerve plates due to foraminal stenosis.

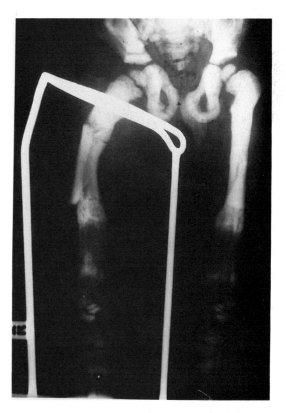

Figure 2.6 Osteopetrosis (Albers-Schonberg disease). Note the pathological fracture of the right femur and the grossly increased density of the bones. Although very hard, these bones are very brittle

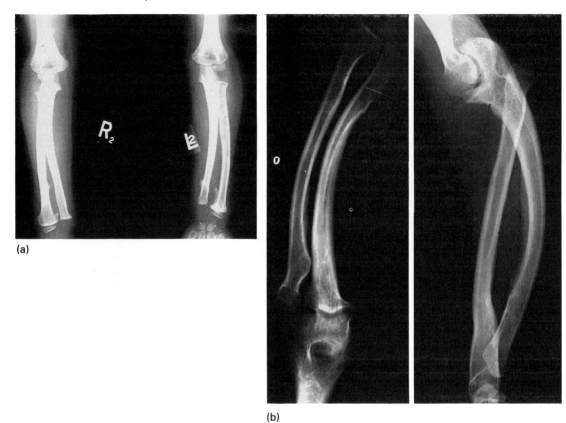

(a)

(b)

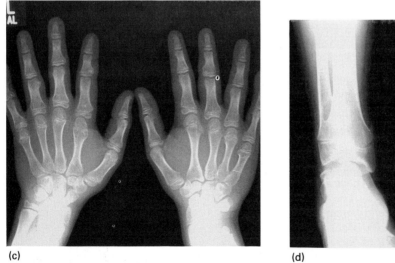

(c)

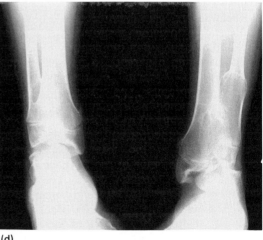

(d)

Figure 2.7 Multiple hereditary exostosis (diaphyseal aclasis). (a) Small osteochondroma in the distal forearm. (b) Same patient, showing later deformity with shortening and bowing of the ulna and dislocation of the radial head. (c) Hands in multiple hereditary exostosis. (d) Deformity at the ankle, due to exostoses

Multiple hereditary exostoses (diaphyseal aclasis)

Diaphyseal aclasis (Figure 2.7) is a familial disease, characterized by cartilage-capped osteomas at the metaphyses or proximal diaphyses, which may grow till maturity. Boys are predominantly affected and there may be moderate retardation of growth.

The condition seems to be due to displacement of a segment of growth plate from its periphery. Once separated, growth continues eccentrically, cartilage being gradually replaced by bone in the usual fashion. If the disturbance is general the result is multiple osteochondromas which migrate distally from a widened, poorly modelled metaphysis, the cartilage cap leading. It is not uncommon to count 20 or more in one patient. Provided that they are viewed in profile, radiographs, readily demonstrate the tumours, which may be pedunculated or sessile. Otherwise they may be seen as sclerotic crescents lying within the boundaries of the bone, simulating cysts.

The effects may be either those of the individual tumours or those of growth plate disturbance, that is retardation or cessation of growth and deformity. Osteochondromas may, by their size or situation, upset function – examples are a small tumour over which a tendon snaps, or a large cauliflower in the axilla preventing adduction of the arm. Rarely, the spinal cord or major nerves and vessels are displaced. In all these circumstances removal is indicated.

The evidence of sarcomatous degeneration is a contentious issue. Jaffe (1958) suggested 11% and others more than 5%. One must assume that they refer to patients and not tumours, but even so the incidence quoted is far in excess of that acceptable from clinical experience. We can recall no such sarcomas developing during childhood in this relatively common disorder (Solomon 1963).

Diseases of the diaphysis

Osteogenesis imperfecta (fragilitas ossium)

Osteogenesis imperfecta is the relatively common variety of brittle bone disease and is essentially congenital osteoporosis – that is to say there is a failure of bone matrix formation. These patients have been shown to have a defect in the formation of Type I collagen. The disease is familial, showing a tendency for severely involved children to be born of parents with mild manifestations. There is a wide spectrum ranging from stillbirth with multiple fractures to apparently normal children prone to fractures from minor violence. The most recent classification is that of Sillence, Senn and Danks (1979) into four main types.

The features in any patient will depend upon the severity of the manifestation, but all display narrow, porotic, long bones, lacking the normal cortical thickness. Many show deformities due to bending of softened bones under physiological stresses – examples being serpiginous ribs (due to negative pleural pressure) and triradiate pelvis. Some deformities predispose to fractures by weakening the architectural stability or the proximal femur bends into varus. Radiographs of the skull usually disclose wormian bones (islands of ossification in non-ossified membrane), bitemporal bulging and platybasia. Some other characteristics include hypotonia and joint laxity, which may contribute to the disability when severe pronated feet or hyperextended knees result. The essential dysplasia may be seen in the teeth, which are small, brown, deformed and carious. Blue sclerotics and deafness may be seen but are by no means always present. It is important to remember the increased capillary permeability which encourages bleeding at operation. Fracture healing is associated with excessive callus formation which may be confused with sarcomatous change. This, though often suspected, in fact very rarely happens. In young patients without blue sclerotics and no family history, fractures in early infancy may be mistaken for non-accidental injury.

In management we are involved in a vicious circle of fracture, immobilization, porosis, predisposing to further fracture and deformity. This pattern of deterioration has been alleviated by the development of the operation in which the deformed bone – often the femur – is cut into multiple segments subperiosteally, which are then threaded over an intramedullary nail (Sofield and Millar, 1959). Union is rapid, and the technique not only provides some increased internal stability to the bone, but, perhaps more important, also corrects deformity which itself invites further fracture.

Nails often need to be replaced as growth proceeds, although the expanding-type nail can reduce this (Bailey and Dubow, 1981; Lang-Stevenson and Sharrard, 1984).

Although nails may be used in any long bone prone to repeated fractures, they have their greatest usefulness in femurs and tibias (Figure 2.8). In general this technique is not suitable for very severely afflicted and bed-ridden children or those with the cystic bone variant of the disease. Errors include failure to appreciate the extent of blood loss due to the capillary abnormality, an insufficient number of segments cut, and the need to ream out those cases with the 'thick boned' variety of the disease. Some bone must be sacrificed in correcting bowing. The nail should pass through the lower femoral epiphyseal plate to reduce the tendency to upward migration and should be replaced immediately if, with growth and deformity, it penetrates the cortex of the supracondylar area. The so-called 'airsplint' developed by Morel in France can be useful as

an external splint once the bones have been straightened.

Medical treatment is unavailing. Studies in hydroxyproline excretion suggested that anabolic steroids might be of value, but early promise has not been realized. Apparent improvement shown by a decreased rate of fracture may be due to many causes – not least a tendency for abatement to a more benign pattern with time. Side effects are serious and seem an unjustified hazard when the benefit is uncertain (Cattell and Clayton, 1968).

Idiopathic osteoporosis

Idiopathic osteoporosis is a curious and unexplained rare condition, afflicting older children and, like Cushing's disease, may present as backache following minor injury. The radiograph shows generalized porosis and vertebral collapse. There is no demonstrable biochemical abnormality and the prognosis is good. Of two personal examples, one presented after a

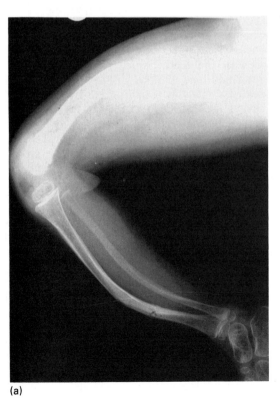

(a)

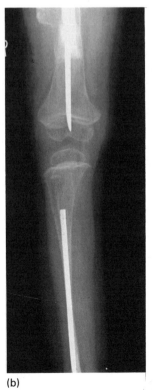

(b)

Figure 2.8 Osteogenesis imperfecta. (a) Bowing of the femur and tibia. Note the thin cortices of the bones, recent fracture of the tibia and signs of an earlier fracture in the femur. (b) Some time after intramedullary nailing. Telescopic nails are much preferable to those used here

fall from a cinema seat, due to unbridled laughter; the other during the transference of a pedicle flap, the spine being necessarily flexed for 3 weeks.

Engelmann's disease (progressive diaphyseal dysplasia)

In Engelmann's disease, there is generalized diaphyseal thickening probably periosteal in origin but of unknown cause. Affected children are poorly, delayed in motor and intellectual achievement, and suffer from bone pains. Prognosis varies from recovery to progressive disability.

Chronic idiopathic hyperphosphatasia

Chronic idiopathic hyperphosphatasia has the features of Paget's disease in the young, with leontiasis ossea as a frequent accompaniment. Juvenile Paget's disease (osteitis deformans) is

an accurate clinical and radiological description of the child with bowed spine and legs. At operation on one patient, the thickened periosteum stripped to reveal a vascular pitted femoral cortex which broke transversely at the tap of an osteotome seeking a histological specimen. The severity of the condition is variable. Some patients are severely deformed and incapacitated; in others, overgrowth of bone may obliterate the nasal passages, cause pressure on cranial nerves and anaemia due to obliteration of marrow cavities.

Craniocleidodysostosis

These intelligent children are somewhat dwarfed and exhibit the ability to approximate the points of their shoulders in front of the chest. This is due to dysplasia of the clavicles which may be absent, either wholly or at their outer ends. Sometimes there is bilateral

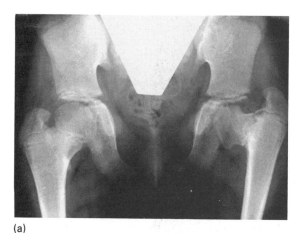

(a)

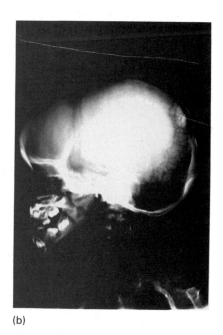

(b)

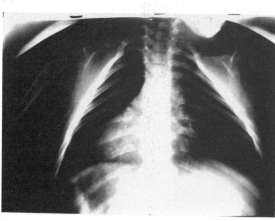

(c)

Figure 2.9 Craniocleidodysostosis. (a) Coxa vara is present on both sides, with a defect of the pubic symphysis. (b) Lateral X-ray of the skull. Note the open fontanelles and numerous wormian bones. (c) X-ray of the chest and shoulders. Note that the clavicles are absent

pseudarthrosis, distinguishing this condition from congenital unexplained pseudarthrosis which is unilateral. The skull, also membranous, is also affected, the frontal bones being prominent and the frontal suture remaining open. The pubic symphysis is defective, resembling that in ectopia vesicae. Care should be taken to exclude infantile coxa vara (Figure 2.9), which is not uncommon, and is treated in the conventional way. This condition is compatible with a normal life.

Melorheostosis

Melorheostosis is readily diagnosed from radiographs because of the well known appearance of dripping candle wax within the bones. Diagnosis, however, is but a stimulus to search for associated abnormalities. Pain usually overlies affected bones, and is a constant symptom of varying severity treatable only by analgesics. Fibrosis is common. When superficial, it is associated with scleroderma; when deep, with joint contractures. Disorders of bone growth may cause inequality of limb length and bony deformity. Treatment is directed towards the correction of progressive disabling deformity (Campbell, Papademetriou and Bonfiglio, 1968).

References

Albright, J. A. (1981) Management overview of osteogenesis imperfecta *Clin. Orthop. Rel. Res.* **159**, 80–87

Bailey, R. W., Dubow, H. I. (1981) Evolution of the concept of an extensible nail accommodating to normal longitudinal growth: clinical consideration and implications. *Clin. Orthop. Rel. Res.*, **159**, 157–170.

Campbell, C. J., Papademetriou, T. and Bonfiglio, M (1969) Melorheostosis. *J. Bone Jt. Surg.* **50A**, 1281

Cattell, H. S. and Clayton, B. (1968) Failure of anabolic steroids in the therapy of osteogenesis imperfecta. *J. Bone Jt. Surg.* **50A**, 123

Fairbank, T. (1963) *General Disease of the Skeleton*. 2nd edn. Edinburgh: Churchill Livingstone

Jaffe, H. L. (1958) *Tumours and Tumorous Conditions of Bones and Joints*. London: Henry Kimpton

Lang-Stevenson, A. I., Sharrard, W. J. W. (1984) Intramedullary loading with Bailey-Dubow extensible rods in osteogenesis imperfecta. *J. Bone Jt. Surg.*, **66-B**, 227–232.

Maudsley, R. H. (1955) Dysplasia epiphysialis multiplex. *J. Bone Jt. Surg.*, **37B**, 228

Rubin, P. (1964) *Dynamic Classification of Bone Dysplasias*. Chicago: Year Book Medical Publishers

Schlesinger, B., Luder, J. and Bodian, M. (1955) Rickets with alkaline phosphatase deficiency. *Archives of Disease in Childhood*, **30**, 265

Sillence, D. O., Senn, A. S. and Danks, D. M. (1979) Genetic heterogeneity in osteogenesis imperfecta. *J. Med. Genetics*, **16**, 101

Sofield, H. A. and Millar, E. A. (1959) Fragmentation, realignment, and intramedullary rod fixation of deformities of the long bones in children. *J. Bone Jt. Surg.* **41A**, 1371

Solomon, L. (1963) Hereditary multiple exostosis. *J. Bone Jt. Surg.* **45B**, 292

Wilson, D. W., Chrispin, A. R. and Carter, C. O. (1969) Diastrophic dwarfism. *Archs. Dis. Childh.* **44**, 48

Wynne-Davies, R., Hall, C. A. and Apley, A. G. (1985) *Atlas of Skeletal Dysplasias*. Edinburgh: Churchill Livingstone

Further reading

Smith, R., Francis, M. J. O., Houghton, G. R. (1983) *The Brittle Bone Syndrome: Osteogenesis Imperfecta*, Butterworths, London

Spranger, J. W., Langer, L. O. and Weidemann, H.-R. (1974) *Bone Dysplasias* Philadelphia, Toronto: W. B. Saunders

Wynne-Davies, R., Hall, C. M. and Apley, A. G. (1985) *Atlas of Skeletal Dysplasias*. Edinburgh, London, New York: Churchill Livingstone

3

Vascular and lymphatic systems

In this chapter we will discuss the main disorders of the vascular and lymphatic systems under three main headings: disorders of the blood vessels, disorders of the blood and disorders of the lymphatic system.

Disorders of the blood vessels

Superficial haemangiomas

The main significance of superficial haemangiomas is as a stimulus to suspect deeper vascular abnormality to be a cause of inequality of limb length or of an obscure tumour of joint or limb. They are usually obvious as fine capillary or flat port wine birthmarks. Sometimes, however, a slight pink flush or brown pigment may be the only clue, but if this is associated with local warmth the implication is clear. They are of singular importance when seen over the spine where they frequently signal an underlying spinal abnormality (dysraphism).

Subcutaneous haemangiomas

As haemangiolipoma, subcutaneous haemangiomas are common tumours in childhood, being often found on the front of the thigh. Apart from swelling, haemorrhage may occur, and pain, bruising and enlargement cause alarm. Although not encapsulated, they are readily removed and do not recur.

In contrast, and rarer, are the infiltrating types which also involve muscle with a tendency to spread widely. Total excision may be difficult and, if incomplete, they tend to recur. They are more properly regarded as hamartomas (Gonzalez-Crussi, Enneking and Arean, 1966).

Deep haemangiomas

The cavernous variety of deep haemangiomas are responsible for local or general gigantism (Figure 3.1). Localized or peripheral tumours may be excised, and sometimes this involves

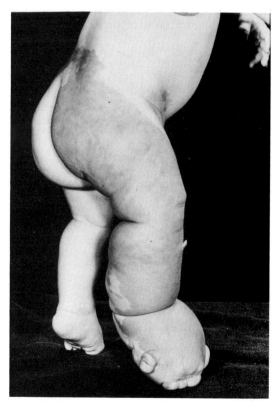

Figure 3.1 Gigantism and haemangiomatosis

15

loss of a giant digit. Diffuse gigantism is a potentially dangerous condition. Repeated deep haemorrhage causes not only an intractable anaemia, but also thrombocytopenia, as the platelets are unequal to the task of repairing the leaks. This compounds the danger, and in one patient urgent hip disarticulation was necessary not only to remove a useless extremity but also to save life. Another baby was found dead in her cot.

Synovial haemangiomas

If diffuse, synovial haemangiomas present as an unexplained, boggy joint swelling, warm to the touch and subject to recurrent effusion and progressive loss of movement, thus resembling a low grade inflammatory lesion or rheumatoid arthritis. The similarity is enhanced by epiphyseal precocity. Phleboliths are a valuable diagnostic clue. Total excision is difficult and postoperative stiffness a hazard, so it is fortunate that they tend to involute with time. It is interesting to speculate upon their relationship to villonodular synovitis, which is rarely seen in young children. The pedunculated variety may cause recurrent haemarthrosis or instability in the manner of a loose body, but are easily excised (Lewis, Coventry and Soule, 1959).

Haemangioma of the bone (disappearing bone disease)

Haemangioma of the bone (Figure 3.2) is a rare but fascinating condition in which there is usually an added lymphoid element. Bones are eroded, fracture, and become radiolucent through loss of mineral content. Later they seem to disappear, resembling somewhat changes in neurofibromatosis. The process reverses with time, and in an ulna radiolucent except for the olecranon, complete restoration occurred. It is therefore important to maintain alignment of fractures by medullary nails. In one case with fractured radius and ulna, a useful forearm resulted from spontaneous healing of the nailed radius. This tumour may be lethal if it develops in vital sites. Thus a cervicothoracic haemangioma killed through chylothorax and finally quadriplegia. Both circular angiomatous bone defects in long bones and the vertebral striated type are exceedingly rare. in children (Gorham and Stout, 1955).

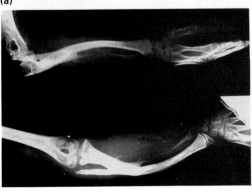

(a)

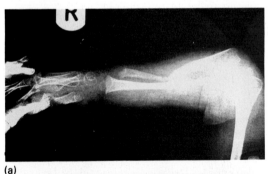

(c)

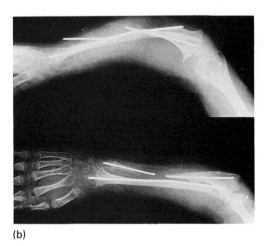

(b)

Figure 3.2 (a) Lateral view of the forearm, showing pathological fracture of both bones in association with haemangioma of the bone. (b) Union of the radius after grafting and fixation; the ulna remains un-united. (c) Cross-union of the ulna to the radius, to stabilize the forearm as a 'one bone' forearm

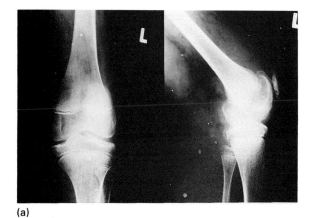

(a)

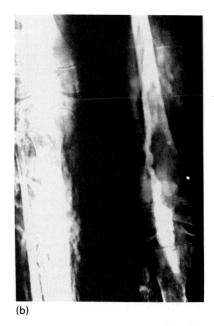

(b)

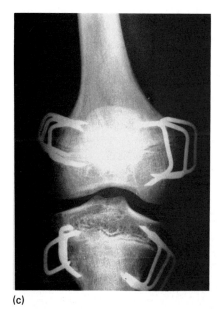

(c)

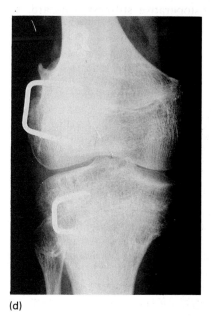

(d)

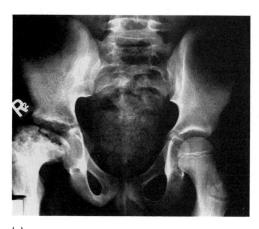

(e)

Figure 3.3 (a) Arteriovenous fistula affecting the knee.
Note the phlebitis and the intra-articular changes. (b)
Arteriogram of the same patient. (c) Staples inserted to try
to control overgrowth. (d) Control of growth is only
partially successful. (e) Perthes'-like changes in the hip,
suggestive of relative ischaemia of the femoral head

Congenital arteriovenous fistulae

Congenital arteriovenous fistulae (Figure 3.3) are usually multiple, and present as unilateral enlargement of a limb, often with some loss of normal contour. The skin is warm, pinkish or naevoid, with prominent superficial veins. Ulceration is common and may be so aggressive that Kaposi's angiosarcoma is simulated. Audible bruits in the line of main vessels, and sometimes the bradycardia phenomenon, complete the clinical picture. Arteriography confirms the diagnosis and demonstrates the position and number of shunts when there is doubt about treatment or diagnosis. Estimation of oxygen content of venous blood is less reliable because intraosseous stasis may cause misleadingly low readings. Multiple shunts are not amenable to surgical correction – indeed, attempts may be followed by gangrene, especially if the main arterial supply is ligated so that blood returns more readily via enlarged venous channels, thus starving the periphery. Heart failure is well recognized and feared, for it may dictate amputation. Nevertheless, this is rare except when the shunts are large and proximal in the limb.

Treatment is mainly a question of leg equalization by epiphysiodesis or leg shortening. Undue haemorrhage need not be feared for postoperative elevation and firm bandaging control it. Localized communications may be multiple, involving part of a limb, as in digital gigantism, or single shunts. It is tempting to treat such apparently isolated fistulae, but in two patients immediate success was spoilt by the subsequent opening of other previously non-functioning communications. There is a variation in which one large shunt is demonstrable, and this can be corrected by surgery or embolization.

Disorders of the blood

Sickle cell anaemia

This familial haemolytic anaemia occurs largely in negroes, but in significant proportion, for 10% of Jamaicans carry the abnormality – haemaglobin S. In most cases there is no demonstrable effect (sickle cell trait).

Symptoms are due to episodes of corpuscular fragility in which sickle cells appear in the peripheral blood, undergo haemolysis, clump and block capillaries by sludging (sickle cell crises). Such children are poorly and leg ulcers are common. Chronic anaemia is reflected in the bones by the generalized porosis due to marrow hyperplasia. This is most marked in the vertebrae, which may collapse as in senile porosis. They are, nevertheless, relatively fit between crises. The crises, which usually occur spontaneously, may be precipitated by anoxia, and so all negroes should be screened preoperatively. The capillary clumping may affect the intestinal tract, brain or kidneys, but most commonly affects the skeletal system.

Bone crises cause severe pain of rapid onset. Local heat, a fever and leucocytosis make the distinction from osteomyelitis very difficult, especially as these children are prone to secondary infection in the affected bones. Further difficulty is caused by ischaemic aseptic sequestra and secondary periostitis. In the absence of infection, symptoms abate and the bone heals, but antibiotics should be given as a precaution against osteomyelitis. Femoral capital necrosis simulates Perthes' disease and behaves similarly (Figure 3.4). Splenectomy is

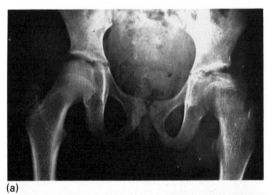
(a)

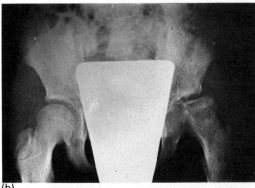
(b)

Figure 3.4 Sickle cell disease (homozygous Ss form). (a) Perthes'-like changes in the left femoral head. (b) Further progression of the change, 18 months later

believed to reduce the incidence of crises, but only if the spleen is enlarged (Golding, 1956, 1959).

Thalassaemia (Cooley's Mediterranean anaemia)

Thalassaemia is also a familial haemolytic anaemia of non-Anglo-Saxons, being common among Eastern Mediterranean peoples. In its 'minor' form the abnormal gene is present, but does not obtrude clinically, being thus analogous to the sickle cell trait.

In the 'major' variety there is a high infant mortality, and survivors have a severe anaemia with exaggerated secondary effects on the skeleton, due to the hyperplastic marrow. In addition to these features (also seen in sickling anaemia) the porotic bones are short with prominent trabeculae, especially in the hands. Hyperplastic haemopoietic marrow may widen bones or cause scalloping of cortices. Sun-ray spicules on the skull vertex are well described as resembling a calcified crew-cut (Middlemiss and Raper, 1966).

Haemophilia

In this well known X-linked recessive disorder, affecting males through females, there is a deficiency of factor VIII. Carrier females are said to be unaffected but often have a low circulating level of factor VIII and therefore may bleed excessively after minor trauma. The severity of the disorder is closely related to the level of factor VIII in the blood. No bleeding tendency is seen if the circulating level is above 50% of normal. Between 25 and 50% of normal bleeding occurs only following major injury. Severe bleeding after minor trauma occurs with levels from 25% down to 1% and only below 1% does spontaneous bleeding occur. This last type of bleeding often affects the musculoskeletal system, with significant orthopaedic implications (Figure 3.5).

Haemarthrosis

Haemarthrosis may present either as acute haemorrhages within relatively normal joints or with the symptoms of repeated episodes in the past. They usually appear for the first time when the child starts to walk. The most common site is the knee, followed by the elbow and the ankle (Houghton and Duthie, 1979).

Acute haemorrhages are usually painless. Sometimes the patient gets a local pricking discomfort, and if he can be given a prophylactic dose of factor VIII at this stage the problem may be rapidly resolved. Minor bleeds therefore, if seen early, can be managed in the outpatient department by prompt administration of factor VIII. However, major bleeds, and all those seen after a period of 12 hours, require treatment by immobilization in a plaster back-slab, compression bandaging and

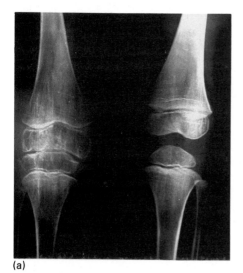 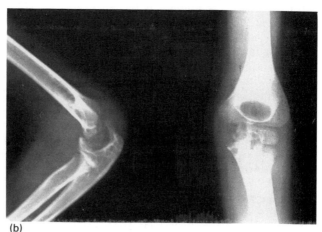

(a)   (b)

Figure 3.5 (a) Haemophilia of the knees, showing degenerative changes and epiphyseal enlargement in the right knee. (b) Haemophilia in the right elbow showing similar changes

factor replacement. If possible, aspiration should be avoided in acute haemarthrosis although it is sometimes used in late chronic haemarthrosis. Following acute haemarthrosis it is most important to rehabilitate the joint carefully with graduated exercises and splintage to regain muscle strength and to prevent the development of joint contracture and deformity.

Late or chronic haemarthrosis

This develops after recurrent acute haemarthroses which have not settled or responded satisfactorily to treatment. They present with a swollen boggy knee due to both haemarthrosis and synovial hypertrophy. Again, the basis of all conservative treatment is compression, immobilization and replacement of factor VIII. This may have to be continued for at least 3–4 weeks followed by a careful rehabilitation programme. If there is persistent swelling, which is largely fluid rather than synovial, there is a place for aspiration. If swelling persists which is largely synovial, synovectomy may be indicated, as it has been shown to lead to a reduction in pain and the number of bleeds. It is most important in all haemophiliac surgery to pay particular attention to haemostasis during the procedure and to have satisfactory coagulation control both during and after it.

Soft tissue bleeds

Spontaneous bleeding into the soft tissues and particularly into the muscles is the next most frequent site of bleeding in haemophilia. The iliopsoas muscle is the most commonly affected, followed by the forearm flexor muscles and the calf. A bleed into the iliopsoas presents with a tender swelling in the iliac fossa, with flexion of both the hip and the knee on the same side (Goodfellow, Fearn and Matthews, 1967). A compression neurapraxia of the femoral nerve can occur in approximately 10% of cases and is often not clinically obvious for at least 24 hours after the onset of the bleed.

Treatment is similar to that for an acute haemarthrosis, with compression, immobilization and factor VIII replacement. A hip spica is applied, often with the hip flexed in a comfortable position, and it is important not to

try to stretch out the flexion contracture too early. The position of flexion may be altered in the spica every 2 to 3 days to slowly reduce the flexion contracture. Once the haematoma has resolved careful rehabilitation with physiotherapy, hydrotherapy and graduated weight-bearing on crutches is undertaken. The neurapraxia of the femoral nerve may take up to 6 months to recover. Similar bleeding into the flexor compartment of the forearm and the calf can result in permanent late contractures which require surgical elongation of the tendoachillis or flexor muscle slide in the forearm.

Haemophilic cysts and pseudotumours

These are rare and occur in patients with little or no circulating factor VIII, often associated with antibodies. They are due to uncontrolled bleeding into muscle, bone or under the periosteum. They gradually enlarge and may become massive, threatening major vessels, nerves and even skin. The differential diagnosis from a neoplasm may be difficult. They should be treated conservatively using the accepted principles of compression, immobilization and factor replacement. Surgery is indicated only if the situation is life-threatening due to uncontrolled haemorrhage, skin ulceration and secondary infection. In the limbs this may mean amputation, but with care excision of even very large cysts has been carried out successfully (Duthie *et al*, 1972).

Disorders of the lymphatic system

Leukaemia

In children leukaemia is usually acute and lymphoblastic, being characterized by delay in the appearance of primitive cells in the peripheral blood (aleukaemic). Anaemia and an abnormal differential white count suggest the need for confirmatory marrow puncture.

Sometimes these children first present themselves to orthopaedic surgeons with ill-defined but troublesome bone pain, lacking the features of growing pains. Backache and a radiograph disclosing multiple collapse of porotic vertebral bodies is a very suspicious combination. The long bones first show unexplained lines of radiolucency in the metaphyses (Figure 3.6), especially of the upper humerus.

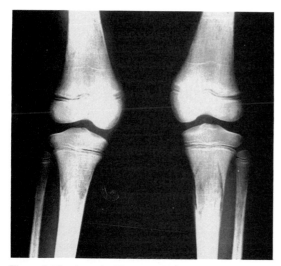

Figure 3.6 Leukaemia. There are destructive lesions on both sides and a fracture through the tibia on one. Note the radiolucent line proximal and distal to the growth plate

Later, widespread destructive lesions, with raising of the periosteum, resemble those of secondary neuroblastoma. Pathological fractures may occur (Caffey, 1967).

Lymphoedema (Kinmouth, Tracy and Marsh, 1957)

Milroy's disease in which lymphoedema is both familial and congenital is extremely rare, but curiously well recognized. Congenital lymphoedema is, on the other hand, relatively common, being due to aplastic lymphatics of varying degree. In infancy it is commonly associated with bulbous oedematous swellings on the dorsum of the hand or foot, later progressing to generalized oedema. The prognosis is poor, but plastic surgeons offer some alleviation.

Lymphoid tumours

Cystic hygromas are familiar in the neck, but they may also, rarely, present in the axilla or groin. Lymphangiomatous tumours are usually multiple and are a cause of, or contribute to, gigantism.

References

Caffey, J. (1967) *Pediatric X-Ray Diagnosis*, 5th edn. Chicago: Year Book Medical Publishers

Duthie, R. B., Matthews, A. M, Razza, C. R. *et al.* (1972) *The Management of Musculo-skeletal Problems in the Haemophiliac.* Oxford: Blackwell Scientific

Golding, J. S. R. (1956) Bone changes in sickle cell anaemia. *Ann. R. Coll. Surg.* **19**, 296

Golding, J. S. R. (1959) Bone changes in sickle cell anaemia and its genetic variants. *J. Bone Jt. Surg.* **41B**, 711

Gonzalez-Crussi, F., Enneking, W. F. and Arean, V. M. (1966) Infiltrating angiolipoma. *J. Bone Jt. Surg.* **48A**, 1111

Goodfellow, J., Fearn, C. B. and Matthews, J. M. (1967) Iliacus haematoma. A common complication of haemophilia. *J. Bone Jt. Surg.* **49B**, 748

Gorham, L. W. and Stout, A. P. (1955) Massive osteolysis: its relation to hemangiomatosis. *J. Bone Jt. Surg.* **37A**, 985

Houghton, G. R. and Duthie, R. B. (1979) Orthopaedic problems in haemophilia. *Clin. Orthop. Rel. Res.* **138**, 197

Kinmouth, J. B., Taylor, G. W., Tracy, G. D. and Marsh, J. D. (1957) Primary lymphoedema. *Br. J. Surg.* **45**, 1

Lewis, R. C. Jr, Coventry, M. B. and Soule, E. H. (1959) Hemangioma of the synovial membrane. *J. Bone Jt. Surg.* **41A**, 264

Middlemiss, J. H. and Raper, A. B. (1966) Skeletal changes in the haemoglobinopathies. *J. Bone Jt. Surg.* **48B**, 693

Steel, W. M., Duthie, R. B. and O'Connor, B. T. (1968) Haemophilic cysts. *J. Bone Jt. Surg.* **51B**, 614

4

Metabolic diseases

Gaucher's disease

In this familial, predominantly Jewish, inborn defect of lipoid metabolism, reticulum cells become filled with glucocerebroside (Gaucher's cells), especially in the enlarged spleen. Some infants die but survival to adult life is more common. Anaemia associated with hypersplenism and marrow depression may improve after splenectomy – which in any case relieves abdominal distension. Other clinical problems are skeletal, and include vertebral collapse, fractures of the femoral neck (leading to coxa vara) and general aching in bones.

The radiological signs reflect bone replaced and often expanded by hyperplastic reticuloendothelial cells. This is seen characteristically in the flask-shaped distal femora.

Major disability is caused by avascular necrosis of the femoral heads (Figure 4.1). One such child became bed-ridden with bilateral hip

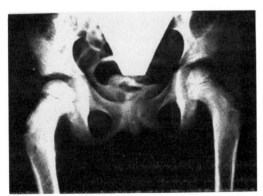

Figure 4.1 Gaucher's disease, showing bilateral ischaemic necrosis of the femoral heads with changes in the femoral shafts

pain which finally responded to radiotherapy. Later, however, deformity developed and corrective surgery was necessary. Sometimes curettage gives symptomatic relief (Askin and Schein, 1948).

Scurvy

Scurvy is now rare but may still occur. It is important to appreciate that scurvy is not seen within the first 3 months – suspicion so soon should prompt a diagnosis of the effects of trauma or congenital syphilis.

Lack of vitamin C causes abnormalities of capillaries and of cell maturation, which is seen most strikingly at the epiphyseal plates. The baby is poorly and prone to intestinal upset. Spontaneous haemorrhage is due to a failure of intercellular capillary cement and may occur anywhere, including the bowel and within the cranium. Conjunctival bleeding is the most conspicuous, for gums bleed only when teeth have erupted.

Diagnosis usually depends on the radiological signs, which are explained by delayed metaplasia of epiphyseal cartilage cells to bone. Generalized porosis is associated with widening of the plate, which sometimes bulges centrally into the metaphysis. The well known white line represents a delay in cartilage maturation at the calcified zone and this may spread peripherally to form spurs.

Subperiosteal haemorrhages are common (Figure 4.2), and are often seen as well demarcated extraosseous calcified shadows. These haemorrhages are painful, palpable and associated with generalized swelling of the

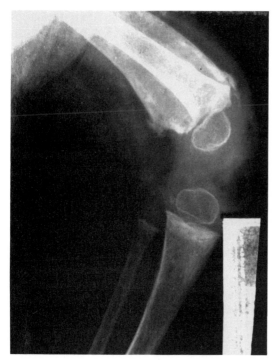

Figure 4.2 Scurvy. Note well marked evidence of subperiosteal haemorrhage and displacement of the lower femoral epiphysis

limbs. 'Pseudo-osteomyelitis' seems more descriptive than the traditional 'pseudoparalysis'.

Pseudohypoparathyroidism

Undue shortening of one finger – usually the little finger or the ring finger – may be due to a short metacarpal. When present, this suggests the possibility of mental defect in a child who is biochemically hypoparathyroid, but in whom the production of the hormone is normal. This is not properly utilized peripherally.

Rickets

The bone changes of rickets, whatever the cause, are the same. They vary only in degree, which is determined by age (the younger the child, the more florid), and the type and extent of the metabolic fault.

Radiologically, there is sometimes diffuse porosis, delay in epiphyseal development, and always cupping with widening of the epiphyseal growth plates due to non-ossification of the zone of provisional calcification in the adjacent metaphysis. These changes are best seen at the wrist and knee. Deformity is due to bending under weight-bearing stress, minor crack fractures and epiphyseal displacement. Deformity is most evident in the legs, when coxa vara and lateral bowing of the femur and tibia are characteristic. Joint swelling may be apparent and the anterior ends of the ribs may be prominent ('rickety rosary'). The prognosis for deformity depends upon the age at which the metabolic disorder is treated. Thus, in nutritional rickets correction is usually good, whereas the prognosis is less good in vitamin D-resistant rickets and renal osteodystrophy, especially when diagnosis is late and control difficult.

The causes of rickets may be classified into five main types: nutritional, vitamin D-resistant, vitamin D-dependent, renal tubular disorders and renal osteodystrophy.

Nutritional rickets

When a child of about 2 years of age presents with bow legs involving the femoral and tibial shafts, rickets is the likely diagnosis (Figure 4.3). Bow legs are otherwise either apparent, being due to tibial torsion, or real, secondary to unequal growth at knee epiphyses. When, in addition, the patient is not thriving, has thickened wrists and costochondral junctions, with protruding abdomen, the radiographs will certainly confirm the diagnosis but not necessarily the cause.

Parents will not always readily confess to depriving their child of the prescribed vitamin D supplement and are less likely to admit to depriving him of sunlight. Thus the cause may not be immediately apparent. Difficulty is increased by the similarity between calcium and phosphorous blood levels in active nutritional and vitamin D-dependent and resistant hypophosphataemic rickets. The plasma calcium is often lowish in nutritional and vitamin D-dependent rickets but normal in vitamin D-resistant rickets. The urine contains some amino acids in the first two but not in resistant rickets. However, a family history or the presence of gastrointestinal malabsorption may be helpful. The latter can be a cause of nutritional rickets when vitamin D intake is adequate. The therapeutic test of 5000 units of

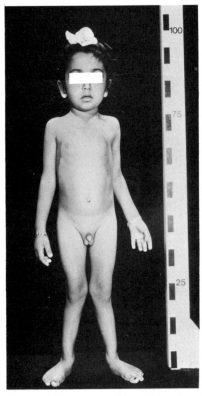

Figure 4.3 Vitamin D-deficient rickets in an Asian immigrant. Note the genu valgum, bowing of the tibiae and chest deformity

Ponseti, 1964). However, other forms of inheritance occur and in some children it occurs as a new mutation.

Blood calcium levels are normal or just below normal, and alkaline phosphatase is high, but the constant and characteristic finding is a low phosphate level which is resistant to treatment. The cause is complex but includes failure to resorb phosphate at renal tubular level, with some abnormality of vitamin D metabolism (lower levels of active vitamin D metabolites than expected) and depressed calcium absorption in the gut. Rickets is due to the combination of these features.

Prompt diagnosis is important, for the sooner the metabolic abnormality is corrected, the less the stunting of growth and the degree of deformity. Deformities in those diagnosed late may be very severe and do not tend to improve with treatment, although they may be arrested (Figure 4.4).

The most effective treatment appears to be a combination of oral phosphate supplementation with either $1,25\text{-}(OH)_2D_3$ or $1\alpha\text{-}(OH)D_3$, which are safer than vitamin D in the doses previously required (50 000–100 000 units per day). The amount needed is controlled by regular estimations of blood calcium, phosphate and alkaline phosphatase levels. Hypercalcaemia is not innocuous and nephrocalcinosis is not an uncommon complication. The need for treatment after skeletal maturity is debatable, but sometimes changes resembling osteomalacia develop in later life. Osteotomy is frequently required to correct deformity. Usually it is possible to achieve this by a single operation (e.g. supracondylar or upper tibial osteotomy for bow legs), but in severe deformity it is sometimes necessary to make multiple osteotomies, threading fragments over a medullary nail.

It is vital to appreciate that surgery in an improperly prepared patient can be very hazardous. Calcium metabolism is labile (especially on high doses of vitamin D) and the combination of osteotomy and immobilization may precipitate dangerous hypercalcaemia. It is important, therefore, to withdraw vitamin D before and after operation. It is prudent to shorten the period of immobilization to the minimum, and it is therefore unwise to operate on both legs at the same time. If hypercalcaemia develops, it may be controlled by

vitamin D daily will usually resolve the problem, for, if nutritional, the hypophosphataemia rapidly climbs to normal, unless malabsorption is present, whereas in the resistant type it is unaffected. Healing is usually followed by steady correction of deformities (unless there has been epiphyseal displacement), so surgery is seldom necessary. Evidence of the pre-existing disease may persist as metaphyseal sclerosis or cortical thickening on the concavity of resolving deformities.

Vitamin D-resistant (hypophosphataemic) rickets

Rickets in children over 3 years of age, or failing to heal when the diet is corrected and a low dose of vitamin D added, is most likely to be of the vitamin D-resistant type. The disease is usually inherited as an X-linked dominant condition, and the family history of shortness with bow-leggedness, especially in the mother, is supportive evidence (Tapia, Stearns and

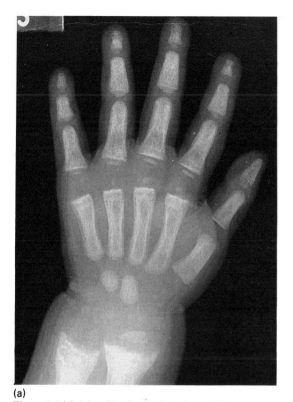

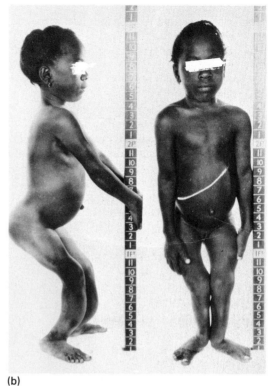

(a) (b)

Figure 4.4 (a) A hand in vitamin D-resistant rickets. Note the marked cupping of the forearm metaphyses and the widening of the epiphyseal plate. (b) Severe deformities in a child in whom diagnosis was delayed

cortisone, but the new short-acting vitamin D products are less of a problem in this respect.

Vitamin D-dependent (Prader) rickets

This is a rare autosomal recessive condition in which there is a specific deficit in 1,25-hydroxylation of 25(OH)D$_3$. This manifests with severe rickets with biochemical features similar to those of nutritional rickets but requiring substantially more vitamin D therapy (but less than vitamin D-resistant rickets) to heal the bones. It is now recommended that 1,25(OH)$_2$D$_3$ be used in physiological doses. In type 1 of this disease there is the hydroxylation defect but in type 2 there is end-organ resistance to vitamin D therapy. This is a much more serious disease and is associated with alopoecia. It requires very high calcium supplements to achieve healing.

Renal tubular disorders (Fanconi syndrome)

Within this category come the group of disorders in which there is a widespread tubular disturbance – predominantly proximal with aminoaciduria, glycosuria, urine sodium and potassium loss, acidosis, phosphaturia and a urine concentration defect. The most common cause in childhood is cystinosis. Treatment is complex but, from the point of view of the rickets, includes phosphate supplements and vitamin D therapy with correction of the electrolyte and acid-base disturbances.

Renal rickets (renal osteodystrophy)

Although renal rickets is evidence of advanced chronic renal failure, these children may sometimes remain untreated until rickets discloses the diagnosis. Any cause of chronic renal failure can be associated with renal osteodystrophy, including renal dysplasia, cystic disease, obstructive uropathy due to urethral valves and neuropathic bladders, reflux nephropathy, chronic glomerulonephritis, tubular disease such as cystinosis, and hereditary nephropathy.

Biochemically there will be hyperphosphataemia with a normal or low plasma calcium and evidence of chronic renal failure.

Radiographs are typical of rickets, frequently with changes of secondary hyperparathyroidism – cysts and erosions – superimposed. The deformities may tempt the surgeon to intervene but, although occasionally necessary, the treatment is essentially medical. This involves the general management of the renal failure but specifically some form of active vitamin D therapy (e.g. $1,25(OH)_2D_3$ or $1\alpha\text{-}(OH)D_3$ plus phosphate binders. The latter commonly used to be aluminium hydroxide but now calcium carbonate is preferred.

Bone disease is not cured by haemodialysis or chronic ambulatory peritoneal dialysis but there is substantial improvement with renal transplantation.

Gargoylism; hypo- and hyperphosphatasia

For gargoylism, hypophosphatasia and hyperphosphatasia, *see* Chapter 2.

Histiocytosis

For histiocytosis, *see* Chapter 8.

References

Askin, A. M. and Schein, A. J. (1948) Aseptic necrosis in Gaucher's disease. *J. Bone Jt. Surg.* **30A**, 631

Tapia, J., Stearns, G. and Ponseti, I. V. (1964) Vitamin D-resistant rickets. *J. Bone Jt. Surg.* **46A**, 935

Further reading

Avioli, L. V. and Krane, S. M. (1978) *Metabolic Bone Disease*. New York: Academic Press

Smith, R. (1979) *Biochemical Disorders of the Skeleton*. London: Butterworths

5

Bone cysts and tumours

There are fundamental differences between both the incidence and the nature of bone cysts and tumours in childhood (under 12 years of age) and their counterparts in adolescence and adult life. Primary and secondary malignant tumours are very rare at this age, being greatly outnumbered by benign tumours and 'cysts'.

'Cysts' are areas of translucency on the radiograph, but are rarely hollow cavities, hence the use of inverted commas.

Tumours of the surrounding soft tissues (Chapter 8) and some tumours of bone are described elsewhere in the book, as indicated by the cross-references.

Bone cysts

The discovery of an area of bone translucency on a radiograph may either be by chance or because swelling or some other symptom has directed attention to the area. In either event the finding promotes discussion about its nature, relevance and management. This is a common and engaging exercise in children.

When the diagnosis is not immediately obvious, the first step is to establish whether the cyst is solitary or one of many, by clinical examination, bone scan and radiographs of the whole skeleton, not forgetting the skull. Clinical examination will, in addition to palpation, include a search for stigmata of general disease, such as coffee patches and the effects, if any, that the lesion may produce locally (e.g. deformity of bone or loss of movement in neighbouring joints).

Multiple cysts

Langerhans' cell histiocytosis (histiocytosis X); multiple eosinophilic granuloma

For Langerhans' cell histiocytosis (histiocytosis X) and multiple eosinophilic granuloma, *see* Chapter 8.

Neurofibromatosis

For neurofibromatosis, *see* Chapter 8.

Subacute osteomyelitis

For subacute osteomyelitis, *see* Chapter 6.

Dyschondroplasia

For dyschondroplasia, *see* Chapter 2.

Secondary neuroblastoma

For secondary neuroblastoma, *see* later in this chapter.

Cystic form of tuberculosis

The cystic form of tuberculosis is not discussed.

Polyostotic fibrous dysplasia (osteitis fibrosa)

Fibrous dysplasia may present as a single cyst (*see* below) or as multiple cysts. The histology is the same. In the multiple form the disease is not present in infancy, though it usually declares itself before the age of 10 years and persists beyond puberty into adult life. The adult patient is never immune to fractures, increasing deformity, and development of fresh lesions, and may develop fibrosarcoma. The disease may present in various ways.

1. Fractures through the cysts may be complete and displaced, but are more usually cracks of the expanded cortex. This commonly happens in the trochanteric area, so pain and a limp are the symptoms. Most cases have fractures at some time and 40% have three or more.
2. Deformities are either due to the effect of body weight on weakened bones, or the result of malunion. Thus coxa vara may reach exaggerated proportions with the femoral head inclined well below the horizontal and the greater trochanter enlarged and abutting on the ilium (shepherd's crook deformity). Anterior tibial and ulnar bowing are also seen which, in the latter, may cause dislocation of the radial head.
3. Discrepancy of leg length may be secondary to deformity and malunion or inherent, when the disease is predominantly unilateral.
4. Asymmetrical enlargement of facial bones.
5. Precocious puberty in girls (Albright's syndrome). The external genitalia are enlarged and menstruation is early – indeed, it may begin within the first year, but is more common at about 6 years of age, when the breasts also enlarge. Although coffee patches are not confined to this variety, they are more conspicuous and may be present at birth. Bone lesions appear early and tend to be extensive.

There is a predilection for certain bones – femur 90%, tibia 80%, humerus 50%, and the hands, feet and ribs may also be involved.

At operation, bleeding from the bone may be profuse and blood transfusion is frequently necessary. The lesion is thin walled and contains gritty, greyish, fibrous tissue resembling potato peelings. The cyst walls are raised by thickened ridges of bone which enclose communicating loculi. Microscopically, fibrous tissue is criss-crossed by thin trabeculae which are undergoing osteoclastic resorption and osteoblastic reinforcement simultaneously.

Radiographs disclose multiple translucencies of ground glass density crossed by thickened ridges and some wide trabeculae. The cortex is thin and expansion modifies normal bone contour. Crack fractures may be visible, being

sometimes signalled by periosteal new bone. The lesions tend to lie at first in the diaphysis near to the metaphysis. Later, several may coalesce and the enlarged area may even spread into the epiphysis in adults. Deformity is common.

Treatment is based on three characteristics. Firstly, the lesions do not heal either spontaneously or following a fracture. Secondly, fractures and osteotomies unite. Thirdly, deformity predisposes to further fracture, as in osteogenesis imperfecta. The principles can be illustrated by reference to the trochanteric area. Crack and complete fractures should be treated by nail-plate fixation or interlocking intramedullary nail to provide a permanent reinforcement and to prevent malunion and deformity. Established coxa vara may be safely (and prudently) treated by abduction osteotomy (Figure 5.1). The contribution of concurrent bone grafting is uncertain. Sometimes healing seems to be encouraged or the calcar femorale is advantageously thickened. We know of a patient with severe tibial disease in whom, as an alternative to amputation, the diaphysis was excised and replaced by a boiled cadaveric tibia. Incorporation was good and a triumph seemed imminent, when the disease

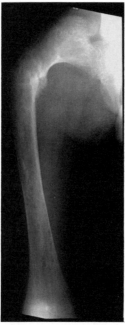

Figure 5.1 Fibrous dysplasia of the right femur with pathological fracture in the subtrochanteric region and gross coxa vara (shepherd's crook deformity)

recurred, gradually replacing the whole of the graft. Extraperiosteal excision might have succeeded (*see* below) (Harris, Dudley and Barry, 1962; Steward, Gilmer and Edmondson, 1962).

Solitary cysts

Monostotic fibrous dysplasia

Solitary cysts are much more common than the multiple cysts (polyostotic fibrous dysplasia). Radiologically the lesions are identical and so is their distribution which again favours femur, tibia, ribs and humerus. Progressive cysts presenting for the first time with a fracture after puberty are not exceptional but there seems a greater tendency to spontaneous arrest than in the multiple form. Treatment is similar, but in situations where the whole bone is expanded to a degree suggesting that the periosteum is involved, curettage or sub-periosteal excision with grafting may fail, whereas an extraperiosteal operation may succeed. Indeed, curettage and grafting or subperiosteal resection has little more than a 50% chance of success (Henry, 1969).

Unicameral bone cyst (simple bone cyst)

Some confusion arises between this and monostotic fibrous dysplasia because the two are often indistinguishable on radiographs and at operation before the cyst is opened. This cyst contains only brown serosanguinous fluid and is lined by a thin fibrous membrane mainly between raised bony ridges, in contrast to the solid fibrous contents of fibrous dysplasia. There is, however, a tendency for it to arise in contact with the epiphysis and, with growth, to move centrally, leaving normal bone between it and the growth plates. It is seen most frequently in the proximal end of the humerus and femur. Expansion is fusiform rather than lobular. The picture is of an unexplained temporary failure of metaplasia of the cartilage of the growth plate to form bone. This recovers in time when normal bone is again laid down (Figure 5.2).

Fractures unite but there is again no apparent following trend towards healing. There is a much greater tendency to spontaneous healing than in monostotic fibrous dysplasia and this is reflected in the higher rate

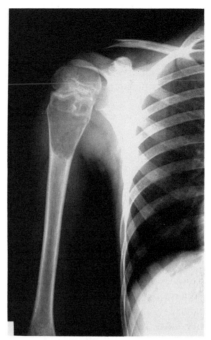

Figure 5.2 Unicameral bone cyst of the right upper humerus. Note the recent fracture through the cyst

of successful operation. This is further encouraged with increasing age of the patient and the distance from the epiphyseal plate. Thus in patients over 10 years of age, with more than a 2.5 cm interval between cyst and plate, failure is rare (Garceau and Gregory, 1954). Local injection of steroid into the cyst has resulted in satisfactory healing in over 90% of cases (Scaglieti, Marchetti and Bartolozzi, 1979).

Non-osteogenic fibroma (fibrous cortical defect)

Although relatively common in adults, non-osteogenic fibroma is occasionally seen in children, usually in the distal femur. The lesion lies at a distance from th growth plate and is placed eccentrically, abutting on the thinned cortex with a well defined sclerotic central margin. There is no expansion and they are harmless unless exceptionally large, when a fracture is possible. They heal in adult life, leaving behind a cyst-like scar.

Cysts derived from pyogenic osteomyelitis

When cysts derive from subacute pyogenic osteomyelitis, they are in the metaphysis with irregular margins, but with growth and chronicity they move towards the diaphysis and the margins become sclerotic (Brodie's abscess). A cyst of any type is rare in the epiphysis unless pyogenic. It may appear as a circular translucency or a defect with a clear-cut semicircular margin.

Single enchondromas

Single enchondromas are largely confined to the hands and feet, appearing as expanding lesions. There is a striking central translucency, occasionally relieved by calcified flakes, enclosed by a dilated wafer-thin cortex.

Solitary eosinophilic granuloma

In cystic form, solitary eosinophilic granulomas are usually in the skull or ilium. In long bones they are less likely to cause confusion. For further discussion, *see* Chapter 8.

Osteochondromas

If osteochondromas grow in such a position that they cannot be seen in profile on standard views, the base of the tumours very closely resemble a bone cyst. Oblique views will provide the answer. These are the condition to consider first in the differential diagnosis of a bone 'cyst' in a child under the age of 12 years. There are other rare causes which will be briefly mentioned below.

Aneurysmal bone cyst

Aneurysmal bone cysts merit consideration between the ages of 12 and 20 years, but very seldom before. In long bones they expand one side at the metaphysis, sometimes eroding the cortex to resemble sarcoma. The epiphyseal plate may be transgressed as they enlarge. In the spine they appear as patchily calcified circular tumours arising from vertebrae – usually the posterior elements. One, arising from the arch of the atlas, closely resembled a calcified cold abscess.

Chondromyxoid fibroma

Chondromyxoid fibroma closely resembles a chondrosarcoma, both radiologically and clinically; only biopsy distinguishes it with certainty.

Osteoblastoma

In osteoblastoma, a central translucency is surrounded by thick sclerotic walls. One patient, with cervical spine osteoblastoma, had pain and torticollis from a lesion which it was not possible to excise completely. There was rapid response to irradiation (Lichtenstein and Sawyer, 1964).

Osteoclastoma and chondroblastoma

These tumours rarely occur in children.

Benign tumours

Solitary osteochondromas

Solitary osteochondromas are by far the most common bone tumours of children, and differ only from those in diaphyseal aclasia (Chapter 2) in being solitary. Thus they are capped by cartilage with growth potential, gradually enlarge and migrate from the growth plate until growth ceases at maturity. In profile they are pedunculated, flat (sessile) or exuberant (cauliflower) (Figure 5.3). Removal is only necessary when they cause symptoms such as unsightliness, interference with joint or muscle action, or parental anxiety. Care must be taken to respect the epiphyseal plate when removing sessile tumours close to it.

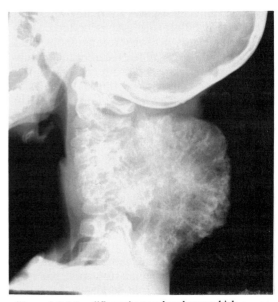

Figure 5.3 A 'cauliflower' osteochondroma which prevented extension of the neck

The danger and fear of malignant change frequently (and usually unjustifiably) worry the surgeon. The incidence as variously quoted lies between 1 and 15%, which does not have a calming influence. Although we have not seen malignant change in childhood, the relation between adult chondrosarcoma and pre-existing and unsuspected osteochondroma is uncertain.

Anxiety is caused by pain, recurrence after operation and exuberant growth. Pain is likely to be due to an overlying bursa, an over-riding tendon or a fracture of the stalk. Recurrence is usually more apparent than real, and is generally seen in the multiple form when a second exostosis develops from the growth plate in a similar situation.

By this time the base of the first should have moved further away from the plate. Exuberant growth is seen most commonly in lesions of the trunk and limb roots, and it is precisely in these situations that adult chondrosarcoma commonly occurs. In practice these tumours are almost invariably ugly or interfere with function and are removed for these reasons. It seems prudent, however, to remove any osteochondroma found in these areas, where they are in any case relatively rare (Jaffe, 1958)

Osteoid osteoma

Whilst not uncommon (about one a year at the Hospital for Sick Children), osteoid osteoma is a curious, painful, benign tumour which presents rather differently in children than in adults. In adults constant bone pain is worse at night, responds to salicylates and is associated with local tenderness. In children, however, pain is likely to be in or around joints and associated muscle spasm and limitation of movement. Regional osteoporosis adds to the suspicion of an inflammatory arthritis. The lesion, which is of unknown cause, consists of vascular osteoblastic tissue with osteoid seams. The radiograph depends on the position of the tumour. If it arises in cancellous bone there will be a circular translucent area less than 1 cm in diameter, sometimes enclosing a small central calcified spot (nidus), but with negligible surrounding sclerosis. If subcortical there is a vigorous periosteal reaction, and cortical thickening which may obscure the nidus in plain radiographs. Tomography discloses some of these. In difficult cases a bone scan and CT

scan can be extremely helpful, when radiographs are equivocal. The trochanteric cancellous bone is the site most favoured in children, and thus the lesion presents frequently as an obscure cause of an irritable hip. We have also seen it twice in the tarsus when the feet were stiff, of almost trophic appearance and deformed by peroneal spasm (Figure 5.4a). The resemblance to tuberculosis is obvious and some cases have been treated as such. If the tumour is central, very careful scrutiny of the radiographs, including oblique and tomographic views or CT scan, may be needed to disclose it. Once seen on the radiograph there is little difficulty in making the diagnosis, for with increasing familiarity it is now unlikely to be confused with a chronic bone abscess or sclerosing osteomyelitis (Figure 5.4b). Calcified bone islands are sometimes mistaken for this tumour.

If untreated, the pain disappears in 2–6 years' time but the radiographic appearances remain. Once recognized, however, symptoms dictate its complete removal, which is confirmed by their immediate and dramatic disappearance. It is best to remove a block of bone containing the nidus with concurrent radiological control. It may be difficult to find the lesion in the excised specimen and it should be remembered that not all are typical – that is to say, bright red nodules in small cavities. Some are white, melon seed in size and have an irritating tendency to pass unrecognized or flip out when the bone is being searched. Recently Szypryt, Hardy and Colton have described an intraoperative technique using a scintillation probe to pinpoint the lesion accurately (Sherman, 1947; Golding, 1954; Spence and Lloyd-Roberts, 1961; Szypryt *et al*, 1986).

Angioma, fibrous and synovial tumours

For angioma, *see* Chapter 3. For fibrous and synovial tumours, *see* Chapter 8.

Primary bone tumours

Osteogenic sarcoma (osteosarcoma)

Although younger patients have been recorded (the youngest at The Hospital for Sick Children was 7 years old), this malignant bone sarcoma occurs most commonly in teenage

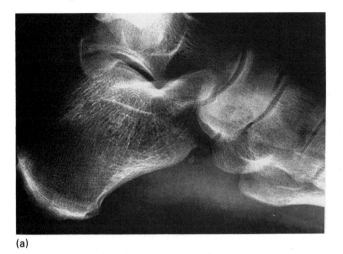

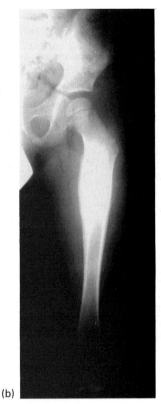

(a)

(b)

Figure 5.4 (a) Osteoid osteoma in the navicular causing peroneal spasm. (b) Osteoblastoma of the femur mimicking osteomyelitis, with large central nidus and florid sclerotic reaction

children. Whilst almost every bone, including skull, jaw, vertebrae, clavicle, rib, scapula and pelvis, has on occasion been the site of the primary tumour, osteosarcoma most commonly develops in the metaphyseal regions of long bones (Figure 5.5), especially around the knee or the upper end of the humerus (Uribe-Botero *et al*, 1977). There are several histological subtypes; the telangiectatic variety has a worse prognosis than the remainder. Multicentric ('multifocal') osteosarcoma is a rare but well defined entity (Mahoney, Spanier and Morris, 1979). Metastases – most commonly in the lung but also in other bones and occasionally in liver and brain – are detectable at diagnosis in only 10–20% of patients but 'micrometastatic' disease is present in the majority. Therefore, before the advent of chemotherapy, almost all patients rapidly succumbed to the effects of widespread metastatic disease. The exceptions were effectively 'selected' by the approach, pioneered by Sir Stanford Cade, in which high-dose radiation therapy was delivered to the primary tumour: patients without evidence of metastatic disease

at 6–12 months after surgery then underwent amputation and a fraction (10–20% of the original total) were apparently cured.

Effective chemotherapy has been the principle factor underlying the dramatic recent improvement in prognosis (Goorin, Abelson and Frei, 1985). Not only have the incidence and frequency of metastatic disease been dramatically reduced over the last 10 years but there has also been a heartening decrease in the need for amputation. Preoperative chemotherapy, for selected tumours with little evidence of soft tissue invasion, allows orthopaedic surgeons the opportunity to attempt local tumour resection with prosthetic replacement (Rosen *et al*, 1979). Recent developments in prosthesis design mean that even young children can have successful bone/joint replacement, the artificial bone being elongated *in situ* to keep pace with growth in the opposite limb (Scales and Sneath, 1987). The success of local excision depends, naturally, on maintenance of effective local tumour control. The efficacy of a particular preoperative chemotherapy regimen can be judged not only

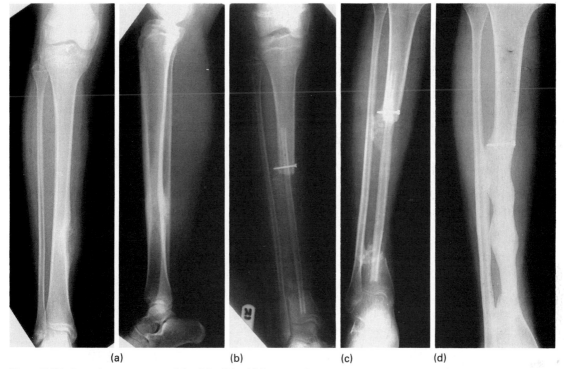

(a)   (b)   (c)   (d)

Figure 5.5 Periosteal osteosarcoma of the right tibia. (a) Preoperative anteroposterior and lateral views. (b) Immediately after treatment by resection and fibular graft. (c) Seven months after the graft. (d) Two years after the graft, showing a stress fracture in the graft

by clinical parameters but also by the histopathological appearance of the operative specimen. A high percentage (> 90%) of necrosis implies that the preoperative treatment has been particularly effective and encourages its continuation postoperatively, whilst a lesser response suggests the need for alternative treatment (Rosen *et al*, 1982).

Although pain relief can be achieved by the use of local radiotherapy, osteosarcoma is not particularly radio-responsive, so the failure – in one large series – of whole lung irradiation to reduce significantly the number of patients developing later lung secondaries is not surprising (Breur *et al*, 1978). By contrast, many recent publications have supported the contention that chemotherapy has a major role to play in management. Several drugs, especially adriamycin (doxorubicin), *cis*-platinum (*cis*-platin) and very high doses of methotrexate are the most active agents and – either individually or in combination, sometimes with other agents – have given 4-year survival rates of up to 75% in unselected series (Goorin, Abelson and Frei, 1985).

Until recently, those sceptical of the value of chemotherapy pointed to results from the Mayo Clinic where, after amputation alone, a 50% 3-year disease-free survival was claimed (Taylor *et al*, 1978). There is no satisfactory explanation for these results, which differ from those of almost every other large centre, but contributory factors could include selective referral, earlier diagnosis or the more aggressive use of pulmonary metastatectomy. An additional theoretical possibility, that the natural history of osteosarcoma had altered and become less 'aggressive' over the last 10 years, was ruled out and the value of chemotherapy finally established once and for all by the results of the prospective randomized multi-institutional international study (Link *et al*, 1986). In this trial, patients without detectable secondary deposits and after surgical ablation of the primary, were randomized to receive chemotherapy either immediately or only after disease recurrence. The trial has conclusively proven that immediate adjuvant chemotherapy reduces the rate of metastatic pulmonary relapse but, with the relatively short follow-up available for the study, it is not yet certain whether or not the proportion of long-term survivors will be different in the two groups. However, because it is easier to eradicate microscopic than macroscopic cancer, it is likely that there will be a survival advantage in favour of the immediate chemotherapy group. In current chemotherapy trials, investigators are attempting to identify the most convenient, effective treatment regimen: in the current Medical Research Council (MRC)/European Organisation for Research and Treatment in Cancer (EORTC)/ International Society of Paediatric Oncology (SIOP) trial (EOI Study 1), for instance, the adriamycin/*cis*-platinum combination is being compared with the more complex, lengthy and costly regimen piloted by Rosen at the Memorial Sloan-Kettering Hospital in New York. Up to one-third of patients developing lung secondaries after chemotherapy may be cured by metastatectomy.

The longer the interval between completion of treatment and the appearance of secondaries, the higher the chance of disease-free survival. In some cases, repeated thoracotomy may be justified (Rosenberg *et al*, 1979).

Parosteal (Unni *et al*, 1976) and periosteal (Hall *et al*, 1985) osteosarcomas have a better prognosis than metaphyseal tumours, being of 'lower grade' and therefore less likely to metastasize. Chemotherapy may not be indicated if surgical margins are clear and lung CT scanning is negative.

Between 1980 and 1984, 9 patients with osteosarcoma were treated at The Hospital for Sick Children with surgery and chemotherapy. One girl, the only patient with pulmonary secondaries at diagnosis, and three patients who developed lung metastases whilst on treatment have died from their disease but five patients (all disease-free) survive at a median of 3.5 years (range 24–60 months) from diagnosis. Five children had amputations. A tenth child with an upper tibial periosteal tumour, was treated with surgery (resection and prosthetic replacement) alone and survives at 40 months after operation.

Ewing's sarcoma

Ewing's tumour is a small, round-cell tumour that most frequently arises in bone (Figure 5.6) but occasionally has a soft tissue origin. The

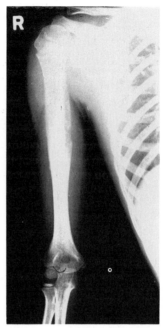

Figure 5.6 Ewing's sarcoma of the upper half of the right humerus. Note the similarity to X-ray changes of osteomyelitis

exact cell of origin is still uncertain (proponents of an endothelial, a mesenchymal, and a haemopoietic origin all regularly express their views in the medical literature) but it is now clear that in most, if not all, Ewing's tumours there is a distinctive karyotypic change, a reciprocal translocation (11;22) (q24;q12) between chromosomes 11 and 22. Interestingly, the same translocation is also seen in the so-called Askin tumour (malignant neuroepithelioma), a tumour that has only recently been recognized as an entity distinct from Ewing's, neuroblastoma and other 'small round-cell tumours of childhood'. Ewing's and Askin tumours can be distinguished by the presence, in the latter, of neurosecretory granules, revealed by electron microscopy.

Contrary to the impression given in some orthopaedic texts, Ewing's sarcomas can arise anywhere in the skeleton with no predilection for axial or limb bones (Jurgens, Donaldson and Gobel, 1986; Wilkins *et al*, 1986). Over the last 5 years, 23 children have been referred to The Hospitals for Sick Children for treatment; their primary tumours were in the orbit (1 case), metatarsal (1), humerus (2), scapula (1), sacrum (5), pelvis (3) and rib (10); during the same time period there were two patients with Ewing's tumours apparently arising in soft tissues. Management is with chemotherapy, to eradicate secondaries and to shrink the primary tumour and surgery and/or radiotherapy for 'local control'; the choice of surgery or radiation depends on the site of the primary tumour. Surgical ablation is the treatment of choice when the bone is 'expendable' (e.g. clavicle, rib) and is favoured where the primary tumour involves the distal part of a limb (e.g. lower end of tibia/fibula or radius/ulna or metatarsal/metacarpal) whilst radiation is usually used when excisional surgery would cause major deformity. Decisions about the best method for local control should be made only after interdisciplinary discussion between orthopaedic surgeon, chemotherapist and radiotherapist, and tailored for each individual patient. Treatment often starts with chemotherapy and 'local therapy' is carried out after several weeks or months. The drugs active in Ewing's tumour include vincristine, actinomycin D, cyclophosphamide, isophosphamide, adriamycin and VP16 (Jurgens, Donaldson and Gobel, 1986). *Cis*-platinum and melphalan and the antimetabolites are not particularly active.

Although there was a lot of excitement about benefits of chemotherapy during the 1970s, long-term results are not particularly encouraging; overall survival figures are between 30–50% for localized tumours and 10% or less for metastatic disease (Jurgens, Donaldson and Gobel, 1986). In survivors who have received high-dose radiation therapy, late sequelae are considerable; growth delay in the irradiated bone is universal and deforming if an epiphysis has to be included in the radiation field, pathological fractures occur and the cumulative risk of second malignancies over 10 years following irradiation has been calculated to be as high as 35% (Strong *et al*, 1979). Given these long-term problems, there has been something of a move, in the last 5 years, back to surgery, with prosthetic replacement where possible, as the local modality of choice in Ewing's tumour.

Non-Hodgkin's lymphoma (old and inaccurate term: reticulum cell sarcoma)

Patients with leukaemia/non-Hodgkin's lymphoma (NHL) often have bone pain because of secondary invasion (*see* 'secondary tumours', below). However, there is a small yet important group of children with histologically proven 'diffuse lymphoblastic NHL of bone' who present with pain at one or more bony sites and have no evidence of disease in lymph nodes, liver, spleen, bone marrow or cerebrospinal fluid. Immunophenotyping of blast cells in all four of such children seen at The Hospital for Sick Children over the last 5 years indicates a 'common' acute lymphoblastic leukaemia (ALL) phenotype, i.e. an early B-cell tumour. Thus, this presentation appears to represent the lymphomatous counterpart of so-called 'common' ALL. Radiologically, the lesions closely resemble Ewing's sarcoma with a primarily lytic lesion and an associated periosteal reaction (Figure 5.7).

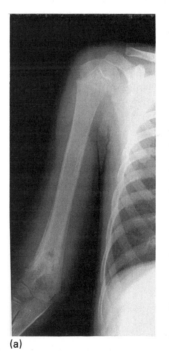 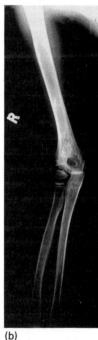

(a)   (b)

Figure 5.7 Acute lymphoblastic leukaemia (ALL) in the lower humerus. (a) Aged 5 years, before treatment; note the similarity to Ewing's sarcoma with associated periosteal reaction. (b) No evidence of recurrence after 2 and a half years of chemotherapy and local radiotherapy

If such children are treated only with local measures (e.g. radiotherapy alone), development of full-blown common ALL inevitably follows after a short interval. Such patients should therefore be treated, from the outset, with combination chemotherapy using a common ALL regimen. If adequate chemotherapy is given, radiation is not indicated. If diagnosed early and treated adequately, the cure rate with chemotherapy alone should be at least 75%.

Secondary tumours

Acute leukaemia, particularly the lymphoblastic variety (common ALL – *see* above), is the most common cause of bone secondaries in children. Identifiable abnormalities are present in the majority of skeletal surveys and bone scans (Clausen *et al*, 1983). Non-Hodgkin's lymphoma (NHL – *see* above) and malignant histiocytosis may also metastasize to bone.

Of the solid tumours, neuroblastoma is by far the most likely to present with skeletal deposits (Figure 5.8). In fact, more children with neuroblastoma present with the symptoms of secondary tumours than of their primary mass. Bony secondaries connote a relatively poor prognosis especially in children over 1 year of age at diagnosis. Although long bones, vertebrae and skull are most often involved, almost any bone may be affected. Since early bone lesions do not always provoke an osteoblastic reaction, skeletal surveys complement bone scanning in staging these children.

^{131}I-mIBG (meta-iodobenzylguanidine) scanning may be more sensitive than either. Although spontaneous 'maturation' of metastatic neuroblastoma has occasionally been documented, the vast majority of children with so-called stage IV disease die within 2 years of diagnosis. The use of combination chemotherapy including vincristine, cyclophosphamide, adriamycin, *cis*-platinum, teniposide (VM-26) and high-dose melphalan prolongs the median survival of these patients but there is as yet little evidence, except in children less than 1 year of age at diagnosis, that the cure rate is improved. Persistent bone scan abnormalities in children on chemotherapy need not necessarily signify active tumour. In The Hospital for Sick Children we have carried out biopsies of bones that are persistently abnormal on isotope scan in six children in clinical remission after combination chemotherapy, and all six have been histologically negative. Thus, many months may elapse before radiological evidence of bone healing is complete.

Other solid tumours may metastasize to bone. Of the several subtypes of Wilms' tumour, one is so likely to produce bone secondaries that it is now known, in Europe, as the 'bone metastasizing renal tumour of childhood' (Marsden *et al*, 1980) (though, confusingly, in the USA, as the 'clear cell renal sarcoma'). The histological appearance of this

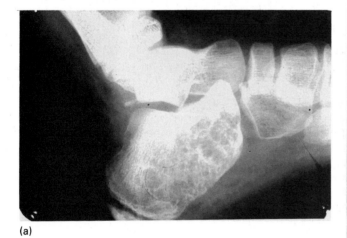

(a)

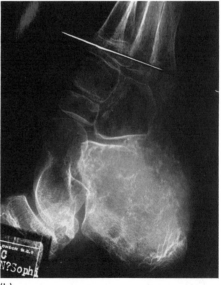

(b)

Figure 5.8 Secondary neuroblastoma: (a) Confined to the calcaneum; (b) enlarged and spread into the soft tissues

tumour is distinctively different from the classic 'triphasic' Wilms' tumour. Bone involvement is exceedingly rare in children with newly diagnosed Hodgkin's disease (Newcomer *et al*, 1982) although we have recently seen one such case. Bony secondaries from other sarcomas, such as Ewing's, rhabdomyosarcoma and malignant germ cell tumours, are unusual at diagnosis but may occur during the terminal stages of the disease. Accurate diagnosis of the cause and source of pain in terminally ill children is essential so that the correct treatment – whether radiotherapy, nerve block, analgesia or a combination of these treatments – can be prescribed.

Orthopaedic consequences of treatment for childhood cancer

As a consequence of judicious combinations of surgery, radiation and chemotherapy, more than 60% of children with cancer are now cured of their disease (Goldman and Pritchard, 1985). Alongside efforts to improve cure rates, there is now major emphasis on modifying successful treatment protocols to reduce morbidity. It is now standard practice, for instance, to include the whole width of vertebral bodies in irradiation fields for thoracic and abdominal tumours; as a result, severe scoliosis is hardly ever seen, the only visible consequence of radiotherapy being a slight shortening of truncal height. Where, to avoid amputation, high-dose radiation is delivered to a long bone of a young child, growth retardation in that limb will result and later reconstructive surgery may be necessary.

Of particular current concern is the increase in the number of secondary tumours arising within previous radiation fields at a mean of 8–10 years from radiation treatment (Mike, Meadows and D'Angio, 1982). The most common histological types of radiation-induced 'second tumours' are fibrosarcoma and osteosarcoma. The occurrence of these second tumours has led to reductions of radiation dosage used in the treatment of several tumour types and the omission of this treatment wherever possible.

References

Breur, K., Cohen, P., Schweisguth, O. and Harts, A. M. M. (1978) Irradiation of the lungs as an adjuvant therapy in the treatment of osteosarcoma of the limbs. *Eur. J. Cancer and Oncology.* **14**, 461–471

Clausen, N., Gotze, H., Pederson, A., Riis-Petersen, J. and Tjalve, E. (1983) Skeletal scintigraphy and radiography at onset of acute lymphocytic leukaemia in children. *Med. Pediat. Oncol.* **11**, 291

Garceau, G. J. and Gregory, C. F. (1954) Solitary unicameral bone cyst. *J. Bone Jt. Surg.* **36A**, 267

Golding, J. S. R. (1954) The natural history of osteoid osteoma. *J. Bone Jt. Surg.* **36B**, 218

Goldman, A. and Pritchard, J. (1985) Current management of chidren with cancer. *Prescrib. J.* **25**, 2

Goorin, A. M., Abelson, H. T. and Frei, E. III (1985) Osteosarcoma: fifteen years later. *New Engl. J. Md.* **313**, 1637

Hall, R. B., Robinson, L. H., Malawa, M. M. and Dunham, W. K. (1985) The natural history of fibrous dysplasia. *J. Bone Jt. Surg.* **44A**, 207

Henry, A. (1969) Monostotic fibrous dysplasia. *J. Bone Jt. Surg.* **51B**, 300

Jaffe, H. L. (1958) *Tumours of Bones and Joints.* Philadelphia, Pa: Lea & Febiger

Jurgens, H., Donaldson, S. S. and Gobel, U. (1986) Ewing's sarcoma. In *Cancer in Children: clinical management*, 2nd edn, eds. P. A. Voute, A. Barrett, H. J. G. Bloom, J. Lemerle and M. K. Neidhardt. Berlin, Heidleberg, New York, Tokyo: Springer-Verlag, p. 300

Lichtenstein, L. and Sawyer, W. R. (1964) Benign osteoblastoma. *J. Bone Jt. Surg.* **46A**, 755

Link, M. P., Goorin, A. M., Miser, A. W., Green, A. A., Pratt, C. B., Belasco, J. B. *et al* (1986) The effect of adjuvant chemotherapy on relapse-free survival in patients with osteosarcoma of the extremity. *New Engl. J. Med.* **314**, 1600

Mahoney, J. P., Spanier, S. S. and Morris, J. L. (1976) Multifocal osteosarcoma: a case report with review of the literature. *Cancer.* **44**, 1897

Marsden, H. B., Lennox, E. L., Lawler, W. and Kinnier-Wilson, L. M. 91980) Bone metastases in childhood renal tumours. *Br. J. Cancer.* **41**, 875

Mike, V., Meadows, A. T. and D'Angio, G. J. (1982) Incidence of second malignant neoplasms in children: results of an international study. *Lancet.* **2**, 1326

Newcomer, L. N., Silverstein, M. B., Cadman, E. C., Farber, L. R., Bertino, J. R. and Prosnitz, L. R. (1982) Bone involvement in Hodgkin's disease. *Cancer.* **49**, 338

Rosen, G., Marcove, R. C., Caparros, B., Nirenberg, A., Kosloff, C. and Huvos, A. G. (1979) Primary osteogenic sarcoma: the rationale for preoperative chemotherapy and delayed surgery. *Cancer.* **43**, 2163

Rosen, G., Caparros, B., Huvos, A. G., Kosloff, C., Nirenberg, A., Cacavio, A. *et al* (1982) Preoperative chemotherapy for osteogenic sarcoma. *Cancer.* **49**, 1221

Rosenberg, S. A., Flye, M. W., Conkle, D., Seipp, C. A., Levine, A. S. and Simon, R. M. (1979) Treatment of osteogenic sarcoma. 2. Aggressive resection of pulmonary metastases. *Cancer Treat. Rep.* **63**, 753

Scaglietti, O., Marchetti, P. G. and Bartolozzi, P. (1979) The efects of methylprednisolone acetate in the treatment of bone cysts. *J. Bone Jt. Surg.* **61B**, 200

Scales, J. T., Sneath, R. S. (1987) The extending prosthesis. In *Bone Tumour Management*, eds. R.

Coombs and G. Friedlander, London: Butterworths, pp. 168–177

Sherman, M. S. (1947) osteoid osteoma: review of the literature and report of thirty cases. *J. Bone Jt. Surg.* **29A**, 918

Stewart, M. J., Gilmer, W. S. Jr and Edmonson, A. S. (1962) Fibrous dysplasia of bone. *J. Bone Jt. Surg.* **44B**, 302

Strong, L. C., Herson, J., Osborne, B. M. and Sutow, W. W. (1979) Risk of radiation-related subsequent malignant tumours in survivors of Ewing's sarcoma. *J. Natn. Cancer Inst.* **62**, 1401

Szypryt, E. P., Hardy, J. G. and Colton, C. L. (1986) An improved technique of intra-operative bone scanning. *J.*

Bone Jt. Surg. **68B**, 643

Taylor, W. F., Ivins, J. C., Dahlin, D. C., Edmonson, J. H. and Pritchard, D. J. (1976) Trends and variability in survival from osteosarcoma. *Mayo Clin. Proc.* **53**, 695

Unni, K. K., Dahlin, D. C., Beabout, J. W. and Ivins, J. C. (1976) Parosteal osteogenic sarcoma. *Cancer.* **37**, 2466

Uribe-Botero, G., Russell, W. G., Sutow, W. W. and Martin, R. G. (1977) Primary osteosarcoma of bone: a clinicopathologic investigation of 243 cases, with necropsy studies in 54. *Am. J. Clin. Path.* **67**, 427

Wilkins, R. M., Pritchard, D. J., Burgert, E. O. Jr and Unni, K. K. (1986) Ewing's sarcoma of bone: experience with 140 patients. *Cancer.* **58**, 2551

6

Infections of bones and joints

Osteomyelitis

In about 80% of acute cases of osteomyelitis *Staphylococcus aureus* is the responsible organism, and this variety will be described first in children, with comments later on the disease in infancy. The subacute and chronic forms together with the effects of other organisms will then be discussed.

Acute staphylococcal osteomyelitis

Natural history

We will first describe the course of a typical untreated infection although this is now rare due to the widespread availability of powerful antibiotics.

A boy of about 8 years of age, from the lower social group, presents with pain of sudden onset around the knee. He may be in poor general health with pyogenic boils, sore throat or septic abrasions. There is frequently a history of recent mild injury to the area – but at this age this is by no means uncommon. There is a rapid deterioration in his general condition due to pyaemia and the toxaemic effects of localized pus under tension, with hyperpyrexia, confusion and rigors. Local pain rapidly increases to great severity and throbbing is common. The limb is motionless and the least disturbance (even noise) is greatly resented. The knee joint will be flexed and often swollen and the overlying skin becomes in turn red and warm, oedematous and indurated. Tenderness is situated over the metaphysis and is indeed exquisite. Finally the skin gives way and pus is discharged, with or without involvement of the joint en route. Survival is likely if and when this stage is reached, but the mortality in the pre-antibiotic era from pyaemia and toxaemia was of the order of 20% around the knee, rising to 80% in the spine.

The patient now begins the long war of attrition – chronic osteomyelitis. Chronic sinus, recurrent abscesses, the discharge of sequestra, and pain with each flare and dressing, combine to undermine his health for many years. Amputation will often be necessary to rid him of an encumbrance which dominates his life, for the sake of his general health or the fear of amyloidosis. Lastly, he may suffer from metastatic abscesses which developed in the early pyaemic phase in brain, lung, perinephric space and so on.

It is obvious that we are dealing with two main factors – firstly generalized toxaemia and pyaemia, and secondly the local effects in the bone.

The local damage and pain are essentially due to the building up of intraosseous tension, for the inflammatory exudate is at first walled in and unable to expand. This developing tension, combined with infection, rapidly causes ischaemia and death of bone. Infective thrombosis in the dilated metaphyseal sinuses adds to the ischaemia. This effect is compounded when pus breaks through the cortex to lift the periosteum over an extensive area, thus compromising the periosteal vessels as well (Clawson and Dunn, 1967).

Diagnosis

To be effective in warning us of the developing and dangerous increase in intraosseous tension, a diagnosis must be made within 48 hours of the onset. Disease in the trunk presents its own obvious and difficult problems, but fortunately these are rare sites and the limbs greatly predominate. Pain at one or other end of a long bone (usually around the knee) and associated with local tenderness over the metaphysis must be regarded as osteomyelitis until proved otherwise. Very soon afterwards the tenderness will increase, the area will be warm and the temperature will rise, as will the neutrophil cell count either absolutely or relatively. It is well known that bone changes are unlikely to be present on the radiograph within the first week but radiographs of a penetration calculated to demonstrate the soft tissues will sometimes disclose the shadow of oedema just outside the periosteum. Otherwise the first sign is a thin white line parallel to the cortex, which represents bone forming in the raised periosteum and is first seen on about the tenth day. This rapidly thickens, and patchy islands of translucency in cancellous bone and erosion of cortical bone follow. A bone scan can be very useful before radiographic changes are seen.

Differential diagnosis

Formerly, acute rheumatic fever and poliomyelitis were the main alternatives to be considered. These are now very rare diseases in the UK.

Cellulitis, when it overlies a metaphysis, is now the most likely deceiver. This, however, is much less painful, and tenderness, being more widespread, does not have the localized and exquisite features seen in osteomyelitis. Redness is diffuse and constitutional signs are less dramatic.

Greenstick fractures are likely to mislead when the history is not forthcoming because the injury occurred during some forbidden activity. Such fractures in patients with diminished sensitivity to pain, such as those with meningomyelocele or hereditary insensitivity to pain, can appear remarkably like osteomyelitis and may even be treated with antibiotics or biopsy for a possible tumour before the true diagnosis of a fracture is recognized.

If there is doubt, none of these conditions will be harmed by exposure to antibiotics.

In infancy there are other considerations which will be discussed later.

Management

Assessment

When acute osteomyelitis is probable, the time and date of onset must, if possible, be established. If less than 48 hours have elapsed, there can be guarded optimism about the outcome, hoping that resolution without permanent damage will follow energetic antibiotic and supportive treatment. If more than 48 hours have passed, operation can be expected to be necessary. If osteomyelitis is only suspected, there is no substitute for the same doctor re-examining the child in a few hours to record changes in tenderness and swelling, and to note a rise in temperature.

Primary treatment

Having made the child as comfortable as possible by pillow, splint or traction (leaving the suspected area exposed), look for evidence of throat or skin infection (impetigo, furunculosis or infected abrasion) and take both a swab and blood for culture. Blood culture may be positive in up to 50% of patients in the pyaemic phase. Sedimentation rate, total and differential white count, and antistaphylococcal antibody titres may not be of immediate value, but are more likely to help in determining response to treatment in the future. Recording the level of haemoglobin and the red cell count may give early warning of progressive anaemia.

Antibiotics should be prescribed forthwith, before the causative organism is isolated. Bactericidal rather than bacteriostatic agents should be used. The majority of infections are likely to be due to *Staphylococcus aureus* which is penicillin resistant, and so a drug such as flucloxacillin or fusidic acid should be used. These should be given parenterally, either by injection or, better, by continuous infusion to avoid the necessity for multiple injections. It is best to combine one or other of these drugs with a broad spectrum antibiotic against Gram-negative organisms, such as ampicillin with flucloxacillin and erythromycin with fusidic acid. New antibiotics develop rapidly and vary in their effectiveness against the staphylococcus, so the advice of a microbiological colleague is of value both at this stage and after the organism is isolated. Once the responsible organism is identified and its sensitivity established, the antibiotic battery is adjusted

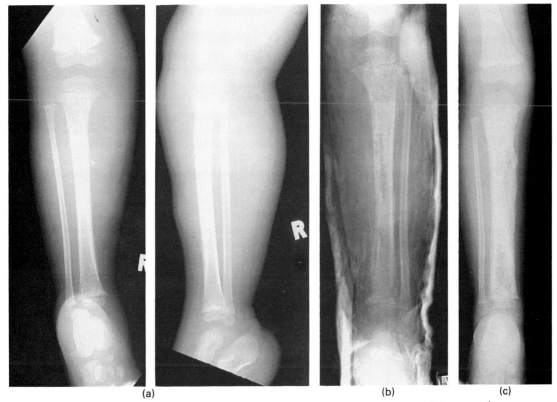

(a) (b) (c)

Figure 6.1 (a) Anteroposterior and lateral views of neglected osteomyelitis of the right tibia in a 2-year-old child. Note that gross soft tissue swelling is the most important sign. (b) After exploration, drainage of pus and drilling 1 week later. Now there is an extensive periosteal reaction. The limb is supported in plaster to protect against the risk of pathological fracture. (c) Three months after drainage. Note the extreme changes throughout the tibia, which subsequently healed with some overgrowth. Fracture and chronic infection were prevented

appropriately. It is also important to remember that analgesia and transfusion for haemolytic anaemia are sometimes needed. Lastly, recall that the term 'resistant organism' is relative to the low concentrations of antibiotic used on the test plate. It is often possible *in vivo* to enable an antibiotic to which the organism is 'insensitive' to become highly effective, by increasing the blood level.

Surgical treatment

The object of surgery is decompression before interference with the blood supply reduces the local concentration of antibiotic, and causes irreversible avascular necrosis. The surgeon is concerned with both the periosteal and the intramedullary circulation. These considerations determine the timing and technique of surgery.

In typical acute infections, surgery should be performed if pain has been present for more than 48 hours before admission. This is, of course, a generalization and as such has its exceptions, but it is undeniable that early surgery, although sometimes not absolutely necessary, is not harmful, whereas delay and procrastination frequently are (Figure 6.1). There are also side benefits, for pain is relieved, the organism isolated with near certainty and the surgeon's mind is at rest. Since decompression is the objective, there is no need for major guttering and saucerization in the acute phase – indeed this may further compromise the blood supply. Longitudinal incision of the periosteum and drilling of the metaphysis is followed by skin closure, usually with closed suction drainage. Drilling should begin near the epiphysis, and if pus is released, this is continued towards the diaphysis until only blood emerges from the hole.

Exceptions to this rule arise when the

infection either seems of low virulence, is poorly localized and there is uncertainty about the exact site, or the diagnosis is in serious doubt. In these circumstances the child must be re-examined by the same surgeon every few hours until a decision is taken.

When antibiotics were first introduced it was hoped that surgery would no longer be necessary in acute osteomyelitis, notwithstanding a similar misapprehension about the sulphonamides. This was soon found to be a false doctrine, but there was hesitation to return to open surgery, for it was still believed that the wound should be left open with the risk of subsequent sinuses and secondary infection. Against this background, aspiration of the subperiosteal abscess was introduced but this did nothing to decompress the bone, if this had not already occurred while waiting for the subperiosteal abscess to form. Trueta and Morgan (1954) were responsible for a more rational approach when they reviewed 100 patients treated by antibiotics and open surgery with very satisfactory results. Blockey has advocated a more conservative approach, using antibiotics and trying to avoid surgical intervention if at all possible (Blockey and Watson, 1970).

Subsequent treatment

Two features need to be considered: the duration of antibiotic treatment, and protection of the bone from stress. There is no certain method of deciding when to stop antibiotics but in uncomplicated osteomyelitis they are usually prescribed for 6 weeks. Harris investigated this problem, but found no certain indications. It seems reasonable (and harmless) to continue for 6 weeks and then stop if the clinical and radiological signs and the sedimentation rate and neurophil/lymphocyte ratio are reassuring. Blockey and Watson recommended much shorter periods of antibiotic treatment. They suggested that if the clinical state had settled, the sedimentation rate was normal or falling and there was no evidence of erosion of the cortex or new bone formation at 10 days then treatment could be stopped. However, we feel that the majority of orthopaedic surgeons would be unhappy to stop antibiotic treatment so early in this condition. Harris found that a persistently high antistaphylococcal titre may indicate that the organism has become resistant to the drugs used.

Involved bones should be protected from full stress for a similar time and until free movement is restored to neighbouring joints. This is because severe osteoporosis often follows even rapidly controlled infection and there is a significant risk of fracture.

The management recommended is an aggressive one. Blockey and Watson are less radical in every respect, and their contrary views are well expressed in their paper of 1970.

Complications

Chronic osteomyelitis and suppurative arthritis are considered later.

Acute osteomyelitis in infancy

In infancy acute osteomyelitis has certain singular and peculiar features which are dependent on the anatomy of the very young. The umbilicus is a common site of origin and readily provides the organism. The bone is soft and pus rapidly breaks through onto the subperiosteal surface. The periosteum, being thick, vascular, markedly osteogenic, and only loosely attached to the bone, is consequently easily stripped up over a wide area in the longitudinal and horizontal plane. The result is copious new bone formation beginning peripherally and spreading in towards the bone surface. By the same token a large area of diaphysis loses its periosteal blood supply. The result is a thick circumferential covering of new bone (involucrum) and frequently the death of part of the diaphysis (sequestrum). Fractures are not infrequent. Lastly, and perhaps most remarkable, is the capacity for repair, for within a year the bone contour may return to normal, and a large sequestrum be partially absorbed and replaced by new healthy bone (Figure 6.2).

The most singular and dangerous feature is the high incidence of spread into neighbouring joints, whether the bone focus be intracapsular or not. Trueta (1959) explained this by showing that there is free communication between the metaphyseal and epiphyseal circulations before bone appears on the epiphyseal side of the growth plate. Later the two become independent and the plate (now the watershed)

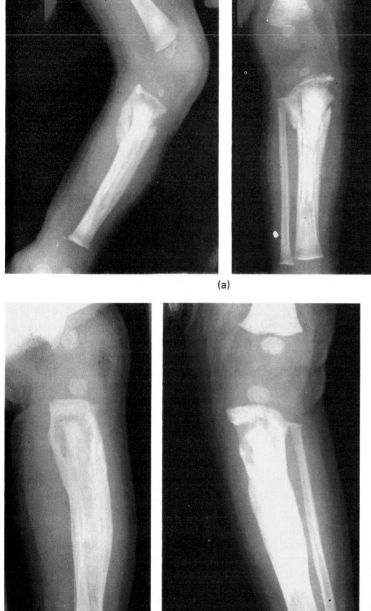

(a)

(b)

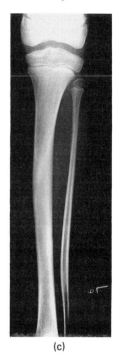

(c)

Figure 6.2 Osteomyelitis in infancy. (a) Neglect of the acute infection has been followed by characteristic thick involucrum, a fracture at the metaphysis and sequestrum of the upper shaft. (b) Sequestrum in a thick-walled cavity supported by the involucrum. (c) Eight years later, showing the quality of repair

demarcates the extent of the lesion. In addition to the joint damage, growth may be inhibited or destroyed either throughout or in part of the growth plate.

The capacity for repair and the rapid development of subperiosteal abscesses should not evoke an expectant attitude, but, if anything, a more aggressive approach than that already described.

The diagnosis may be difficult and understandably delayed in a very ill baby with septicaemia, who may display few signs drawing attention to the bones and joints. Localized swelling, failure to move a limb and apparent pain or tenderness on movement should alert the doctor to the possibility of bone infection. Later NAI (non-accidental injury), Caffey's disease (cortical hyperostosis) described in Chapter 8 and possibly scurvy (Chapter 3) are the main consideration today, whereas syphilis used to be the great deceiver. Radiological signs are quicker to appear in infancy, and subperiosteal bone may be seen within 3 days of the onset.

Acute osteomyelitis in special situations

Spinal acute disease is fortunately very rare, for most are subacute. The child is probably extremely ill when first seen and therefore difficult to examine. If neurological involvement is lacking, referred pain and possibly paralytic ileus are most misleading, and a justifiable diagnosis of an acute abdominal emergency is likely without thought of the spine. Paraplegia of rapid onset, with or without root pain, may be due to an acute extradural abscess and is, of course, a surgical emergency of the first order.

Femoral trochanteric osteomyelitis has a disturbing tendency to be gradual in onset, difficult to diagnose, and pass gradually into a chronic stage without causing alarm. Unfortunately, however, the blood supply to the capital epiphysis is specially vulnerable (as in children's fractures in this region) and necrosis of the femoral head may follow. This is not necessarily associated with spread of infection to the joint. Decompression is indicated as soon as trochanteric disease develops.

In the pelvis, diagnosis can be very testing and delay enables infection to spread widely in the cancellous bone, to become chronic and exceptionally difficult to eradicate. Bone and CT scanning are again very helpful in these diagnostic dilemmas.

In the ribs and scapula the same observations apply, but chronicity is more easily dealt with by excision of areas of residual infection.

Primary subacute osteomyelitis

Primary subacute osteomyelitis implies that bone infection develops without known previous acute disease. The assumption is that the staphylococcus (again the commonest infecting organism) is of low virulence or the victim's resistance is high. This variety is more common than the acute in East Africa, but is now being seen (or being recognized) with increasing frequency in other parts of the world. Although it is believed that this is not simply acute osteomyelitis modified by antibiotics, it is possible that in Great Britain some are the result of their use in undiagnosed fevers. Nevertheless, there are significant differences, notably in that it affects adults as frequently as children.

This is essentially an exercise in the diagnosis of constant though increasing pain in a patient who is apyrexial and well. The resemblance to neoplastic disease is obvious; local tenderness and swelling, often with inconclusive changes in the peripheral blood, add to the difficulty. Furthermore, the radiographs, although always abnormal, do not by any means always immediately suggest bone infection. Bone scanning, CT scanning and magnetic resonance imaging (MRI) can be very valuable in these cases.

In children there are three ways in which this usually presents – bone abscess, osteolytic lesions of long bones, and disc space involvement of the spine. These lesions are also seen in adults, but in addition there are two other forms usually involving the diaphysis, which occur less commonly in children – Garre's sclerosing osteomyelitis and subcortical diaphyseal lesions.

Bone abscess

Bone abscess is probably the lesion described by Benjamin Brodie in 1836, but 'Brodie's abscess' is now used to describe any abscess of bone including this primary form. Usually in the metaphysis, it may be seen on tomography and CT to transgress the growth plate or to be entirely in the diaphysis. It is relatively small and circular, with a thin sclerotic border contrasting with the irregular, larger and thick-walled cavities seen in chronic osteomyelitis (Figure 6.3). Curettage plus antibiotics are usually all that is needed to relieve symptoms.

Osteolytic lesions

Metaphyseal, osteolytic lesions are larger, more irregular and without defined edge, but

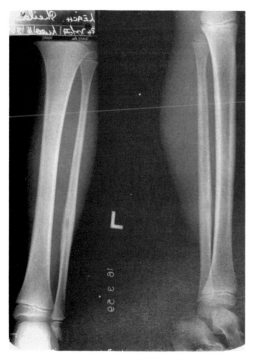

Figure 6.3 Brodie's abscess in the left fibula. Note the central cavity and the surrounding sclerosis

are also sometimes seen to cross the growth plate. Most respond to rest plus antibiotics if the surgeon has the confidence not to do a biopsy.

Spinal lesions

A spinal lesion lies in the upper and anterior quadrant of a vertebral body which is usually in the lower thoracic or upper lumbar spine. The symptoms and signs, however, are very often determined by irritation of the nerve roots arising from that level. Appendicitis, pyelitis, diseases of the chest and hip are all likely to be diagnosed, for there is often little to direct attention to the spine. Indeed, diagnosis, is incidental to pyelography or plain abdominal or chest radiography in any cases.

Examination often reveals a slight prominence of one spinous process (gibbus) and angular scoliosis beginning at this point. Movement is limited and there is tenderness. The radiograph discloses sclerosis of the opposing margins of one intervertebral disc which is apparently narrowed, and a sharp, but minimal, kyphosis and scoliosis. Imaging demonstrates a lesion in the vertebral body which

is much larger than expected and usually has a sclerotic margin. It is often noted that the disc space height is better preserved than it seems on the plain films. Although rare, there may be a small anterior abscess, which, together with the preservation of the disc and sclerosis, helps to distinguish pyogenic infection from tuberculosis.

Rest plus antibiotics is usually followed by healing and loss of symptoms. Stability is restored by fibrous, rather than bony, ankylosis, so a few patients with persisting pain require arthrodesis.

Diaphyseal lesions

Garre's sclerosing non-suppurative osteomyelitis is characterized by diffuse cortical thickening which both enlarges the bone circumferentially and encroaches on the marrow cavity. Erosions may be seen but pus, cavities and sequestra are absent. Subcortical diaphyseal lesions are probably the result of infection carried by the nutrient artery. Part of the surface of the cortex may sequestrate and deep to this the bone may be eroded while subperiosteal new bone is laid on the surface. The similarity to Ewing's tumour or eosinophilic granuloma is obvious (Menelaus, 1964; Harris and Kirkaldy-Williams, 1965; Harris, 1967).

Chronic pyogenic osteomyelitis

In an ideal world in which prompt diagnosis was followed by effective surgery and potent antibiotics, chronic pyogenic osteomyelitis would disappear, but we are at present far from this happy state. Chronic osteomyelitis, though far less frequent, remains a cause of invalidism in children and a problem for surgeons.

The clinical manifestation today is usually of recurrent 'flares' of pain, fever and sometimes discharge from a bone previously acutely inflamed. Chronic sinuses are now less common. The radiograph is a mixture of cortical and medullary sclerosis and thickening, erosions, translucencies and sequestra. Drainage and antibiotics will usually bring relief from the existing attack, but do little to prevent recurrence.

There are three common presenting patterns, modified by the age at which the acute infection occurs and the bone affected. When the lesion occurs in an expendable bone such as a rib or fibula, total excision is possible, but these are rare situations and so, fortunately, today, is the need to sacrifice a limb.

Localized lesions in the metaphysis

Localized lesions in the metaphysis follow disease in children rather than infants and consist of thick-walled chronic bones abscesses with or without sequestra. Removal of a sequestrum and the greater part of the thick avascular sclerotic wall of the abscess, together with thorough curettage of granulation tissue, will cure many, but fails in some. However, the organism and its sensitivity should be known by now. In well covered bones such as the femur with ample skin and vascular surrounding muscles, a further operation during a quiescent phase excises all scar tissue inside and outside the bone. The resulting partially saucerized cavity may safely be filled with cancellous bone and the skin sutured with closed suction drainage, using the appropriate antibiotics both parenterally and locally by instillation of irrigation (Compere, Metzger and Mitra, 1967; Taylor and Maudsley, 1970). More recently, gentamicin beads have been employed.

Subcutaneous bones such as the tibia can seldom be so treated because the overlying skin is thin, avascular and adherent. New full-thickness skin transferred either by pedicle or by free graft with vascular anastomosis should precede definitive bone surgery.

Generalized disease of the greater part of a bone

The principles of treatment of generalized disease remain the same in deep bones, but excision must be radical and should be inhibited only when the stability of the bone is in peril. Postoperative protection is always needed. In superficial bones radical excision may allow closure by healthy skin without tension (Bryson and Mandell, 1964), but when this is unlikely new skin must first be introduced. An alternative is a two-step operation in which saucerization and excision is the first, and split skin grafting of the resulting covering granulations the second (Evans and Davies, 1969).

Defects of the metaphysis or diaphysis

Defects of the metaphysis or diaphysis usually follow mishandled disease in infancy. Late diagnosis encourages sequestration and if this is removed too radically or too soon – that is, before the involucrum is stable – a defect is probable. This is particularly unfortunate as sequestra in infancy frequently absorb and are replaced by normal bone.

Defects of the metaphyses of paired bones such as tibia or lower radius are filled with cancellous bone – an operation which may need to be repeated as the gap progressively closes. Length is maintained by fibula or ulna. In unpaired bones treatment is as for non-union of an infected fracture with excision, shortening, and prolonged splinting in carefully applied plasters.

When the diaphysis has been excised in paired bones it is best to bypass the defect by using the normal bone as a graft, and accepting the loss of rotation in the arm (Griffiths, 1968). We have fortunately not met this problem in unpaired bones, however, repair has been attempted in such situations using either internal fixation with intramedullary nail or plate, or an external fixator to provide stability and to retain length. The intra-bone lengthening technique pioneered by Ilizarov has added another method of closing large gaps in bone.

Uncommon infections of bones and joints

Infections other than tuberculosis

We have seen only one child with congenital syphilis. This was of the osteoperiosteal variety in which the cortex is thickened by periosteal bone. There was therefore a resemblance to Caffey's disease, pyogenic osteomyelitis and the effects of injury. The virtual disappearance of congenital syphilis and the changing pattern of disease, is emphasized by reference to Jones and Lovett's book (1929), in which as many pages are devoted to syphilis as to osteoarthritis of the hip.

Streptococcal and pneumococcal osteomyelitis favour the very young and, once identified, the organism is usually very sensitive to antibiotics. *Escherichia coli* is similar in its presentation to staphylococcal disease. Brucellosis of bones and joints has not been seen by us in children, but in adults the radiological features are similar to those of tuberculosis in joints and subacute osteomyelitis in bones. Salmonella infection has been seen in association with sickle cell anaemia with multiple lesions and direct spread into joints in some cases. One case of actinomycosis presented as a dactylitis indistinguishable radiologically from pyogenic or tuberculosis infection. The phalanx was greatly thickened with discharging sinuses from which the organism was identified. The caecum and liver were also involved but the finger responded satisfactorily to penicillin and potassium iodide in very large doses. Smallpox can produce joint changes which resemble neuropathic arthropathy, especially bilaterally in the elbows (Cockshott and MacGregor, 1958; Zammitt, 1961; Huckstep, 1962; Mendelsohn, 1965; Caffey, 1967).

Tuberculosis

Clearly, from so limited an experience of the disease in children we can no longer write with authority about a disease which is still common elsewhere. It is sometimes held that it is useful for those working in areas where the disease is still prevalent to have access to our views on this subject. This is not only presumptuous but there are also two valid reasons why our opinions are of doubtful value. Firstly, recollection (always fickle) may be positively misleading in this context for at the time when the disease in children was becoming a rarity here, we were only beginning to appreciate fully the impact of antibiotics. Indeed, we have only just reached the stage at which a surgeon no longer forfeited his reputation for soundness if he conceded that antibiotics had changed the principles of treatment. Secondly, the virulence of infection and the resistance of the victim vary greatly in different parts of the world.

Tuberculosis in children is still rarely seen at The Hospitals for Sick Children, although there has been a marked increase in bone and joint tuberculosis in the adult population in this country in the past few years.

The surgeon who works in areas where the disease remains a problem would be better advised to read the observation of those currently treating the disease, preferably in his own region.

Pyogenic arthritis

The staphylococcus is again predominantly responsible, but its effects on joints differ fundamentally between infants and children, so they will be discussed separately. *Haemophilus influenzae* should be considered under the age of 2 years.

Children

The infection usually reaches the joint from a focus of osteomyelitis within the joint capsule, for if the metaphysis lies without, the growth plate is an effective barrier in acute disease. In subacute osteomyelitis, progress is so slow that in spite of breaching the plate the infection remains localized to the bone. Thus the hip is at greater risk than the knee, for although the suprapatellar pouch overlies the metaphysis it is attached below it. Sometimes there is no evidence of bone infection and then one must assume either a direct blood stream infection or very rapid resolution of a bony focus leaving no stigma behind.

Pus and articular cartilage are incompatible. Lack (1959) developed Phemister's observations (1924) upon the digestive action of pus in which he demonstrated a proteolytic enzyme derived from degenerating neutrophils. Lack described a further mechanism whereby blood plasminogen is converted to cartilage-eroding plasmin by an activator, staphylokinase, present in pyogenic pus. Articular cartilage is rapidly digested and, having little or no power of regeneration as such, a fibrous and possibly a bony ankylosis develops later. It must be emphasized that pus rather than infection is the important factor, for articular cartilage seems to resist infection well provided that pus formation is prevented. To be sure, synovial adhesions are probable, but the cartilage remains intact. The implication is obvious. Pyogenic arthritis must be treated with the utmost vigour to prevent pus formation.

Diagnosis

The child may be toxic, febrile and ill, with a raised neutrophil count. A superficial joint will be swollen, warm and possibly red, but these signs are not evident in deep joints. However, in both, there is deformity due to muscle spasm (flexion of knee, flexion adduction of hip) and attempted movement from this position is not only painful but also aggravates muscle spasm.

There are two common diagnostic problems, one in superficial joints (the knee) and the other in deep joints (the hip).

Osteomyelitis around the knee is usually accompanied by an effusion into the joint which, although seldom infected, nevertheless causes anxiety. Aspiration at a distance from the suspected site of bone infection is indicated, but the findings must be interpreted with reserve. Somewhat opalescent fluid with some neutrophils on microscopy does not necessarily indicate infection of the joint. However, cloudy fluid with a neutrophil count of more than $4000/mm^3$ and raised protein is significant, and in these a positive culture is probable.

Hip infection is difficult because of its initial similarity to an 'irritable hip'. Of these the majority are innocuous, being merely transient non-specific synovitis of which some are febrile. However, the irritability tends to be more marked than usual, the patient is suspiciously toxic and the neutrophil count may be raised. Urgent exploration of the hip is indicated, as aspiration of a deep-seated joint such as this is frequently unsuccessful and unreliable.

Acute rheumatic fever is now very rare, but sometimes juvenile rheumatoid arthritis develops rapidly and acutely in one joint. Lastly, children are forever falling on their knees and puncture wounds are not uncommon as portals of entry.

Early treatment

The urgency and the need for joint aspiration on suspicion have already been mentioned. General management is as for osteomyelitis, but traction will relieve much of the pain in the leg joints and maintain the joint space.

If aspiration yields suspicious fluid, systemic administration of antibiotics is started while the fluid is cultured. In theory, one should also deal with the primary bone focus, but in practice this is rarely possible, for by discharging into a joint it has decompressed and has, moreover, already done its worst. Furthermore, decompression removes those signs which make accurate localization possible until radiological changes develop.

If the joint fails to settle then open operation or arthroscopy in suitable joints such as the knee and shoulder is indicated, to thoroughly explore the joint and wash out any pus or debris. This is especially likely to be necessary in the hip.

There is an unnecessary fear of opening infected joints which stems, no doubt, from the pre-antibiotic era, when to do this almost inevitably sacrificed movement forever. Today joints are opened or arthroscoped to preserve movement and this should not be delayed when aspiration is inadequate.

The joint is incised and pus and as much fibrin as possible are removed. Loculi should be broken down. It is generally advised that the synovia and capsule be closed, but we have not found this practicable nor do we think it specially desirable, particularly in the hip. Other layers are loosely closed with suction drainage.

Late treatment

Late treatment will depend upon the damage inflicted. In only the most neglected will the growth plate be damaged or the hip dislocated. One has usually to deal with the effects of articular cartilage destruction, fibrous adhesions either between the joint surfaces or in the joint cavity, and deformity. Unlike osteomyelitis, recrudescence of infection is excessively rare. A well managed patient should have no deformity at the end of primary treatment, but this tends to develop later, together with progressive stiffness. In spite of this it is of the utmost importance to delay for as long as possible irrevocable decisions such as performing arthrodesis, for these joints sometimes have a remarkable capacity to develop useful painless movement over the years. Furthermore, arthrodesis is more likely to succeed when maturity is approaching, and corrective osteotomy less likely to be followed by recurrence of deformity. The exception is seen in the hip when the femoral head has become avascular, crumbles and is painful (Watkins, Samilson and Winters, 1956; Harold, 1960).

Infants

For reasons already given (*see* 'Acute osteomyelitis in infancy'), joint involvement is commonplace and often very serious. The hip is the likely site, possibly because of its relation to the umbilical circulation. The knee is next in frequency, followed by any major joint.

Diagnosis

Infection of superficial joints is obvious, but serious difficulties arise in the hip. If the baby is very ill with septicaemia he will be flaccid, and if in addition he is plump there will be no indication that the hip is involved until an oedematous swelling is noted over the adductors. Even awareness and careful examination may be unrewarding and the radiograph is unlikely to be helpful before the hip dislocates.

Early treatment

Early treatment is on the lines already described for joints other than the hip. Positive aspiration from the hip should be followed by drainage with skin closure, if the dangerous tension which is in part responsible for further destruction is to be relieved. Furthermore, distension of the capsule, destruction and flexor-adductor muscle spasm combine to cause dislocation, so the hip is splinted in 90 degrees of abduction as soon as the diagnosis is made.

Late treatment

If permanent injury is inflicted there is usually one of four possible problems with which to contend. These are partial or complete damage to either an epiphysis or the growth plate. Lesser damage with survival of the epiphysis with subsequent ankylosis is very rare.

Epiphyseal lesions

Total destruction when seen in the hip means that the capital epiphysis has either been absorbed or, if the neck is fractured, incorporated in the acetabulum. Dislocation is inevitable. Partial destruction is more difficult, for if dislocation is present it cannot be distinguished during infancy from the total form by radiography.

Partial destruction is well displayed in the knee where the radiograph may show 'loss' of one femoral condyle and its underlying growth plate (Figure 6.4). On examination, however, the condyle is palpable, the knee is stable and movement is good. The illusion is due to persistent decalcification rather than loss of condyle. In the knee no great harm is taken if nothing is done, for recovery is not now dependent on treatment. This may be undertaken later, usually to correct deformity. In contrast, an expectant attitude when the hip is dislocated but not destroyed may prejudice for ever any prospect of salvage (Lloyd-Roberts, 1960).

It is, therefore, our practice to explore all hips at about 1 year of age. Total destruction may be alleviated by using the greater trochanter in place of the femoral head (Weissmann, 1967; Freeland *et al*, 1980). In partial destruction, enough may be preserved for the hip to be stabilized in some way. Sometimes the head is intact and a routine open reduction is possible.

Lastly, undisplaced pathological fractures of the femoral neck are amenable to abduction displacement trochanter osteotomy. At worst, these operations place the hip in a favourable position for arthrodesis later; at best, they restore stability and a variable range of useful movement (Figure 6.5).

Growth plate lesions

These are usually seen in the knee. Total loss of growth potential throughout the plate with resulting gross shortening is very rare. Partial loss is more common, and causes obstinate, progressive deformity. These problems are treated on conventional lines. Often growth is only inhibited on one side or throughout, so that growth is slowed and deformity develops gradually. The results of surgery are then more favourable.

Loss of the femoral capital growth plate is usually associated with dislocation, which is the major cause of shortening. The epiphysis of the greater trochanter contributes to longitudinal growth and the true length of the femur may be little reduced. Hence the importance of stabilizing the upper end of the femur by

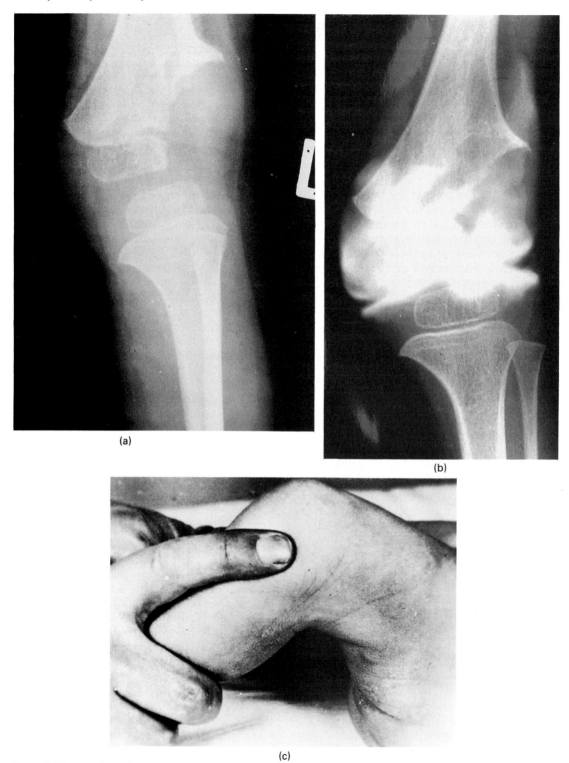

(a)

(b)

(c)

Figure 6.4 Suppurative arthritis of infancy. (a) Apparent total destruction of the lateral femoral condyle. (b) Arthrography shows that the condyle is damaged and smaller than usual but still present. (c) Clinically the condyle is palpable and movement is free and stable

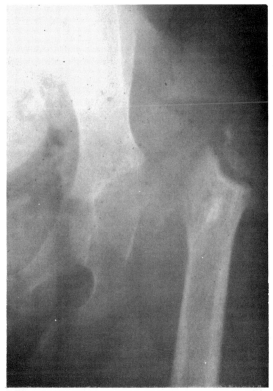

(a)

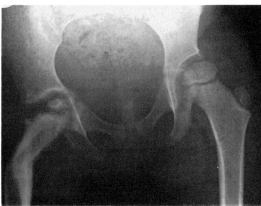

(b)

Figure 6.5 Septic arthritis of the hip. (a) Loss of the head and neck of the femur. If this is not stabilized, progressive shortening will occur. (b) The result of trochanteric arthroplasty and subtrochanteric osteomy with gluteal advancement. Note that the greater trochanter is stable in the acetabulum, which is remodelling

trochanteric arthroplasty, if possible, to preserve both the stability and length. This is also a helpful feature when late arthrodesis is under consideration (Eyre-Brook, 1960; Obletz, 1960).

References

Blockey, N. J. and Watson, J. T. (1970) Acute osteomyelitis in children. *J. Bone Jt. Surg.* **52B**, 77

Bryson, A. F. and Mandell, B. B. (1964) Primary closure after operative treatment of gross chronic osteomyelitis. *Lancet.* **1**, 1179

Caffey, I. (1967) *Syphilis in Pediatric X-ray Diagnosis*, 5th edn. Chicago: Year Book Medical Publishers

Chapchal, G. (1979) (Editor) *Pseudarthroses and Their Treatment*. Stuttgart: Georg Thieme

Clawson, D. K. and Dunn, A. W. (1967) Management of common bacterial infections of bones and joints. *J. Bone Jt. Surg.* **49A**, 164

Cockshoot, W. P. and MacGregor, M. (1958) Osteomyelitis variolosa. *Q. Jl. Med.* **27**, 369

Compère, E. L., Metzger, W. I. and Mitra, R. N. (1967) Clinical irrigation with non-toxic detergent and antibiotics. *J. Bone Jt. Surg.* **49A**, 614

Evans, E. M. and Davies, D. M. (1969) The treatment of chronic osteomyelitis by saucerisation and secondary skin grafting. *J. Bone Jt. Surg.* **51B**, 454

Eyre-Brook, A. L. (1960) Septic arthritis of the hip and osteomyelitis of the upper end of the femur in infants. *J. Bone Jt. Surg.* **42B**, 11

Freeland, A. E., Sullivan, D. J., Wilbur Westin, G. (1980) Greater trochanteric hip arthroplasty in children with loss of the femoral head. *J. Bone Jt. Surg.* **62A**, 1351–1361

Girdlestone, G. R. (1965) *Girdleston's Tuberculosis of Bone and Joint* revised by E. W. Somerville and M. C. Wilkinson. London: Oxford University Press

Griffiths, J. C. (1968) Defects in long bones from severe neglected osteomyelitis. *J. Bone Jt. Surg.* **50B**, 813

Harris, N. H. (1967) Infections of bones and joints. In *Clinical Surgery*, volume 13, *Orthopaedics*. London: Butterworths.

Harris, N. H. and Kirkaldy-Willis, W. H. (1965) Primary subacute pyogenic osteomyelitis. *J. Bone Jt. Surg.* **47B**, 526

Harrold, A. J. (1960) Acute infective arthritis. In *British Surgical Practice*. London: Butterworths.

Huckstep, R. L. (1962) *Typhoid Fever and Other Salmonella Infections*. Edinburgh: Livingstone

Ilizarov, G. A. and Deviatov, A. A. (1971) Operative elongation of the leg. *Ortop. Traumatol, Protez.* **32**, 820

Jones, R. and Lovett, R. W. (1923) *Orthopaedic Surgery* 1st edn. London: Hodder & Stoughton

Klemm, K. (1980) Clinical experience with Septopal chains in West Germany. In *Proceedings of a Symposium held at the Royal College of Surgeons, London*, p. 21

Lack. C. H. (1959) Chondrolysis in arthritis. *J. Bone Jt. Surg.* **41B**, 384

Lloyd-Roberts, G. C. (1960) Suppurative arthritis of infancy. *J. Bone Jt. Surg.* **42B**, 706

Menelaus, M. B. (1964) Discitis. *J. Bone Jt. Surg.* **46B**, 16

Mendelsohn, B. G. (1965) Actinomycosis of a metacarpal bone. *J. Bone Jt. Surg.* **47B**, 739

Obletz, B. E. (1960) Acute suppurative arthritis of the hip

in the neonatal period. *J. Bone Jt. Surg.* **42A**, 23

Phemister, D. B. (1924) The effect of pressure on articular surfaces in pyogenic and tuberculosis arthritides and its bearing on treatment. *Ann. Surg.* **80**, 481

Seddon, H. J. (1976) The choice of treatment in Potts' disease (editorial) *J. Bone Jt. Surg.* **58B**, 395

Taylor, A. R. and Maudsley, R. H. (1970) Instillation-suction technique *J. Bone Jt. Surg.* **52B**, 88

Trueta, J. (1959) The three types of acute haematogenous osteomyelitis. *J. Bone Jt. Surg.* **41B**, 671

Trueta, J. and Morgan, J. D. (1954) Late results in the treatment of 100 cases of acute osteomyelitis. *Br. J. Surg.* **41**, 449

Watkins, M. B., Samilson, R. L. and Winters, D. M. (1956) Acute suppurative arthritis. *J. Bone Jt. Surg.* **38A**, 1313

Weissman, S. L. (1967) Transplantation of the trochanteric epiphysis into the acetabulum after septic arthritis of the hip. *J. Bone Jt. Surg.* **49A**, 1647

Zammitt, F. (1961) *Brucellosis in Tropical Radiology.* London: Heinemann Medical

Further reading

Gillespie, W. J., Nade, S. (1987) *Musculoskeletal Infections*. Melbourne: Blackwell Scientific Publications

7

Disorders of the central nervous system

There must be something of a neurologist in every orthopaedic surgeon, but when his practice includes children there should be a particularly acute awareness of the close relationship between the two specialties. Many motor disorders have a neurological background, and disability arising from neurological disease frequently has an important skeletal component. This close association has been emphasized by a number of authors (e.g. Sandifer, 1967; Samilson and Perry, 1975).

Having confirmed an underlying neurological abnormality, rational management of the motor effects depends on the diagnosis, since with that comes some idea of the prognosis. For this one must often turn to the specialist neurologist for guidance.

Disorders presenting in infancy and childhood

The floppy infant

The first question to be asked when confronted with a floppy baby is: is there weakness with incidental hypotonia, or is there hypotonia without significant muscle weakness (Dubowitz, 1980). Whether or not the baby can move his limbs against gravity is helpful in deciding the answer.

Conditions with weakness

Spinal muscular atrophy

Severe form (Werdnig-Hoffman disease)

Fetal movements may be reduced, but onset is sometimes later although always within the first 3 months of life. Survival beyond the first year is rare. The infant lies in a frog position with abduction and external rotation of the legs. There is little spontaneous movement and reflexes are absent. Tongue fasciculation and hand tremor may be present. Bulbar and respiratory muscles are involved.

Intermediate forms

The onset of weakness is usually in the second half of the first year of life, although in retrospect it may have been present earlier but mildly. Proximal muscles are weaker than distal ones, and respiratory but not bulbar muscles may be involved. Survival into adolescence or adult life is the rule and these children therefore present considerable problems of orthopaedic management. Close attention is necessary to try to prevent the development of scoliosis and contractures. Many can become ambulant with the aid of lightweight long leg calipers and sticks.

Mild form (Kugelberg–Welander disease)

Early motor milestones are usually normal but walking may be a little delayed, waddling and flat footed, with weakness evident then, mainly around the hips. Deterioration is very slow.

Congenital myopathies

Many but not all of these disorders are progressive. They are not usually distinguishable clinically, and their diagnosis depends upon specialized investigations such as electromyography, nerve conduction studies, muscle biopsy with full histochemical analysis, blood creatine kinase estimation etc. A few of these conditions (e.g. the glycogenoses) have a known metabolic basis and can be diagnosed with specific enzyme estimations. Many affected patients are likely to develop secondary complications requiring orthopaedic intervention. An example of one such condition is congenital fibre-type disproportion and our experience of it in this hospital has been recorded (Cavanagh *et al*, 1978).

Other neuromuscular conditions

This group includes *myotonic dystrophy* (dystrophia myotonica) which may be suspected in a weak floppy infant with an expressionless face, respiratory difficulties and skeletal deformities such as talipes, and confirmed in nearly 90% of cases by the elicitation of myotonia in the mother. Other disorders are the various forms of *congenital muscular dystrophy* where congenital contractures are common, the various forms of *myasthenia*, and some of the *hereditary motor and sensory neuropathies*. Rarely, *Duchenne muscular dystrophy* may present early with hypotonia.

Conditions without significant weakness

These comprise a heterogeneous group of disorders which Dubowitz (1980) has usefully subdivided into a number of broad groups:

1. Disorders affecting the central nervous system of which the most notable are probably Down's syndrome and birth trauma.
2. Connective tissue disorders.
3. Metabolic.
4. The Prader–Willi syndrome – hypotonia, characteristic facies, later onset obesity, mental retardation, cryptorchidism etc.
5. Benign congenital hypotonia; this last group may not be a real entity at all, but simply a repository for cases with hypotonia, no weakness and no specific abnormality on aetiological investigation.

General comments

Nearly all the conditions referred to above are genetically determined. A careful family history is therefore important for management.

The question whether or not a child has a progressive condition will be answered by knowledge of the diagnosis, but assessment of deterioration in any one patient will depend upon a full developmental history and the awareness that progressive deterioration in early life may be masked by natural maturation.

The diagnosis of arthrogryposis cannot be easily considered under any of the categories mentioned so far. This is undoubtedly a clinical description of a heterogeneous group of disorders characterized by extreme stiffness, joint contractures, and fixed deformities such as dislocated hips, talipes, scoliosis etc. (Wynne-Davies and Lloyd-Roberts, 1971). The cases are usually sporadic, in children of normal intelligence, and show no progression. There appears to be an association with Potter's syndrome, oligohydramnios and breech presentation. Abnormalities of spinal anterior horn cells have been described although it is uncertain whether these are primary or secondary.

Cerebral palsy

The syndromes which are collectively described as cerebral palsy comprise the effects of brain injury (congenital or acquired) during birth, early infancy or in early childhood. Although the obvious 'positive' features are spasticity, rigidity, athetosis and ataxia, there are also significant 'negative' phenomena such as the absence of postural reflexes that have an equally important bearing upon prognosis.

Cerebral palsy is a frequent cause of motor disability. It is probable that 2 out of every 1000 children of school age are affected. About half have normal or above normal intelligence and about one-quarter become entirely self-supporting in adult life. In addition to the disorder of posture and movement which is the essence of cerebral palsy, it is common to find evidence of other disabilities, for example of vision, language, hearing and behaviour, and also for there to be epilepsy. Factors other than the physical handicaps do significantly affect outcome (Wortis and Cooper, 1957). The colloquial designation 'spastic' is unsatisfactory because it emphasizes one aspect to the exclusion of others and because it has a derogatory connotation.

Classification and diagnosis

Classification and diagnosis are traditionally based upon an anatomical and neurological description of peripheral motor impairment. This ignores the more subtle features of damage at higher levels, but is used *faut de mieux*, with the understanding that the total disability in each group is the quotient of the motor and intellectual disturbances.

Monoplegia (probably very rare and usually a hemiplegia), *diplegia* (both legs involved but often some hyperreflexia and minor functional disabilities in the upper limbs), *hemiplegia* (arm more involved than leg) and *quadriplegia* (all four limbs involved, the arms more than the legs) are descriptions based on the limbs affected most. These terms are usually combined with others that have more neuroanatomical and functional implications: *spasticity* (exaggerated reflexes, clonus, extensor plantar responses developing after infancy, and increased muscle tone in one direction only – e.g. supination of the forearms, dorsiflexion of wrist or ankle); *rigidity* (muscle tone increased in all directions); *dyskinesia* (irregular and involuntary movements that may be choreoid, athetoid or dystonic and involve some or all muscle groups); *ataxia* (which may be characterized by hypotonia, intention tremor, truncal disequilibrium or, particularly in the young child, by excessive misery and tendency to cling to adults).

The pathogenesis of cerebral palsy is still not understood. A number of factors may be involved, including anoxia, acidosis, hypoglycaemia, all of which may lead to brain swelling, poor cerebral perfusion, vascular infarction or to various forms of intracranial bleeding. A history of infection, drug ingestion or irradiation during pregnancy or of fetal distress, prolonged or precipitate delivery, breech delivery, caesarian section or prematurity may be significant, but many children with cerebral palsy do not appear to have experienced any of these early problems. Whether any of these factors is directly causal or if they are simply indications of pre-existing fetal abnormalities, due perhaps to an underlying abnormality of reproductive capacity in the mother, is still not known.

Whereas there is no mistaking the established signs of an upper motor neuron disorder in the young child, the clinical features in infancy may be quite subtle. Inertia and inactivity are as much evidence of physical as of intellectual damage. Hypotonia is common, especially in incipient athetosis, and, if the arm bears the brunt, may simulate an obstetrical injury to the brachial plexus. Sharing a common cause they may in fact coexist. Supporting signs are failure to relax the grasping reflex at 4 months, and reflex adduction of the hips and equinus of the ankle on suspension. After walking begins (this is usually delayed), other more familiar signs appear, such as tiptoe gait and the important abducted flexed arm (bat wing arm). Indeed, the gait alone is usually diagnostic. Tiptoeing is either unilateral or bilateral with knees flexed. In contrast, dynamic or structural shortening of the heel cord may be overcome by hyperextension of the knee and eversion of the heel which can then touch the ground. Adduction or flexion or internal rotation at one or both hips will contribute additionally to the walking pattern. Lastly, valgus of the heel, if confined to one side, may well signal unilateral spasticity.

General management

In ideal circumstances diagnosis should be followed by reference to a cerebral palsy unit in which a neurologist is supported by physiotherapists and occupational therapists with special experience, a psychologist, speech therapist, audiologist, ophthalmologist and social worker. The function of the group is to try to assess the child's handicap as accurately and as early as possible and then to anticipate physical, intellectual and emotional problems before, or as soon as, they appear – including the problems of the parents.

Treatment other than the prevention of deformity by stretching, appropriate seating and disciplined splinting has a secondary role in the management of the motor disability – indeed, many children need no more than this. The elaborate systems of treatment advocated by sectarian mystics are, in general, time consuming for the parents and of little apparent value to the child. The often repeated claim that, given a child in infancy, 'the system' will work wonders is suspect, because in infancy an accurate prognosis is seldom possible. Consequently the effects of treatment cannot be assessed on the basis of the performance of older children who have had such treatment. Furthermore, it is virtually impossible to match infant patients for controlled trials, and, if it were possible, by the very philosophy advanced the control patient could not be left untreated.

It cannot be emphasized too strongly that a brain-damaged child will improve in his motor achievement as he grows, in a manner related to the quotient of his intellectual and physical handicaps, regardless of treatment or the lack of it, provided that deformity is prevented and his emotional and intellectual needs are met. In treatment one can offer no more than prevention of some problems before they arise by intelligent anticipation, and alleviation of some of the effects which one is unable to control.

One of the concerns of those working in the cerebral palsy assessment units is the selection of the appropriate educational environment most suited to the individual need of the child. Some children need to go to special schools for the mentally retarded, others who are intellectually unimpaired to a school for the physically handicapped. Of equal importance is the assessment unit's role in ensuring that there is continuity of medical, psychological and physiotherapeutic care wherever the child goes for day-to-day care.

The work of assessment centres is exacting at all times, especially when the parents are resentful or ill equipped to co-operate in management. Many different specialties are involved and some centres rely upon case conferences with the various specialists present. This multidisciplinary approach (as contemporary jargon has it) does not necessarily benefit the child more than separate assessment by individual specialists co-ordinated by the physician in charge of the patient. The busy person may be wise in being cautious in accepting an invitation to join such a group. The conferences are often lengthy, and as relatively few patients concern all those attending, boredom is prone to set in and cross-fertility becomes low.

Orthopaedic management of the motor component of cerebral palsy

This may be divided into three phases: first, stretching, splinting (orthotics) and education

of child and parent; second, selection of those needing surgical treatment and the exclusion of those unsuitable, and third, the practice of surgery. Although somewhat artificial because the three phases overlap and merge into each other, this is a useful generalization especially because it introduces broad time factors – phase one being from birth to about 5 years, phase two from 5 to 8 years and phase three from then on.

Stretching, splinting and education

All joints exposed to the risk of deformity are moved firmly and repeatedly through their fullest range twice daily. The parent must therefore be taught to do this at home. To establish the system we must provide constant instruction, encouragement and support, which are often best offered in a day centre. Splinting (orthoses) should be simple – such as metal or plastic gutter knee and foot splints – and in general used only at night, after the evening stretching. There is relatively little place for walking calipers or irons. They are an added encumbrance, yield to the spasm they are meant to control and do not correct deformity. It is most unfortunate that the model of a child used to draw attention to the collecting box of a well known charity for cerebral palsy is displayed wearing long leg calipers with pelvic band – a device calculated to make walking virtually impossible for anyone who is not the victim of flaccid paraplegia.

Education of the child in walking or manual skills requires nice judgement, for at this age the development of a functional, if ungainly, gait, may be of greater value as the key to independence than the slower, more difficult, but orthodox progression pleasing to some physiotherapists.

In this phase fixed deformities should not develop, but if they do, correction by serial plasters is usually adequate.

Surgery is rarely indicated except to prevent hip dislocation, or occasionally, to control rapidly recurring deformity in spite of satisfactory splintage.

Selection and rejection of patients for operation

This diffuse and somewhat contentious subject may be discussed from three aspects: contraindications, relative contraindications and indications.

Contraindications

Patients with severe mental defect with or without severe physical handicaps, which make the prospect of independent living remote, often disqualify themselves. Others are so emotionally labile that even admission to hospital is hazardous. Those with severe athetosis, ataxia or atonia are excluded, apart from rare exceptions. In those who are mildly affected and have good function, surgery is ill advised.

Relative contraindications, suggesting that decision be postponed

Examples of these patients are those with lesser degrees of mental deficiency, who with time may achieve limited independence. Others are emotionally disabled, demonstrated by deterioration when admitted to hospital or by an inability to co-operate or by a lack of will to improve. Some patients have a poor sense of balance, preventing standing, holding onto a coat or some walking device. Children with rigid cerebral palsy are disappointing for they fail to achieve that degree of improvement we would expect if their deformities were due to spastic palsy. Lastly, deformity may be an advantage, as when mild equinus encourages knee extension and thus stability in the hemiplegic.

Indications

The essential indications are found among patients who, with certain provisos mentioned above, fail to improve under the influence of good non-operative treatment, and who in addition have a disabling deformity (structural or dynamic) similarly uncontrolled, which surgery can correct or improve. In borderline decisions good balance and determination strongly support operation. Other factors must sometimes be considered if there is doubt. There may be parents who are overdemanding or overindulgent, coexisting and unsuspected disease, and of course the possibility that the diagnosis of cerebral palsy is wrong.

Preventive surgical measures are sometimes used – for example, to prevent hip dislocation (commonly) or (rarely) progressive genu recurvatum.

Additional indications are rare. They include pain due to deformed toes – especially the big toe – and displaced hips made painful when degenerating and subject to uncontrolled movement in athetosis.

Operative surgery in cerebral palsy

General considerations

The correction of deformity is so important a part of surgery in this disease that a consideration of its causes merits discussion. Deformity may be structural and persisting under anaesthesia, or dynamic, when an abnormal posture, adopted only during activity, disappears under anaesthesia. Obviously the types may be mixed, and the dynamic, if uncontrolled, become structural. The distinction is important if only to protect physiotherapists from the frustration of trying to correct established fixed deformity in the conscious patient by stretching.

Deformity is due to inequality of muscle power between opposing muscle groups, the effect being sometimes reinforced by gravity, growth and an overall pattern of movement. For example, a foot controlled by spastic invertors and plantar flexors, and weak evertors and dorsiflexors will at first lie in equinovarus, but is correctable by pressure (dynamic deformity). Later, muscle shortening will establish fixed deformity and this is aided by gravity and the bed clothes. Later still the bones will grow abnormally (much as a tree grows away from the prevailing wind) so that bony operations are needed for correction, whereas in the earlier stages stretching or soft tissue procedures will succeed.

We must be prepared to accept some temporary deterioration in function and emotional instability in a proportion of children for a variable time after operation, and should warn the parents of this.

Relatively few children are likely to be helped by surgery – perhaps 10% of those attending a mixed cerebral palsy clinic – but in so common a disease this proportion represents an important part of orthopaedic surgery at childhood.

Lastly, and of such importance that a platitude is justified: surgery is but an incident in the continuing care of the child, which is concerned not only with his motor problems but also with his intellectual, emotional and other abnormalities.

The surgery of deformity and other disabilities

The upper limb

Opportunities to use surgery helpfully are extremely few in the upper limb. In a recent review from a special clinic for upper limb cases, approximately 50 out of over 500 patients were considered eligible for surgery, and in the majority of these the surgery was found to be of cosmetic rather than functional benefit (Bell, Baker and Sergiov, 1988).

In quadriplegia brain damage is so diffuse that few are suitable, and there remain only hemiplegics and the occasional diplegics with adequate intelligence.

Congenital amputation of one hand in an otherwise normal child is compatible with virtually full function. The same principle applies in hemiplegia when the disabled hand, lacking precision, is used at best to grasp while the other works on an object, or at worst is an activated paper weight. This lack of precision is permanent, quickly recognized by the child, and not amenable to improvement by training. It is too much trouble to use the hand as a prime mover and no amount of encouragement will persuade him otherwise – indeed there are grave risks of disturbing the emotional equilibrium if those responsible are too demanding. The same effect is sometimes seen after operation.

Consideration of the upper limb should start with assessment of the shoulder. Operation is rarely, if ever, indicated. However, the child should have reasonable control of the shoulder before considering surgery more distally. At the elbow, fixed flexion can be a considerable functional and cosmetic problem. This can be released by the Max Page type of flexor muscle slide which can improve the position of both the elbow and the wrist (White, 1972).

This operation is in general preferable to arthrodesis of the wrist which sacrifices movement at the wrist and should be used only if a very carefully controlled trial of rigid splinting of the wrist shows that hand function is clearly improved when the wrist is rigidly held. Transfer of the flexor carpi ulnaris to the extensor carpi radialis can correct wrist flexion, particularly when, on grasping, the hand is palmar flexed and ulnar deviated. This operation can also strengthen dorsiflexion and supination (Green and Banks, 1962). Excessive pronation of the forearm can be improved

by the pronator teres tendon transfer originally described by Robert Jones (1921) and assessed more recently by Colton, Ransford and Lloyd-Roberts (1976).

Finally, persistent adduction of the thumb into the palm can be improved by a so-called Matev release of the insertions of the adductor pollicis, flexor pollicis brevis and the distal two-thirds of the adductor pollicis brevis at their insertion (Matev, 1963). This can be combined when necessary with transfer of the extensor carpi radialis longus or brevis to the base of the first metacarpal or to the over-stretched abductor pollicis longus and extensor pollicis brevis to increase the abduction power of the thumb.

The spine

Spinal deformity, particularly scoliosis, is being increasingly recognized in patients with cerebral palsy. In hemiplegia it is rare, despite the unilateral involvement. However, in quadriplegia and particularly those children who develop the so-called 'windswept' position (Figure 7.1), serious and progressive spinal deformity is frequently seen. In the past, little attention was paid to this, and it often led to very severe deformities which made the management of these extremely handicapped patients very difficult. It is most important to refer any patient with increasing spinal deformity in cerebral palsy to a special scoliosis clinic as soon as it is recognized, rather than waiting until the deformity becomes gross and correction a very difficult and sometimes hazardous procedure (*see also* Chapter 12).

The hip joint

Dislocation and subluxation

The predisposition to dislocation and subluxation dominates the hip joint. Flexor and adductor spasm produce deformity which, at first dynamic, becomes fixed with time. The pelvis then tilts, the femoral head is partially uncovered, subluxates and finally dislocates. This sequence may be rapid but, being common, should be anticipated by regular radiographs, which are particularly indicated in the severely handicapped quadriplegic.

When the femoral head is at risk, being adducted and incompletely covered, division of

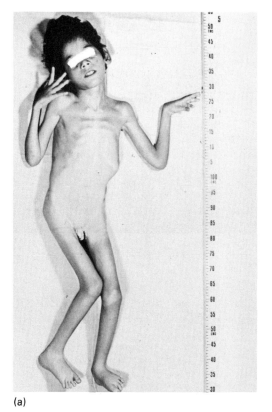
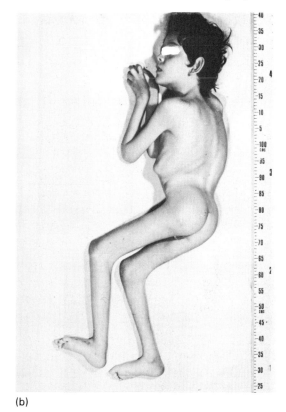

(a)   (b)

Figure 7.1 Severe quadriplegia (total body involvement – Bleck). Note the windswept posture of the legs and the developing scoliosis. (a) Anterior view. (b) Side, lying view

gracilis, adductors longus and brevis, and sometimes anterior obturator neurectomy followed by complete splinting in abduction for 6 weeks will usually restore congruity.

In quadriplegics with severe subluxation or recent dislocation, a similar operation adding iliopsoas tenotomy through the same incision is indicated.

Established irreducible dislocation is usually seen in severely handicapped children who do not walk. If possible, this situation should be prevented by earlier surgery (Figure 7.2). In a few cases, open reduction of the hip combined with open adductor release and iliopsoas tenotomy together with femoral osteotomy or pelvic osteotomy, if indicated, may be necessary to achieve stabilization (Figure 7.3). Anterolateral iliopsoas transfer may be helpful in stabilizing these hips.

In later life pain may demand relief, especially when degenerative arthritis is aggravated by the involuntary movements of atheto-sis in a patient unable to walk. Excision of the femoral head and neck and the upper end of the femur to below the level of the lesser trochanter can provide a mobile hip which is reasonably pain free. This operation is particularly indicated when there is anterior subluxation or dislocation of the hip with fixation in extension (Figure 7.4). It should be used only as a last resort when all other methods have failed. This type of surgery is especially valuable in the severe quadriplegic patient who will require continuing nursing care throughout life.

Deformity

Flexion and adduction without dislocation are first treated on the lines already described. Severe adduction may require more radical adductor section occasionally including part of the magnus and the pectineus, but complete

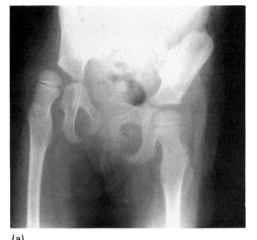

(a)

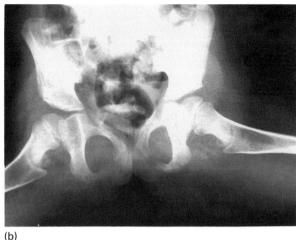

(b)

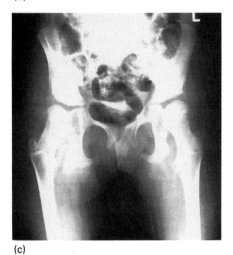

(c)

Figure 7.2 Subluxing right hip with tight adductors. (a) Preoperatively, the right hip is at risk. (b) After open adductor tenotomy and anterior obturator neurectomy. Note the wide abduction obtained. (c) After operation, showing subluxation (lateral displacement) of the hip reduced; however, there is still coxa valga

obturator neurectomy should not be performed lest fixed abduction follow. Fixed flexion deformity persisting after iliopsoas tenotomy may occasionally require an extensive anterior release, or even trochanteric osteotomy.

Internal rotation, when a handicap, can be difficult to analyse, and therefore manage. In theory the anterior gluteus medius and medial hamstrings (semitendinosus and gracilis) are dynamic deforming forces but do not seem to shorten structurally. Fixed deformity is therefore more likely to be skeletal, due to torsion of the shaft or anteversion of the femoral neck. It is often difficult to confirm this clinically without doing an examination under anaesthetic. Radiological measurement of anteversion is rarely necessary although CT scanning and ultrasound can be used. Soft tissue procedures

to correct the deformity have rarely been successful. At the knee, lateral transfer of the semitendinosus is sometimes helpful, but can have rather a variable result. Steel (1980) has described advancement of the insertion of gluteus medius and minimus to correct this deformity with good results in 26 patients.

This is probably a useful procedure in younger children before they have developed significant structural abnormality. Once significant structural abnormality *has* developed, an external rotation osteotomy of the femur will be necessary, either at the upper end if there is significant valgus as well as anteversion or at the lower end if there is simply rotation deformity. It is important not to perform such bone surgery under the age of 10 or 11 years of age, otherwise deformity may well recur and a further osteotomy be necessary.

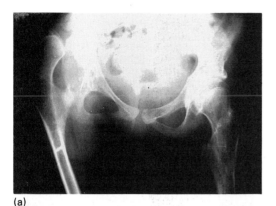

(a)

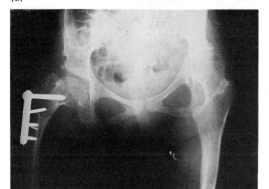

(b)

Figure 7.3 (a) Dislocated right hip in a 13-year-old diplegic who can still walk. The hip is painful. (b) X-ray after open reduction, femoral osteotomy with shortening, adductor release and iliopsoas transfer

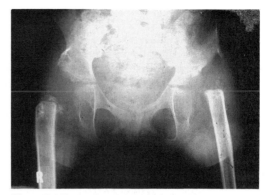

Figure 7.4 X-ray after excision of the upper quarter of both femurs for stiff anteriorly dislocated hips in severe quadriplegia

The knee joint

Flexion

This is the most common deformity requiring treatment, but it must be emphasized that it may not arise primarily in the knee. Equinus of the foot and flexion of the hip may be compensated for by a bent knee, as may contralateral adduction causing apparent shortening. Furthermore, in diplegia both knees may be flexed equally when walking but the less spastic may be flexed in sympathy and therefore straighten when the more spastic is corrected. Fixed flexion deformity is best corrected by a distal elongation of the hamstrings. The original operation (Eggers, 1952) in which the hamstrings were transplanted to the distal end of the femur was soon found to be too radical, leading to loss of flexion which makes stairs difficult and hyperextension common. A simple distal elongation of the hamstring tendons, combined with serial plas-

ters if it is not possible to straighten the knee fully under anaesthetic at the first operation, will usually correct most deformities. Only very occasionally is a supracondylar extension osteotomy required. This should be done at or near maturity. The patient should be immobilized in plaster and encouraged to walk as soon as possible. It is best to allow him to remain in plaster for 6 weeks so that the hamstrings are fully healed before removal. It is often necessary to use a back slab temporarily until the quadriceps apparatus, which has been chronically stretched, is able to control the knee satisfactorily.

Proximal hamstring release (Seymour and Sharrard, 1968) is only useful for the occasional patient who has no fixed flexion deformity at the knee, who walks with a short stride with pelvic rotation, whose passive straight leg raising is 30 degrees or less and who cannot sit up with the knees extended but can sit with the knees flexed. Attempts to apply this operation to patients with more serious flexion problems have failed.

Hyperextension

Strangely, hyperextension rarely progresses to a degree which causes handicap, in spite of the extended knee gait of hemiplegia with tendo Achillis shortening. It may, however, follow overenthusiastic hamstring transplant, posterior capsulotomy and recession of the origins of the gastrocnemius. For these reasons these procedures have fallen out of favour. If necessary, it can be controlled by a caliper or knee brace.

Other deformities

Genu valgum secondary to hip adduction may need correction after the hip has been dealt with. External tibial torsion is commonly seen in association with persistent femoral anteversion and should be taken into account when correcting internal rotation in the femur.

The feet

Equinus

In cerebral palsy, equinus is by far the commonest deformity. Operation is much more likely to be required in hemiplegic cerebral palsy than in diplegia. In diplegia it is often secondary to fixed flexion at the hip and knee (Figure 7.5). If in this latter case the

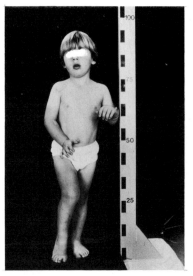

Figure 7.6 Characteristic stance in hemiplegia. Note equinus of the right foot

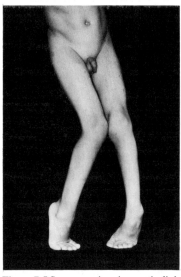

Figure 7.5 Severe equinus in spastic diplegia. It is essential that the proximal hip and knee deformities are corrected first

tendo Achillis is unwisely lengthened, then, although the heels come to the ground, the patient assumes an even more crouched posture, much to the alarm and despondency of this parents, his physiotherapist and his surgeon. In hemiplegia the leg is frequently slightly short and the equinus may compensate very well for this shortening. In this case lengthening tendo Achillis will not improve the gait and will often make it worse. However, if there is significant fixed equinus or severe dynamic equinus with complete loss of a

heel–toe gait then elongation of tendo Achillis can be very helpful (Figure 7.6). In the young child under the age of 5 years, it is frequently better to control early dynamic or structural equinus by serial plasters. These can be applied under general anaesthetic and retained for 6 weeks, changing them if necessary at 3 weeks. It is often surprising how much correction can be obtained, although frequently the equinus will recur over the next 2–3 years. However, if surgical lengthening of tendo Achillis is done before the age of 4 or 5 there is a greater tendency for the deformity to recur with growth and need repeat surgery at a later date (Graham and Fixsen, 1988). There are several ways of lengthening the tendo Achillis. In the presence of fixed equinus under general anaesthetic, we prefer the slide method described by White (1943) in which the proximal and medial part of the Achilles tendon is divided in the calf and distal part anteriorly near its insertion. Two mnemonics have been suggested for this: 'Peter May dislikes Australians' and 'DAMP' (distal, anterior, medial, proximal).

The ankle is dorsiflexed and the tendon elongates without the necessity for any internal stitches. A below-knee plaster is applied unless there is a particular need to control the knee. The child is allowed to walk within 48 hours and the plaster is retained for 4 weeks. In most series approximately 10–15% of such tendo

Achillis lengthenings require repeat surgery. It is rarely possible to repeat a slide and a formal 'Z' lengthening of the tendo Achillis is necessary, occasionally with capsulotomy, re-suture in the neutral position (0 degrees) and plaster for 6 weeks. By contrast with the equinus of older children with club feet, correction is always possible. In the presence of dynamic equinus but no fixed deformity, a gastrocnemius recession, as described by Strayer (1950) can be used.

Subcutaneous tenotomy of tendo Achillis can be performed in certain cases, but in our hands has proved less reliable. The Silfvers-kiold (1923/24) procedure has proved unreli-able and it tends to cause genu recurvatum. For many years the so-called Silfverskiold test in which the equinus is assessed with the knee extended and the knee flexed has been used to try to differentiate between gastrocnemius and soleus contracture. However, Perry and col-leagues (1974) showed by electromyographic studies that this test is not reliable.

Equinovarus

Equinovarus is normally a handicap and is commonly progressive. Treatment with an iron and T-strap or moulded orthosis can hold the deformity only rather ineffectively. It is most important to correct any fixed or dynamic equinus before correcting the varus. If the tibialis posterior is clearly overacting then split tibialis posterior transfer is the safest method of correcting the varus. It is tempting to transplant the tendon through the interosseus membrane, but it is extremely easy to develop overcorrection into valgus with time (Figure 7.7). In older children with fixed bony deformi-ty, calcaneal osteotomy, plantar strip and occasionally triple arthrodesis may be neces-sary.

Valgus

Valgus heels and pronated feet are particularly common in diplegia and quadriplegia. In general, function is good in the early years, but can lead to severe deformity and marked rocker-bottomed feet in later life. Simple lengthening of the Achilles tendon will not correct the deformity because the subtalar joint is basically unstable. In the early stages, conservative measures with a medial arch

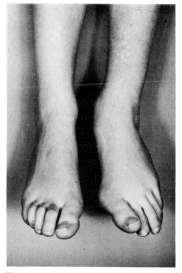

Figure 7.7 Overcorrection into valgus following tibialis posterior tendon transfer on the left for previous severe varus

insole and an outside iron and an inside T-strap or moulded orthosis will help to support the medial side of the foot. However, with time it is often necessary to stabilize the subtalar joint by a Grice subtalar arthrodesis combined with elongation of tendo Achillis once the subtalar joint is stable, and also sometimes elongation of the peroneal tendons. The Batchelor modifi-cation described by Brown in 1968 is very attractive, using a fibular graft, but there have been problems with graft breakage and dis-turbance of the growth of the fibula. More recently, Dennyson and Fulford (1976) have described an attractive method using a single screw to obtain immediate internal fixation, combined with autogenous cancellous grafting to achieve solid fusion (Figure 7.8). Transfer of the peroneus brevis to the tibialis posterior has been advocated but, like all tendon transfers in cerebral palsy, it is difficult to get the balance exactly right and has proved unreliable.

The toes

The toes are frequently the cause of pain and minor disability. Hallux valgus – interpha-langeal or metatarsophalangeal – can be corrected by arthrodesis (Figure 7.9). Howev-er, in hallux valgus of the latter type it is difficult to position the toe exactly right and a first metatarsal osteotomy combined with

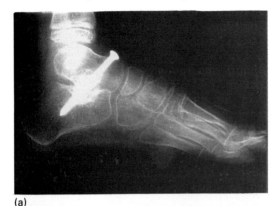

(a)

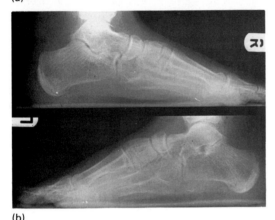

(b)

Figure 7.8 Extra-articular subtalar arthrodesis using screw fixation. (a) Aged 7 years. (b) Aged 15 years; the screw has been removed

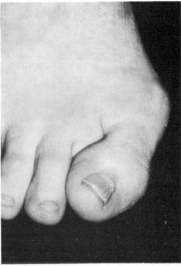

Figure 7.9 Hallux valgus in spastic diplegia. Note the severe deformity and the rotation of the toe, causing pressure on the medial side of the big toe

operate at one, two or three levels in some cases.

Myelomeningocele (Figure 7.10)

Myelomeningocele is by far the commonest manner of presentation. The spinal cord and nerve roots are enclosed within, and adherent to, a membranous sac, or lie exposed on the surface. The leaking cord is open like a book on the hinge of its central canal with nerve roots streaming from it (myeloschisis). The lesion is commonest at the lumbosacral level

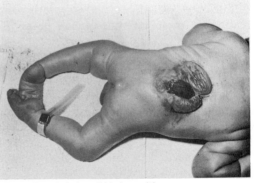

Figure 7.10 A 1-day-old infant with open myelomeningocele. Note the neural plaque exposed in the centre of the lesion and the severe lower limb deformities

division of the adductor hallucis can give satisfactory results without sacrificing movements at the metatarsophalangeal joint. The clawing of the lesser toes can be corrected by arthrodesis rather than by flexor-to-extensor transfer.

These deformities have, necessarily, been discussed in an artificial localized way, but their interrelationship must be considered. Thus equinus may cause knee and hip flexion or vice versa, and hip abduction dispose to genu valgum, eversion and pronation of the foot and contralateral knee flexion to compensate for apparent shortening. It is vital to determine which are the primary deformities and which the secondary before embarking on surgery.

Gait analysis at present is only available in a few centres in the UK. It emphasizes the complexity of the situation and the necessity to

but may appear at any level in the spine. Myelodysplasia is almost constantly present and the neurological deficit will depend upon the upper level of this in the spinal cord. Hydrocephalus is common, usually prompt in its appearance and increasing in frequency in relation to the spinal lesion from below upwards. Curiously, however, cervical lesions carry the best prognosis from every aspect.

General management in infancy

In the early 1960s the results of early and of delayed treatment of the back reported by Sharrard and his colleagues from Sheffield (1962) suggested that early closure improved muscle function and preserved neurology. As a result, a policy of early closure was accepted in many centres. However, the results of this policy presented by Lorber in 1971 were so disappointing that he (Lorber, 1971) put forward certain criteria which appeared to be associated with a poor prognosis and suggested that these be used as a basis for selection. The criteria were: gross paralysis of the legs; thoracolumbar or thoracolumbosacral lesions; kyphosis or scoliosis; hydrocephalus with a head circumference of 2 cm or more above the 90th percentile; intracerebral birth injury and other gross congenital anomalies. In Edinburgh and Melbourne a policy of selection had always been practised and the results of this selection policy were reported by Stark and Drummond (1972) and Smith and Smith (1973). Of those patients not selected for treatment, the great majority died in the first year of life. Of those treated, 70% survived at least 5 years. The majority of the survivors will have only mild or moderate handicap.

The question of selection will always remain a difficult one. The orthopaedic surgeon is rarely primarily involved with this, although he may be asked to give an opinion about the patient's probable locomotor function in later life. The results reported by Lorber (1971) in his unselected series are extremely helpful in advising about these patients as they were classified according to the neurological levels. It is clear that unless a child has good musculature under voluntary control down to the knees he is unlikely to remain an active walker.

The tragedy of failure is emphasized by the contrast between the victim as a baby and as a young adult. As a baby he lies relatively inert with wet nappy, and must be carried from place to place. He differs little from others. As a young adult he is usually in a wheelchair, having abandoned the struggle for independence by rejecting the calipers and crutches. Obese, acneform, odoriferous and impotent, he contemplates a sorry future with understandable melancholy.

The musculoskeletal system in infancy

Where possible, it is wise to postpone operative treatment until the first year has passed. This is because the majority of those destined to die in the early years do so before they are 1 year old, and also because assessment, including charting of muscle power, is likely to be more accurate later.

With some exceptions, the first year is spent on assessment of paralysis and correction of deformity by stretching and simple splinting – a programme in which the mother should share. The emphasis is on fixed flexion of hips and knees and equinovarus deformity of the feet. The possible exceptions include talipes equinovarus and hip dislocation (*see* below).

Management of the first year

During the preliminary period most babies with significant weakness will be found to have one of three grades of paralysis, depending upon the upper level to which the cord is damaged.

Group 1

These cases of paralysis have virtually a flaccid paraplegia, the level extending to the first lumbar or twelfth thoracic segment. There may be weak psoas action insufficient to cause hip dislocation or deformity, and there are no active deforming forces operating lower in the legs.

Group 2

These cases of paralysis have the first three lumbar segments intact and have, therefore, strong hip flexors and adductors but no abductors or extensors. Knee extension is present to an extent dependent on the third lumbar representation. Hip deformity and dislocation are likely to occur.

Group 3

In these cases of paralysis all the lumbar segments are in action and the paralysis is largely below the knee.

The following concept was elaborated and refined by Sharrard (1964). Fixed deformity may be present at birth or develop later. Neonatal deformity is the quotient of the effects of paralysis and the position imposed by the intrauterine posture. Thus, in a baby with flaccid paraplegia the hips and knees may be flexed because this is the close-packed fetal position from which, because of paralysis, he cannot escape. In contrast, a baby with group 2 paralysis may be born with adducted and flexed hips, but extended knees reflecting the position adopted when the antagonists are paralysed. When treatment begins the contrast is even more striking, for those deformities imposed by the accident of fetal positioning upon flaccid joints do not recur after correction, whereas those for which unopposed muscle action is responsible tend to recur.

We must accept these fundamentals in planning treatment, and the approach is therefore different in dealing with total, as opposed to partial, paralysis. In total paralysis we aim to correct deformities sufficiently to allow boots and calipers to be fitted, by stretching or minor operation (usually tenotomy). Daily stretching effectively prevents relapse. In partial paralysis, however, we have to both correct the deformity and maintain the correction by measures designed to restore muscle balance. When calipers are needed, it is usually futile to introduce them to a child who is not showing spontaneous efforts to pull himself up or clearly enjoys being stood in a standing frame.

Treatment of individual deformities

The hip joint

Deformity and dislocation may appear separately or together, or the former may lead to the latter.

Deformity without dislocation is usually in flexion and adduction, and is associated with either unopposed muscle action or pelvic obliquity secondary to lumbar scoliosis.

Subluxations or dislocations are more likely to be present at birth. If weak, there may be no subluxation (as in the group 1 type of lesion) but it is best to try to protect the hip by regular passive stretching and, if necessary, simple tenotomy of the deforming muscle. Subluxations and dislocation are more difficult, for one must decide whether to treat the dislocation and the deformity, or the deformity only. If bilateral, the vast majority should be left alone (Menelaus, 1976). However, the inevitable flexion deformity should initially be treated by stretching and positioning; subsequently, soft tissue release and even extension osteotomy may be required if it is clear that the child is going to be able to stand and use calipers.

When dislocation is unilateral, reduction (usually by open operation) is indicated, provided that the child is clearly going to be a reasonable walker.

Timing and technique are important. We prefer to postpone operation for at least a year to see how the child is developing generally. The vast majority will require open operation and will not respond to conservative measures. If the child is treated in an abduction harness or plaster for a long period in the first year, severe abduction and flexion contractures can develop.

The technique is largely governed by the power of the muscles around the hip. Thus, if flexors and adductors are relatively weak, simple tenotomy of the adductors and iliopsoas may allow the hip to be replaced in the socket. If there is severe valgus of the femoral neck, varus osteotomy may be necessary. Iliopsoas transplant, introduced by Mustard (1952, 1959) and modified by Sharrard (1964), was initially very popular. However, as Carol and Sharrard reported in 1972, unless the patient has very strong hip flexors and adductors, weak abductors, good quadriceps power and a lesion of the lower motor neurone type, the results prove disappointing.

The most common reason for failure, not only of iliopsoas transfer but also of other muscle transfers in the lower limbs of myelomeningocele patients, is that it is not realized that fewer that half of them have a simple lower motor neurone lesion. This was pointed out by Stark and Baker (1967), who showed that there were two basic types of neurological lesion. In about one-third of patients there was complete loss of spinal cord function below a certain segmental level, resulting in sensory loss, flaccid paralysis and absent reflexes below this level. In the other two-thirds there was interruption of the corticospinal tracts but preservation of purely reflex activity in isolated distal segments. If the more common pattern of innervation is not recognized by the orthopaedic surgeon, his muscle transfer surgery is likely to fail and simple tenotomy of the over acting or reflexly acting muscles is much more likely to be successful.

The knee joint

In grade 1 paralysis, flexion due to uterine positioning usually responds to stretching and splinting, but hamstring tenotomy is sometimes needed and, rarely, posterior capsulotomy. In grade 2 paralysis, the knee may be straight due to flexor paralysis with good extensor power. This gives a stable knee, which seldom develops into genu recurvatum severe enough to warrant treatment. Fixed flexion at birth obscures extensor power, but this will become evident as the knee straightens. The danger of recurvatum will be increased if posterior support from tendons and capsule is ruthlessly removed. In grade 3 paralysis, flexion deformity is less likely, but if present and resistant, the flexor tendons should be lengthened rather than divided. Sometimes neglected hip adduction causes troublesome knee valgus. This can be treated in older children by supracondylar osteotomy. However, the temptation to treat recurrent or resistant flexion deformity by supracondylar osteotomy in the younger child should be resisted, because this can give rise to a very ugly and disabling anterior angulation of the lower end of the femur as the child grows. Supracondylar osteotomy for flexion deformities of the knee should be reserved for the child nearing skeletal maturity.

The foot

In grades 1 and 2 paralysis, the object is to produce a plantigrade foot which will fit into a boot and which has no high points of pressure liable to ulceration. Most have equinovarus or calcaneovalgus deformity and respond to conventional methods of treatment – sometimes aided by tenotomy of obstinate and otherwise functionless contracted tendons. It is hard for the orthopaedic surgeon to resist surgery in the first year of life, when he is used to treating congenital talipes equinovarus as early as possible. However, if early surgery is performed and is not followed by persistent long-term splintage, the deformity will inevitably recur unless the child is ready to get on to his feet. We therefore recommend leaving surgery on these deformities until the child is ready to start standing, with or without calipers, because so often very early surgery has to be repeated because of the difficulty in maintaining adequate splintage posture. Talectomy remains a useful operation for the rigid arthrogrypotic-like deformity sometimes seen in the meningomyelocele foot.

Grade 3 paralysis is variable in distribution and depth, so the deformities actively produced are equally variable. They range from mild pes cavus with claw toes developing in adolescence to obstinate and early equinovarus and calcaneovalgus (Figure 7.11). They are similar in cause and effect to those seen in poliomyelitis and are managed by the same techniques of correction, tendon transplantation and stabilization. It is becoming increasingly obvious that a plantigrade foot without high pressure areas is essential for those meningomyelocele patients who remain active walkers in adult life. Otherwise, trophic ulceration will ensue, leading to complete breakdown of the foot, sometimes even requiring amputation (Figure 7.12 and 7.13).

The spine

Deformity of the spine is becoming increasingly recognized as one of the most serious problems in meningomyelocele patients. This is particularly noticeable in those with thoracolumbar sacral lesions who have survived, with or without selection, but also can occur with devastating effects in children with low lesions and good lower limb function. Sharrard (1968) advocated osteotomy in patients with severe kyphosis, to aid primary closure, but unfortunately the recurrence rate of the kyphosis is very high. If a kyphosis is stable, has good cover and is not causing any problems, it probably can be left alone. If, however, there are persistent problems with ulceration and with collapse when sitting, excision of the kyphos combined with anterior and sometimes posterior fusion to stabilize the spine may be required.

Scoliosis may progress rapidly and become severely disabling. It is being increasingly realized that the combination of anterior and posterior fusion is the best method of dealing

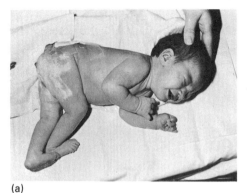

(a)

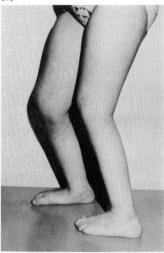

(b)

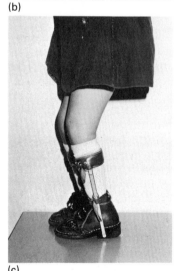

(c)

Figure 7.11 Patient with innervation to L4, with calcaneus feet and active quadriceps muscles. This patient has a good chance of walking with below-knee orthoses or even no orthoses. (a) At birth. (b) At 18 months, following simple tenotomy of the overacting dorsiflexors of the feet. (c) Ankle/foot orthoses to help stabilize the ankles

with these difficult progressive paralytic deformities (Osebold *et al*, 1982).

Variant manifestations

Paralysis may be entirely or predominantly confined to one side, usually associated with so-called hemimeningomyelocele. These patients can be very difficult to treat because the lower limb abnormalities are so asymmetrical. Shortening is often marked and the deformity on the affected side can cause significant problems in management.

Spasticity, due to autonomous reflex action in isolated cord segments, is often a disadvantage. Recognition is important for it will greatly influence treatment.

Progressive paralysis suggests spinal dysraphism (*see* below), tethering and sometimes a syrinx of the cord.

It is most important to make a realistic assessment of the child's potential. Early in life, orthopaedic management should aim to correct and prevent deformity if possible by conservative stretching and strapping. When the general prognosis is clear and the functional ability of the child has been assessed reasonably accurately, then those deformities which are preventing him from functioning to his maximum ability should be corrected with the minimum number of surgical procedures (Menelaus, 1976).

The influence of abnormalities of other systems on orthopaedic surgery

Genitourinary

Few patients with significant peripheral paralysis escape sphincteric paralysis, but the responsibility for these problems rests elsewhere. The orthopaedic surgeon is affected when uncontrolled leaking contaminates wounds or urinary diversion to the abdominal wall is contemplated, although this is now less popular since intermittent catheterization has been introduced, particularly for girls. It is imperative that the genitourinary and the orthopaedic surgeon co-operate so that hip surgery is completed before diversion (Figure 7.14). Spinal osteotomy may be indicated where kyphosis reduces the affected abdominal surface.

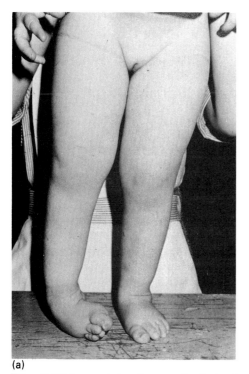

(a)

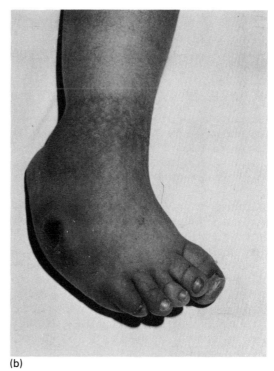

(b)

Figure 7.12 Uncorrected equinovarus despite bracing in a child who is a good walker. (a) Standing position. (b) Trophic ulceration over high-pressure area on the fifth metatarsal base

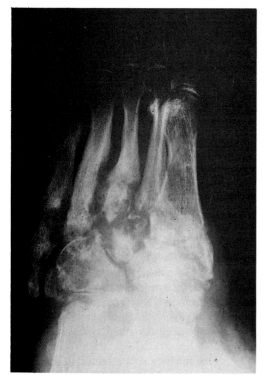

Figure 7.13 Gross Charcot-like changes in a spina bifida foot in adult life

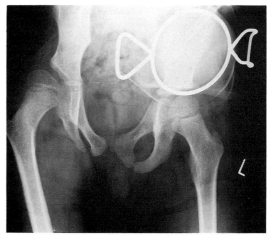

Figure 7.14 Subluxating hip. Urinary diversion, now very much less commonly used, has unfortunately been performed and this may compromise hip surgery

Bowel

Training is usually successful, and as colostomy is very rarely indicated there are no common problems.

Trophic effects

Surgical wounds of tissues lacking sensibility heal like any other, but plasters or splints that have been applied carelessly are a frequent cause of ulceration. It is curious that ulcers are otherwise rare in children under 10 years of age. Nevertheless, deformity such as equinovarus must be prevented, for the feet are then prone to lateral ulceration. Established chronic ulcers occur most frequently over the heel, the fifth metatarsal and the ischial tuberosity. Radical surgery, with removal of enough bone and the fashioning of flaps from healthy skin to provide full thickness cover, is necessary. Amputation is sometimes the only solution.

Trivial injuries cause fractures, especially after periods of immobilization. If joints are involved, neuropathic changes may develop. Lack of pain may obscure the diagnosis when, for example, a warm swollen knee is due to a supracondylar fracture. Exuberant callus is common. Operations such as Colonna arthroplasty, which involve injury to articular cartilage, should be avoided.

Cerebral

Varying degrees of mental defect are due to hydrocephalus, some of the worst cases being vegetative. The emotional problems of these children frequently influence their response to treatment.

Meningocele

In meningocele, the spinal hernia is covered by skin or membrane, has a cry impulse and contains no neurological elements, so repair is simple and there are no neurological sequelae. Certain distinction from myelomeningocele is not possible at birth without operation, and its rarity adds to the difficulty. The diagnosis is, in fact, usually retrospective, being based on the absence of cord or nerves in the sac and the lack of subsequent paralysis. Associated abnormalities may be present from which cord compression may arise later (spinal dysraphism).

Spinal dysraphism

The spinal dysraphism syndrome includes the effects of malformations of vertebrae, nerve roots or spinal cord, which are unlikely to be recognized at birth. They may, of course, be suspected if skin changes are present, but their consequences appear later and ordinarily affect the nervous system with secondary skeletal manifestations. They may be static but are commonly progressive.

This is one of those remarkable conditions which although only relatively recently defined with clarity (James and Lassman, 1960) is now so frequently recognized that its management has become a significant part of the work of neurosurgeons engaged in paediatric practice. It is astonishing that symptoms such as delayed urinary incontinence without genitourinary abnormality or the development of a foot deformity with shortening but without evidence of poliomyelitis should have defied diagnosis for so long. This is in many ways analogous to the delay in recognizing prolapsed lumbar intervertebral discs as the commonest cause of sciatica. Both, with the wisdom of hindsight, seem so obvious.

Orthopaedic surgeons must be alert to the syndrome for they are frequently the first to see the patient. Commonly one foot is small and may be deformed or the leg slightly shortened or diminished in girth. Trophic sores on toes or lateral border are significant. Attention to the spine may disclose midline skin dimples, scars, capillary naevi, hairy patches or mild scoliosis – all are significant. Plain radiographs should include the whole spine and are invariably abnormal. The signs range from spina bifida occulta to widening of the pedicles with vertebral fusion and a central bony spur (diastematomyelia). Myelography, CT scanning and MRI if available are useful in the investigation.

Laminectomy is indicated when there is evidence of a progressive neurological deficit, an expanding lesion and a low conus with local tethering. This may also cause a traction lesion when a diasematomyelic spur divides the spinal cord at a higher level. The findings at operation are variable, often multiple, and include (in order of frequency) tethered conus, split cord and lipoma. The aim of surgery is to prevent deterioration rather than to improve the existing situation for this seldom happens.

There is therefore an urgent indication to investigate these children.

Lastly, it must be remembered that the more florid manifestations of congenital defect of the neuraxis are not immune from late neurological deterioration due to mechanical causes rather than spreading gliosis It is easy to be blind to progressive neurological deterioration if the changes in the periphery are always accepted as due to the quotient of static paralysis and growth. Repeated muscle charts are of great value in this context.

Spina bifida occulta (Figure 7.15)

This may occur at any level in the spine but is found most commonly at the lumbosacral level, where an incidence of 17% was reported in a survey of 3000 spines (Brailsford, 1928). Obviously, most are harmless but the lesion is not infrequently significant when associated with other spinal or lower limb abnormalities.

Sometimes it explains deformity in the feet (notably pes cavus) or the reason for disappointment when a club foot fails to respond to expert and dedicated care. In these circumstances the paralysis is non-progressive, but the effects may be. When it is suspected that the neural deficit is progressive, lumbosacral spina bifida is of great importance, for it may indicate that there is another and more sinister congenital lesion at a high level. Lastly, there may be associated abnormalities such as spondylolistheses or congenital scoliosis. Operative treatment may then need to be modified because of the inadequately protected spinal canal.

Neurological conditions usually presenting in childhood

Ataxia

Delay in walking or in the acquisition of the motor skills expected at a given age may, if not due to cerebral palsy, be ataxic in origin. The orthopaedic surgeon is most likely to meet this in a child already walking but with an obvious lack of assurance. The gait is staggering and unstable, with forward inclination, in part compensated by lumbar lordosis, and abducted hips. The arms seek support from the air like a tightrope walker. The causes being varied and

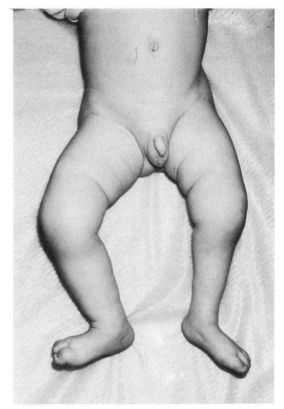

(a)

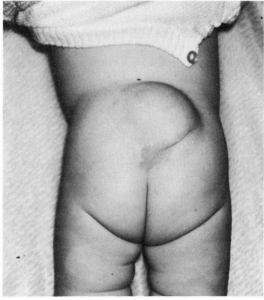

(b)

Figure 7.15 Spina bifida occulta. (a) Anterior view showing waste of the left leg, asymmetry and shortening. (b) Posterior view, showing lipomeningocele and naevus over the lumbosacral area

complex, neurological help is obviously necessary. However there is one condition – Friedreich's ataxia – that should be mentioned here because of the associated skeletal abnormalities. Onset of this autosomal recessively inherited condition can be early in the first decade, and in 5% of cases with scoliosis. However, the most constant presenting features are limb and truncal ataxia and absent reflexes. Pes cavus and, rarely, finger and knee contractures may develop. A wheelchair existence by the age of 25 years is common.

It should not be forgotten that cerebral tumours, which are not necessarily confined to the cerebellum and posterior fossa, may present with ataxia.

Clumsy children

Children are sometimes seen who, for no apparent reason, have been noticed to lag behind their fellows at games, to be prone to fall repeatedly and hurt themselves and to be forever dropping things or bumping into the furniture. Not all awkward people are abnormal and here, as elsewhere, the dividing line between normality and abnormality is ill defined.

Examination may reveal a definite, unsuspected neurological disorder, such as early muscular dystrophy or mild cerebral palsy. Others have a recognizable skeletal abnormality of which persistent femoral anteversion with secondary external tibial torsion (Chapter 13), if not the most obvious, is certainly the most common.

Many defy diagnosis and merit further attention. Abnormality may be confirmed by the patient's performance in the gym under the scrutiny of a physiotherapist. Minor degrees of brain injury without demonstrable signs in the nervous system may be suspected if there is a history of perinatal abnormality. This may be supported by irregular scholastic performance and confirmed by intellectual assessment. Others may have dyslexia – the inability to appreciate the spatial relationships of letters, words or numbers, or even to distinguish left from right – or apraxia and agnosia – failure to synthesize the components of movement or sensory input. Yet others may be demonstrating in protest against some extraneous situation with which they cannot contend.

Non-progressive flaccid paralysis

Polyneuritis (Guillain–Barré syndrome)

Most children with this condition recover without sequelae. A few may die in the acute phase or after a chronic illness, and a few may survive with chronic neurological handicap. The cause is not known, although it usually occurs a short time after a non-specific viral illness. Characteristic features of the condition include the sudden onset of an ascending symmetrical paralysis, painful paraesthesiae, cranial nerve palsies, involvement of the respiratory muscle and, on examination of the cerebrospinal fluid, a raised protein without significant pleocytosis.

Management of the paralysis involves prevention of deformity by the judicious use of splints and passive movement in the early phase. Muscle charting is vital, for only thereby can relapse, improvement or stability be recognized. When apparent stability is reached and the general well-being suggests that the process is quiescent, reparative surgery may be undertaken on conventional lines.

Mononeuritis (neuralgic amyotrophy; Spillane's syndrome)

In mononeuritis, pain of rapid onset is usually felt around the shoulder and is difficult to explain, because (as in herpes) the diagnostic sign of muscle weakness does not appear for a few days. Osteomyelitis or acute arthritis are likely misdiagnoses. The nerves to deltoid and serratus anterior are those most commonly affected, and full recovery is the rule.

Anterior poliomyelitis

Textbooks should reflect contemporary patterns of disease. Because the victims of this wretched crippling disease are becoming fewer, we feel justified in foregoing a detailed description. The reader is referred to a review by Sharrard (1979) and for details of the many operative techniques to *Campbell's Orthopaedics* (Crenshaw, 1971) and James' *Poliomyelitis: Essentials of Surgical Management* (1987).

The significance of poliomyelitis, like syphilis, is now a matter of remembering the possibility in differential diagnosis of some neurological diseases such as polyneuritis and spinal dysraphism. The legacy is valuable, for the techniques developed over the years are of value in the surgery of other causes of handicap, such as myelomeningocele, peripheral nerve lesions and peripheral neuritis.

Peripheral nerves

Some lesions are peculiar to, or most common in, children – for example, obstetrical lesions of the brachial plexus (Chapter 9). Similarly, high sciatic palsy may follow injections of noxious substances, such as nikethamide, into the umbilical vessels. The damage is due to its passage into the nerve via the inferior gluteal artery, which is disproportionally large at birth. Injections to subdue status epilepticus may be misdirected on the moving target and, once again, injure the sciatic nerve.

The femoral nerve may be compressed in haemophilia (*see* Chapter 3) and any nerve compressed by ganglia or other tumours, especially osteochondromas. Ischaemic neuritis frequently accompanies muscle contracture in Volkmann's syndrome.

Congenital indifference to pain

Congenital indifference to pain may be conveniently included here, in spite of our ignorance of the exact site or nature of the cause. The loss of pain sensibility, although specific (other sensory modalities being intact), is not necessarily absolute. The presenting symptoms usually arise from a neuropathic joint, secondarily infected with discharging sinuses. Fractures may be ignored and develop non-union and, similarly, corneal abrasions ulcerate and dental caries runs riot. The neuropathic joints and fractures resemble those sometimes seen in myelomeningocele, but are otherwise unmistakable, for syringomyelia, leprosy and diabetes in childhood do not present in this way.

Progressive flaccid paralysis

Peroneal muscular atrophy (hereditary motor and sensory neuropathy types I and II)

Electrophysiological studies have shown that peroneal muscular atrophy first described by Charcot and Marie Tooth can be divided into two distinct groups based on nerve conduction velocity. In type I the velocity in the median nerve is below 38 metres per second, in type II it is above. Although type I presents earlier, both forms do appear in childhood with symptoms which often take them first to orthopaedic surgeons who are commonly called upon to treat them.

Progressive pes cavus, equinovarus and footdrop beginning at the age of 6 years or thereabouts (Figure 7.16) should arouse suspicion and stimulate enquiries about the family, among whom other members may be affected. Weakness begins in the peronei, spreading to the dorsiflexors and sometimes to all the muscles below the knee. The ankle jerk soon disappears. Spread to hand and arm below the elbow and sensory changes do occur. Ataxia may be a feature and scoliosis can develop.

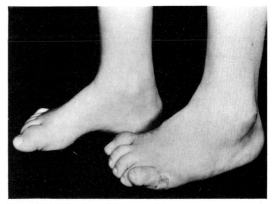

Figure 7.16 Clawing of the toes with pes cavus in hereditary motor and sensory neuropathy type 1 (previously known as peroneal muscular atrophy)

Most cases are very slowly progressive, so surgery is helpful. In the young, medial release, plantar strip, transplantation of toe tendons, tibialis anterior and tibialis posterior (through the interosseous membrane to reinforce dorsiflexion) may be used individually or together. Coleman's block test (Chapter 15) is most useful in assessment. Older children with established fixed deformity may need wedge tarsectomy or triple arthrodesis, with the addition, where possible, of a suitable tendon transplant. Provided the feet are stabilized and plantigrade, disability may be negligible, because power is retained proximally.

Duchenne muscular dystrophy

This X-linked condition is remorselessly progressive and survival beyond 21 years of age is rare. Death is from respiratory or heart failure.

Boys with this condition often have slightly below average intelligence and consequently may show global developmental delay. Concern is not usually felt until he starts to walk, when he appears to trip frequently. Within the next 2–3 years it becomes clear that he has never learnt to run, that he tires easily and that he has difficulty climbing stairs. By 10–12 years of age he becomes so weak as to become confined to a wheelchair. Weakness is at first most evident around the hip joint, but eventually all muscles become involved. Calf enlargement is noticeable early. Reflexes may be depressed but not abolished and often the ankle reflexes are relatively brisk. Deformities, notably scoliosis, hip and knee flexion and equinovarus, develop later.

Diagnosis is confirmed by finding very high levels of serum creatine kinase and by the characteristic appearance of the muscle biopsy.

Early genetic counselling is important and is based upon a carefully taken family history and maternal creatine kinase estimations and DNA analysis.

Surgery offers some alleviation. Prevention of deformity or correction by simple procedures, such as tendo Achillis tenotomy, can prolong independence by enabling calipers to be worn. Once chairbound, scoliosis often makes sitting difficult, and early operative treatment is helpful. Effective seating is most important.

Other less rapidly deteriorating neuromuscular disorders

Facioscapulohumeral dystrophy defines itself. Deterioration is very slow and remains localized to the shoulder girdle. Scapulothoracic arthrodesis developed by Howard of Norwich is of great benefit in this extremely rare disorder (Copeland and Howard, 1978).

Polymyositis frequently arrests with or without steroid therapy, and certain sequelae., such as weakness and deformity due to muscle contracture, require surgical correction. When confronted by an unexplained deformity such as equinus due to 'idiopathic' shortening of the Achilles tendon it is prudent to consider the less florid form of polymyositis as a possible cause.

Non-progressive spastic paralysis

Cerebral palsy is of course by far the most common example of non-progressive spastic paralysis. There is also a familial type of spastic diplegia, absent at birth and presenting later, with slow progress.

The remainder are due to arrested spinal neurological disease, such as transverse myelitis, injuries to head or spine, surgically treated neoplasms or hydrocephalus, and inflammatory diseases of which tuberculosis was at one time common. Congenital lesions are rare, except for non-progressive spinal dysraphism and reflex activity in isolated cord segments associated with myelomeningocele.

Progressive spastic paralysis

Progressive spastic paralysis demands urgent investigation, for although there is a group of progressive cerebral and spinal degenerative diseases, most are mechanical in origin and are therefore often amenable to treatment. The causes are congenital, neoplastic and inflammatory, which may arise within the cranium or within the spine, sometimes encroaching upon it from nearby.

Intracranial lesions need concern us no more, but spinal abnormalities must.

Spinal dysraphism (page 70) is the most common cause, followed by spinal tumours such as neurofibromas (extramedullary) or ependymomas (intramedullary). The spine may be invaded by a neuroblastoma or compressed by an extradural abscess, now more likely to be staphylococcal than tuberculous. Congenital lesions of the vertebrae and idiopathic scoliosis are surprisingly rarely to blame, in spite of the severe deformity that may follow. There are, however, certain dangerous varieties. These include absence of the odontoid process, Klippel–Feil deformity (the responsible lesion is often a dermoid in the posterior fossa), severe congenital cervicothoracic scoliosis and congenital anterior hemivertebra (Chapter 12).

Whatever its cause, progressive spasticity (and this includes bladder dysfunction) demands most urgent investigation.

References

Bell, M. J., Baker, R. H. and Sergiov, S. P. (1988) The results of surgery in the upper limb in cerebral palsy. *J. Bone Jt. Surg.* **70B**, 338

Brailsford, J. F. (1928/29) Deformities of the lumbosacral region of the spine. *Br. J. Surg.* **16**, 562

Brown, A. (1968) Simple method of fusion of the subtalar joint in children. *J. Bone Jt. Surg.* **50B**, 369

Carol, N. C. and Sharrard, W. J. W. (1972) Long-term follow-up of posterior iliopsoas transplantation for paralytic dislocation of the hip. *J. Bone Jt. Surg.* **54A**, 551

Cavanagh, N. P. C., Lake, B. D. and McMeniman, P. (1976) Congenital fibre type disproportion myopathy. A histological diagnosis with an uncertain clinical outlook. *Archs. Dis. Childh.* **54**, 735

Colton, C. L., Ransford, A. O. and Lloyd-Roberts, G. C. (1976) Transposition of the tendon of pronator teres in cerebral palsy. *J. Bone Jt. Surg.* **58B**, 220

Copeland, S. A. and Howard, R. C. (1978) Thoracoscapular fusion for facioscapulohumeral dystrophy. *J. Bone Jt. Surg.* **60B**, 547

Crenshaw, A. H. (1986) (Editor) *Campbell's Operative Orthopedics*, 7th edn. St Louis, Mo: Mosby

Dennyson, W. G. and Fulford, G. E. (1976) Subtalar arthrodesis by cancellous grafts and metallic internal fixation. *J. Bone Jt. Surg.* **58B**, 507

Dubowitz, V. (1980) *The Floppy Infant*, 2nd edn. Clinics in Developmental Medicine, no. 76. London: SIMP/ Heinemann Medical; Philadelphia: Lippincott

Eggers, G. W. N. (1952) Transplantation of the hamstring tendons to femoral condyles. *J. Bone Jt. Surg.* **34A**, 827

Graham, H. K. and Fixsen, J. A. (1988) The White slide technique for lengthening the calcaneal tendon. *J. Bone Jt. Surg.* **70B**, 472

Green, W. T. and Banks, H. H. (1962) Flexor Carp: ulnaris transplant. *J. Bone Jt. Surg.* **44A**, 1343

Grice, D. F. (1952) Extra-articular arthrodesis of the subastragalar joint for correction of paralytic flat feet in children. *J. Bone Jt. Surg.* **34A**, 927

James, C. C. M. and Lassman, L. P. (1960) Spinal dysraphism. *Archs. Dis. Childh.* **35**, 315

James, J. I. P. (1987) *Poliomyelitis: essentials of surgical management.* London: Edward Arnold

Jones, R. (1921) Tendon transplantation in cases of musculospinal injuries not amenable to suture. *Am. J. Surg.* **35**, 333

Lorber, J. (1971) Results of treatment of myelomeningocele. *Develop. Med. Child Neurol.* **13**, 279

Lorber, J. (1971) Spina bifida cystica: results of treatment of 270 consecutive cases with criteria for selection for the future. *Archs. Dis. Childh.* **47**, 854

Matev, I. (1963) Surgical treatment of spastic 'thumb-in-palm' deformity. *J. Bone Jt. Surg.* **45B**, 703

Menelaus, M. B. (1976) Orthopaedic management of children with myelomeningocele. *Devel. Med. Child Neurol.* **18**, suppl. 37, 3

Mustard, W. T. (1952) Iliopsoas transfer for weakness of the hip abductors. *J. Bone Jt. Surg.* **34A**, 647

Mustard, W. T. (1959) A follow-up study of iliopsoas transfer for hip instability. *J. Bone Jt. Surg.* **41B**, 289

Osebold, W. R., Mayfield, J. K., Winter, R. B. and Moe, J. H. (1982) Surgical treatment of paralytic scoliosis associated with myelomeningocele. *J. Bone Jt. Surg.* **64A**, 841

Perry, J., Hoffer, M. M., Giovan, P., Antonelli, D. and Greenberg, R. (1974) Gait analysis of the triceps surae in cerebral palsy. *J. Bone Jt. Surg.* **56A**, 511

Samilson, R. L. and Perry, J. (1975) Orthopaedic assessment in cerebral palsy. *Clin. Devel. Med.* **52/53**, 35

Sandifer, P. (1967) *Neurology in Orthopaedics.* London: Butterworths

Seymour, N. and Sharrard, W. J. W. (1968) Bilateral proximal release of the hamstrings in cerebral palsy. *J. Bone Jt. Surg.* **50B**, 274

Sharrard, W. J. W. (1964) Posterior iliopsoas transplantation in the treatment of paralytic dislocation of the hip. *J. Bone Jt. Surg.* **46B**, 426

Sharrard, W. J. W. (1968) Spinal osteotomy for congenital kyphosis in myelomeningocele. *J. Bone Jt. Surg.* **50B**, 466

Sharrard, W. J. W. (1979) *Paediatric Orthopaedics and Fractures,* 2nd edn. Oxford: Blackwell Scientific

Sharrard, W. J. W., Zachary, R. B., Lorber, J. and Bruce, A. M. (1962) A controlled trial of immediate and delayed closure of spina bifida cystica. *Archs. Dis. Childh.* **38**, 18

Silfverskiold, N. (1923/24) Reduction of the uncrossed two joint muscles of the leg to one joint muscle in spastic conditions. *Acta Chir. Scand.* **lvi**, 315

Smith, G. K. and Smith E. D. (1973) Selection for treatment in spina bifida cystica. *Br. Med. J.* **4**, 189

Stark G. D. and Baker, G. C. W. (1967) Neurological involvement of the lower limbs in myelomeningocele. *Devel. Med. Child Neurol.* **9**, 732

Stark, G. D. and Drummond, M. (1972) Results of selective early operation for myelomeningocele. *Devel. Med. Child Neurol.* **14**, suppl. 27, 155 [summary]

Steel, H. H. (1980) Gluteus medius and minimus insertion advancement for correction of internal rotation gait in spastic cerebral palsy. *J. Bone Jt. Surg.* **62A**, 919

Strayer, L. M. Jr (1950) Recession of the gastrocnemius: an operation to relieve spastic contracture of the calf muscles. *J. Bone Jt. Surg.* **32A**, 671

White, J. W. (1943) Torsion of Achilles tendon: its surgical significance. *Archs. Surg.* **46**, 784

White, W. F. (1972) Flexor muscle slide in the spastic hand (the Max Page operation). *J. Bone Jt. Surg* **54B**, 453

Wortis, H. and Cooper, W. (1957) The life experience of persons with cerebral palsy: a study of 63 histories. *Am. J. Phys. Med.* **36**, 328

Wynne-Davies, R. and Lloyd-Roberts, G. C. (1971) Arthrogryposis multiplex congenita. Search for prenatal factors in 66 sporadic cases. *Archs. Dis. Childh.* **51**, 618

Further reading

Bleck, E. E. (1987) *Orthopaedic Management in Cerebral Palsy.* Oxford: MacKeith Press/Blackwell Scientific; Philadelphia: J. B. Lippincott

Drennan, J. C. (1983) *Orthopaedic Management of Neuromuscular Disorders* J. B. Lippincott, Philadelphia

Galasko, C. S. B. (1987) *Neuromuscular Problems in Orthopaedics.* Oxford: Blackwell Scientific

Menelaus, M. B. (1980) *The Orthopaedic Management of Spina Bifida Cystica,* 2nd edn. Edinburgh, London, New York: Churchill Livingstone

Schafer, M. F. and Dias, L. S. (1983) *Myelomeningocele: Orthopedic Treatment.* Baltimore, London: Williams & Wilkins

8

Miscellaneous conditions

Histiocytosis X (eosinophilic granuloma and its variants)

Langerhans' cell histiocytosis (histiocytosis X)

As a result of the activities of the newly formed Histiocyte Society, the proposal that the disorders previously known as 'histiocytosis X' should be renamed 'Langerhans' cell histiocytosis' (LCH) (to differentiate them from the non-Langerhans' cell group of histiocytic disorders) is gaining ground. The term LCH has the advantage of defining the cell type considered pathognomonic of this group of disorders, whether the lesion is solitary ('eosinophilic granuloma') or one component of a multi-system disorder. In LCH patients, the skeletal system is more commonly involved than any other; skull, vertebrae and long bones are most frequently affected. In young children, the radiological appearance of lesions in long bones can closely and alarmingly mimic malignancy, especially Ewing's sarcoma. Spontaneous fractures can occur.

Either solitary or multiple bone lesions can be managed expectantly unless their anatomical location (e.g. cervical vertebra, roof of acetabulum) threatens to cause morbidity. Figure 8.1 shows a striking example of spontaneous healing after biopsy alone. Other therapeutic options include curettage, intralesional steroids (100–200 mg hydrocortisone) or systemic treatment with steroids (prednisone), VP16 or *Vinca* alkaloid (vincristine or vinblastine). The use of combination chemotherapy and of radiotherapy is now discouraged.

There is virtually no mortality in patients with 'single system' LCH but 10–20% of patients with multi-system disease eventually succumb to lung, liver or bone marrow failure. In our experience, bone involvement – even as a component to multi-system disease – confers a favourable prognosis.

Eosinophilic granuloma localized to bone (LCH, single system disease, solitary or multiple)

Eosinophilic granulomas localized to bone may be single or multiple. They are seen most commonly in the skull and femur, and thereafter in the ribs. In the skull and flat bones, such as the ilium, the lesions are discrete, circular and punched out. In the long bones the appearances are different, for localized expansions with cortical erosions are ensheathed by layers of subperiosteal new bone. The lesions involve the metaphysis or diaphysis and are usually sufficiently characteristic for a confident diagnosis – except in some diaphyseal deposits, which in older children may resemble Ewing's sarcoma.

The lesions may present either as a lump with mild aching or by chance on a radiograph. In either event a bone scan should be done to identify any other lesions which would support the diagnosis.

Individual lesions usually heal and it is therefore difficult to know the indications for, or the contribution of, curettage and grafting to the outcome. Biopsy will be necessary when doubt exists. A yellowish granuloma is disclosed and, if the stability of the bone is thought to be at risk, grafting follows curettage. Sometimes defects in perilous positions such as the acetabular roof (Figure 8.2) invite

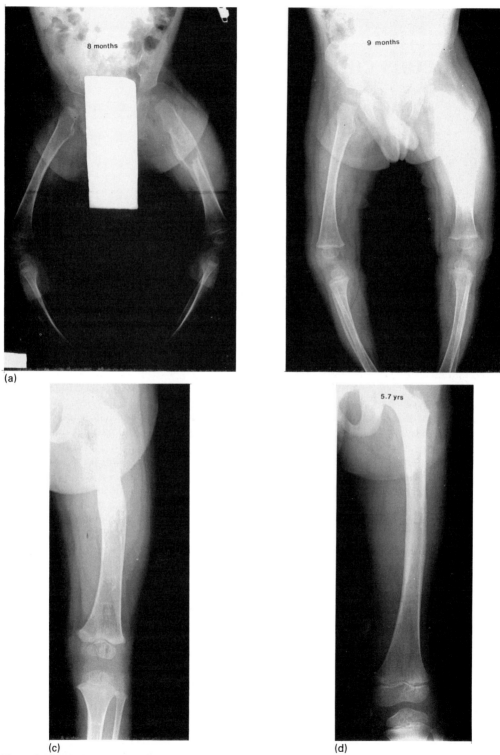

(a)

(c)   (d)

Figure 8.1 Langerhans' cell histiocytosis: solitary eosinophilic granuloma lesion in the left femur. (a) At 8 months of age; note the aggressive appearance of the lesion. (b) One month later; note the rapid extension of the lesion. (c) At 20 months; note regression of the lesion following biopsy only at 10 months. (d) At 5 years 7 months; healed

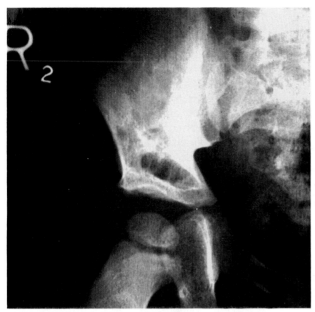

Figure 8.2 X-ray of a right hip showing lytic lesions due to eosinophil granuloma above the acetabulum

grafting. We have recently tried local injections of steriod, as for simple bone cysts (Scaglietti, Marchetti and Bartolozzi, 1979) with remarkably good results. Rib lesions are especially liable to cause diagnostic uncertainty, but lend themselves to excision biopsy (McGauran and Spady, 1960).

Calve's disease (vertebra plana)

In Calve's disease, backache demands a radiograph with shows that one vertebral body is flattened, appearing as a sclerotic plaque. Symptoms resolve with rest and sometimes, a plaster jacket. Later the body returns to a near-normal contour with a small residual opaque centre. The commonest cause is eosinophilic granuloma (solitary LCH disease). The diagnosis may be aided by the presence of the small smooth shadow of the granuloma expanding in front of the body (Fripp, 1958).

Hand-Schuller-Christian disease

The full triad of skull lesions, exophthalmos and diabetes insipidus is rare. However, other systems are variably involved, including enlargement of the liver and lymph glands, scaly red rash and anaemia. Pulmonary infiltration is dangerous both on its own account and because of secondary infections.

The bone lesions, although similar to those of the localized type, seem more aggressive, and pathological fractures and coxa vara have been seen. The radiographs may in fact resemble secondary neuroblastoma.

Ehlers-Danlos syndrome

Friable and overstretchable skin are the obvious features of the Ehlers-Danlos syndrome, but the associated joint laxity is responsible for many of the disabilities. The laxity is presumably present *in utero*, for it is frequently familial. Being autosomal dominant, it carries a high risk of transmission. It is not surprising, therefore, that congenital club feet and dislocated hips are not infrequently present at birth, for both include laxity among their probable aetiological factors. Later, hypotonia combines with laxity, thus causing predisposition to recurrent dislocations of joints (especially the patella), severe relaxed flat feet and scoliosis. Minor degrees of joint instability produce recurrent effusions and encourage the development of degenerative arthritis.

Hypermobile skin is prone to tearing, and scars and ulcers are common, especially around the knees. Congenital cardiac malformations are also described (Beighton and Horan, 1969).

Ligamentous (joint) laxity

Abnormal joint laxity is frequently associated with hypotonia, which is discussed further in Chapter 7. Sometimes, however, it exists as an isolated joint phenomenon which then has important clinical implications. The cause may be hormonal or familial.

The hormonal type is transitory and, being due to relaxin produced by the maternal uterus spilling over into the fetal circulation, is short lived. It may, however, be an aetiological factor in congenital dislocation of the hip.

The familial variety is permanent, being transmitted by a dominant gene as an isolated phenomenon or in association with Marfan's and Ehlers-Danlos syndromes or osteogenesis imperfecta; such children may join the rest of the family in professional acrobatics, others are prone to recurrent dislocations of patella and shoulder, disabling flat feet and minor joint derangements. Normal standards of joint range are available (Carter and Sweetnam, 1959; Carter and Wilkinson, 1964).

Tumoral calcinosis

In tumoral calcinosis deposits of calcium phosphate, visible as calcified irregular masses on the radiograph, appear in the neighbourhood of joints. The clinical presentation is of a mass, fixed deeply to periarticular structures, but surprisingly not associated with significant limitation of movement. There is a familial distribution confined to siblings, but in spite of this there is no demonstrable biochemical abnormality except occasional hyperphosphataemia of uncertain significance.

The lack of symptoms usually contraindicates surgical removal in most, for the recurrence rate is high. It may be necessary to interfere when joint movement is limited, if the tumour is unsightly, or for ulceration and secondary infection. Recurrence is common and should be treated by early re-excision (Baldursson *et al.*, 1962).

Juvenile chronic arthritis (juvenile rheumatoid arthritis, Still's disease)

In juvenile chronic arthritis (previously known as juvenile rheumatoid arthritis, and commonly called Still's disease) it has been shown that the prognosis is related to the time elapsing between onset and diagnosis. Thus the orthopaedic surgeon must be alert to this possibility, for he is frequently the first to see the patient.

The juvenile disease varies in many ways from that in adults: for example, nodules are rare and the hands are involved relatively infrequently and then only late in the disease. The presentation is variable. Some are not ill, with one swollen joint (usually the knee), whereas others who are ill, with polyarthritis, fever, rash splenomegaly and lymphadenopathy, present no difficulty in diagnosis.

Problems arise when it appears that only one or two joints are involved. A careful search for arthritis elsewhere, especially in the subastragaloid joints and wrists, is frequently rewarding. A history of recurrent stiff neck (otherwise unusual in children) is significant. Anaemia and a raised sedimentation rate are helpful but it must be emphasized that serological tests are very seldom positive in the young. It is essential to realize that the onset is usually before the age of 5 years and frequently below the age of 2 years.

The prognosis in overlooked and badly managed children with florid disease is likely to be poor, with progressive ill-health, emotional disturbance, inhibited growth, blindness from iridocyclitis (8%) and possible death, with amyloidosis contributing. The joints develop progressive deformity with fibrous and, later, bony ankylosis. Premature epiphyseal closure sometimes occurs.

In contrast, of those coming for treatment within a year of onset and reviewed 5 years later, two-thirds were inactive and half had no joint sequelae.

The Taplow Centre proposed certain diagnostic criteria to differentiate between these children and those suffering from other forms of arthritis, such as systemic lupus, polyarteritis nodosa and juvenile ankylosing spondylitis; at least four joints should be affected for more than 3 months or, if less than 3, there should be a positive synovial biopsy.

Treatment is directed in part against the general manifestations and in part towards the joints. General measures include the judicious use of rest, alternating with controlled activity and correction of anaemia which may be aggravated by salicylate intestinal bleeding.

Steroids are now rarely ever indicated, except in life-threatening situations, because of their side effects – porosis, vertebral collapse, stunting and obesity – which are formidable. Salicylates are effective if the dosages required can be tolerated. Other anti-inflammatory drugs such as ibuprofen are useful, and gold, penicillamine and cytotoxics have been used, but all have serious side effects.

The care of joints involves prevention and correction of deformity by splinting. Deformity is prevented by bivalved plaster splints retaining affected joints in neutral or functional positions. The joint should be moved throughout its painless range daily. Established deformity of relatively recent onset will usually respond to serial plasters followed by graduated movement, muscle development, hydrotherapy and splinting at rest periods and during the night. Prone nursing or traction may be needed for hip flexion. These principles are the sheet anchors of early treatment, for in children synovectomy remains of unproven value.

Periods of activity are as important as periods of rest, and this should be remembered when an incidental fracture or operation requires prolonged immobilization which, if not modified, may cause intractable stiffness. Thus internal fixation allowing movement has much to commend it in fracture treatment.

Surgery has a place when deformities fail to respond to non-operative treatment, and for the late relief of severe joint stiffness and pain (Arden and Ansell, 1978). The operations are those conventionally used for similar problems arising in other conditions. Joint replacement has a place in some of these very severely handicapped children and adolescents.

Stress fractures

Although stress fractures are familiar in adults, these are not well recognized as occurring in children too. They are important, not so much as a cause of unexpected leg pain and limp, but because they may be readily confused with osteomyelitis and malignant tumours. Diagnosis is aided by the rapidity and profusion with which callus forms, in comparison with adults. For the same reason the fracture line may be soon obscured. Although they may be seen elsewhere, the proximal tibia and distal fibula are by far the commonest sites. Protection by rest is followed by rapid healing (Devas, 1963).

Non-accidental injury (NAI), child abuse, the battered child syndrome

Child abuse can appear in many forms, both mental and physical. The management of the abused child and the abuser is a complex and difficult situation. Every hospital and district should have guidelines laid down by the Area Review Committee for the management of these patients by a team including doctors, social workers, the local authority and the police.

From the medical point of view the major load falls on the consultant paediatrician. The orthopaedic surgeon's role is to recognize the possibility of abuse when presented with fractures and injuries, to manage these injuries and to alert the Child Abuse Team. Child abuse should be suspected in any fracture in a child under walking age, unless there is a clearcut history of accidental injury. Fifty per cent of child abuse fractures occur under the age of 1 year, 80% under the age of 2 years. Delay in bringing the child to hospital and an unsatisfactory history of trauma are also common. The child must be examined fully. Soft tissue injuries, bruising and abrasion, particularly intraoral bruising, a tear of the frenulum, nail marks, bilateral bruising, particularly of varying ages are always suspicious. It is now recognized that diaphyseal fractures of the humerus and femur are the commonest single presenting fracture, whereas the metaphyseal impaction and buckle fractures although very characteristic are less common (Figure 8.3).

Epiphyseal injuries are rare. Rib fractures are uncommon in children under the age of 18 as an accidental injury but are the commonest fractures seen in this age group due to non-accidental injury.

Fractures to the skull, which led to Caffey's original description in 1946, usually occur in the occipital or temporal region. Commonly they are multiple and may be associated with widening of the sutures.

Fractures of different ages and at different stages of healing are the cardinal sign of abuse. Osteogenesis imperfecta must always be considered in the differential diagnosis particularly because of its wide spectrum of severity, and variable inheritance. It is particularly true of the so-called 'white eye' type 4 disease described by Sillence *et al*, (1979) where the patient appears relatively normal with normal sclerotics and yet has fractures in the first year of life. It is essential in the management of child abuse to help both the abused and the abuser. It is most important to recognize the condition as soon as possible and refer the patient to the Child Abuse Team.

Infantile cortical hyperostosis (Caffey's disease)

Caffey's disease (Figure 8.4) affects babies who are less than 6 months old, most commonly at about 2 months. The presenting feature is a brawny indurated swelling (sometimes several), fixed deeply in the plane of bone. Irritability, fever, raised sedimentation rate and malaise combine to simulate osteomyelitis and this error is further supported by the radiographic signs. In contrast with osteomyelitis, however, there is neither local heat nor redness.

The bones usually involved are the mandible, scapula or clavicle, but others are not immune and multiple lesions are common. The radiographic signs are pathognomonic, although they may not be seen when the indurated areas first appear. New bone appears on the surface of the partially absorbed cortex of the diaphysis and spreads outwards until the shaft is ensheathed in an oval mantle of new bone, the original architecture lying ghost-like in the centre. On the scapula this may resemble a chondroma.

Differentiation from osteomyelitis, scurvy (the age helps here) and trauma is based on diaphyseal rather than metaphyseal predilection, and the development of new bone from the centre outwards towards the periphery rather than the opposite.

The course is generally benign, being in most cases limited to about 6 months, though some relapse briefly. The bones may take some years to restore their normal corticomedullary rela-

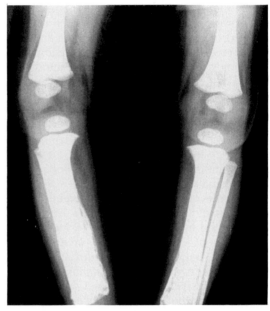

Figure 8.3 Non accidental injury in a newborn. Note thickening of both tibiae with periostitis. There is avulsion of a chip from the lower medial metaphysis

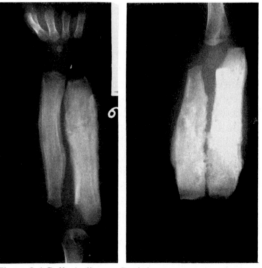

Figure 8.4 Caffey's disease. Both forearms are involved in asymmetrical fashion. The shafts of the bones are visible in the centre of exuberant periosteal new bone

tions and contours, but do so eventually. Treatment is seldom necessary, but severe mandibular involvement may demand feed aids. Cortisone is said to encourage rapid resolution (Caffey, 1967).

Pigeon chest and funnel chest (pectus excavatus)

Pigeon and funnel chests are not infrequently first seen by orthopaedic surgeons. In pigeon chest the sternum is proud and in funnel chest it is depressed. Sometimes when the deformity is severe the parents will request correction on cosmetic grounds or because of recurrent respiratory problems. This somewhat formidable operation – in relation to a purely cosmetic indication – is not without risk, and the result is somewhat marred by the likelihood of keloid scarring in the vertical presternal incision. Some boys unable to sport an appropriately manly torso on the beach and elsewhere become abnormally obsessed, and in these cases operation is sometimes justified, together with those few cases with exceptional deformity.

Nail–patella syndrome

In the nail–patella syndrome the nails are dystrophic or absent and the patellae are absent or displaced laterally. The nail dystrophy is the most prominent sign, being confined to the hands in decreasing severity from thumb to little finger.

There are, in addition, other features which, with one exception, are not disabling. The exception is cubitus valgus, which is due to dysplasia of the capitellum and a disordered radiohumeral joint. The diverting and unique curiosity is the development of iliac horns. These arise at a distance from the apophysis, below and behind the summit of the iliac crest. They may be palpable and even visible on the surface.

The importance of the syndrome is twofold. Firstly, there is a liability to congenital nephropathy and, in some, death from uraemia in middle age. One baby who presented with 'funny nails' at 18 months was found to have proteinuria. Secondly, it is inherited as an autosomal dominant linked with the blood group so that those members of the family affected have the same blood group.

Chromosome abnormalities

The analysis of chromosome arrangement is a relatively new development, and this science is becoming increasingly important in our understanding of the causation of several multifocal congenital anomalies. Turner's syndrome (ovarian dysgenesis) displays webbing of the neck and, among many congenital deformities, cubitus valgus. In Klinefelter's syndrome (testicular dysgenesis) multiple congenital deformities are accompanied by mental deficiency of varying degree.

These syndromes indicate the type of patient in whom chromosome studies may be revealing. They are those with multiple deformities associated with mental defect or abnormalities of the genitalia.

Mongolism (Down's syndrome), the commonest known chromosome disorder, combines mental deficiency with multiple anomalies, including a high incidence of club foot and hip dislocation which can occur late in childhood for which associated hypotonia and joint laxity are possibly the responsible factors (Bennet *et al*, 1982).

Neurofibromatosis (von Recklinghausen's disease)

Neurofibromatosis is responsible for a variety of curious abnormalities involving several systems, and is transmitted as a non-sex-linked dominant.

The manifestations in the skin are the most conspicuous, and, of these, multiple pigmented areas with well defined edges (*cafe au lait*) are the commonest. Usually light brown, they may be darker and hairy. Rarely, the skin is thick and in loose folds (elephant skin). Mobile subcutaneous fibromatous nodules sometimes become pedunculated, and associated superficial haemangiomas may be seen.

It is important to appreciate that the characteristic superficial lesions sometimes develop later, so their absence should not prejudice the diagnosis in a young child with some other typical manifestation. Coffee patches also occur in polyostotic fibrous dysplasia and phaeochromocytoma, and may of course exist alone with no sinister implications.

Peripheral nerves, as the name suggests, are frequently affected and display discrete tumours which are often central or diffuse enlargements. In both types of tumours nerve bundles run intact through the fibromatous overgrowth, so neural transmission is unimpaired unless the tumour is excised or there is

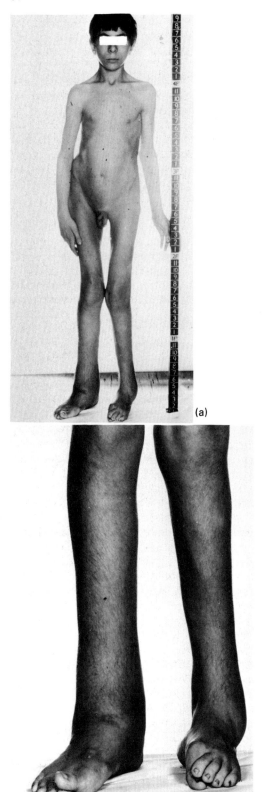

(a)

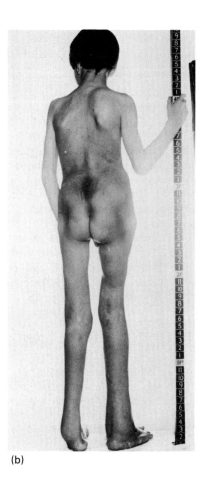

(b)

(c)

Figure 8.5 Patient with neurofibromatosis: (a) anterior view; (b) posterior view; (c) view of the legs. Note the asymmetrical limb deformity, spinal deformity and skin lesions

sarcomatous change. This last is rare and is likely to have the characteristics of a malignant schwannoma rather than a neurofibrosarcoma, so the prognosis after excision is correspondingly better.

The central tumours may arise in cranial nerves (acoustic neuroma) or from spinal nerve roots causing cord compression. Curiously, both these and the large intrathoracic or retroperitoneal tumours are infrequently associated with obvious skin lesions.

Peripheral diffuse neurofibromatosis is a cause of gigantism of the whole or part of a limb or even a digit. The limb is irregularly enlarged and deformed (Figure 8.5) by diffuse subcutaneous fibromatous tissue, through which normally small and invisible peripheral nerves run thickened and tortuous. There are frequently diffuse lymphangiomatous malformations which feel like soft lipomas and contribute to the bulk. Lengthening is associated with angiomatous malformation, the bones becoming somewhat slender but of normal contour.

Amputation of a digit or painstaking excision sparing the main nerves improves some cases, but in others this is not practicable and if pain, unrelieved by excision of tender nodules, is prominent, amputation is the best policy. Lengthening, if it warrants treatment, is best corrected by bone shortening or epiphyseodesis.

Radiographs disclose some of the other features. There is commonly subperiosteal cortical thickening and erosion from parosteal tumours which may penetrate, giving the appearance of bone cysts, similar to non-osteogenic fibroma. The distal ulna, fibula or clavicle may absorb and resemble angiomatosis of bone. The tibia may be kyphotic and subsequently fracture (Chapter 14), and scoliosis (Chapter 12) is present in up to half the patients. Intervertebral foramina are enlarged if tumours arise from the spinal roots. Vitamin D-resistant rickets is a rare concomitant. In short, one should remember neurofibromatosis when there is a curious atypical lesion in a bone (McCarroll, 1950, 1956; Murray and Jacobsen, 1971).

Myositis ossificans

Post-traumatic myositis, once a common complication of elbow injury overenthusiastically treated, is now rare, but still follows crushing injuries to muscle. It may develop following operations, especially on the hip joint, and mar the outcome. Ectopic bone of traumatic origin, when mature and bridging a joint as an extra-articular arthrodesis, may be excised with guarded optimism.

Myositis ossificans may occur in children as in adults, in acquired neurological disease, particularly if there is spasticity.

Myositis and dermatomyositis show patchy muscular calcification accompanied by fever, rash and extreme muscle tenderness and weakness. Contractures develop later to cause joint deformity.

Myositis ossificans progressiva is a progressive familial disease resulting in premature death from respiratory inefficiency. The familial factor is evident in shortness of the first metacarpal or metatarsal which precedes the onset of myositis. At first there are deep, indurated, hot tender swellings around the shoulders which later calcify and then ossify, spreading to encircle the chest and involve the limb roots, resulting in generalized rigidity and deformity. Although steriods seem to alleviate the symptoms they do not prevent the recurrence of excised bone (Harris, 1961).

Arthrogryposis multiplex congenita (amyoplasia congenita)

In amyoplasia, multiple deformities are present at birth (Figure 8.6). These are due to absence, fibrous replacement or weakness of muscles. In spite of appearances, intelligence is almost invariably above average.

The nature is obscure but the syndrome probably represents the end product of arrested intrauterine neuromuscular disease, and is therefore non-progressive. Deformities reflect the intrauterine posture from which the infant cannot escape, thus resembling myelodysplasia when the legs are involved, but when the arms are also involved, arthrogryposis is likely.

Studies of twins in whom only one may be affected dispose of intrauterine compression as a prime factor. A recent study (Wynne-Davies, Williams and O'Connor, 1981) has suggested that its instance was sporadic and not genetic in origin in man. The Akabane virus in cattle, sheep and horses is known to produce anterior

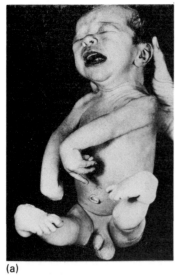
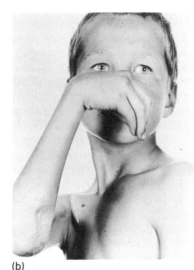

(a)   (b)

Figure 8.6 Arthrogryposis multiplex congenita. (a) In infancy: the child shows multiple deformities, and may be regarded as mentally subnormal. (b) In childhood: following operations to restore elbow flexion. Note the bright, intelligent expression

horn cell degeneration and arthrogrypotic-like appearances, as do meningomyelocele, sacral agenesis and benign hypotonia with contractures. When investigating a patient with arthrogrypotic appearances the chromosomes, the creatine phosphokinase, an X-ray of the whole spine and skull, EMG, muscle biopsy and possibly a CT head scan should be considered.

Most patients live to be adults, but some die in infancy of respiratory dysfunction. The deformities in likely survivors should be treated by stretching and splinting from birth, and these measures alone may correct fingers, wrist, hip, elbow and knee flexion contractures, but are unlikely to influence equinovarus feet, internally rotated shoulders and dislocated hips. Splinting of corrected deformity must continue for many years, using night splints and calipers for the legs. Assiduous and prolonged stretching is equally important, so the mother must become involved from the beginning and be aware of the object and sequence of treatment.

After a first year of non-operative treatment, an assessment can be made of the residual deformity and disability requiring operative treatment. The only absolute contraindication is hypotonia so severe that correction would be valueless. As with non-operative treatment, prolonged stretching and splinting must follow operation.

The legs are treated first. If rigid in equinovarus, the feet are recalcitrant to conventional methods and require astragalectomy with partial excision of the calcaneal tendon. Other deformities may be left for triple arthrodesis later. Flexed knees should not be corrected by supracondylar osteotomy which elsewhere, as here, is only of transient benefit in the very young. Posterior capsulotomy is successful in most cases.

Hip flexion deformity frequently relaxes once the knees are straight, and the child can be nursed prone with abducted legs joined by a cross-bar. Hips, if both stiff and dislocated bilaterally, should remain untreated once fixed flexion is overcome, but, if mobile or unilateral, they are best reduced by operation. Recently Staheli (1987) has reported good results with the medial approach in bilateral dislocated hips.

Decisions about the treatment of arm disability are best postponed for some years. The problems are more complex and it is possible to do harm by interfering with effective substitution patterns of activity. One can also prejudice walking, when rising from a chair or using a crutch depends upon a stiff, straight elbow. Furthermore, stiff fingers and flexed wrists demand that both hands function together as a prehensile coupling for lifting or eating, and interference with this adaptation may be unhelpful.

In general, surgery of the arms is planned around enabling a child to get a relatively good hand to his mouth. This may require all, or some, of the following: anterior capsulotomy of the wrist; posterior capsulotomy of the elbow (to convert whatever passive flexion there is to a more useful range), external rotation osteotomy of the humerus (internal rotation places the hand on the opposite shoulder when the elbow flexes), and, lastly, some type of elbow flexorplasty.

Finally, the adaptability and intelligence of these children ensures that any advantage one can give them is fully exploited, so treatment is often both rewarding to the patient and flattering to the surgeon (Figure 8.6b) (Mead, Lithgow and Sweeney, 1958; Friedlander, Westin and Wood, 1968; Lloyd-Roberts and Lettin, 1970; Williams, 1978).

Fibrous tumours

This group of tumours presents great difficulties to the pathologist, and consequently their classification and individual prognosis are confused. Indeed, the precise diagnosis of a fibrous tumour may depend upon its behaviour over the course of time rather than its histological appearance, which in any case may vary between different blocks cut from the same tumour. The situation is similar to the more familiar problem of cartilaginous tumours in adults. In childhood they generally present in one of three ways. Very young children tend to have fibroblastic tumours (juvenile aponeurotic fibromas) whereas in the older children desmoid tumours and fibrosarcomas predominate.

Fibroblastic tumours

A child aged 1 year was noticed to have a lump on the volar aspect of the forearm, which on palpation was hard, fixed to deep structures, and occupied the middle third of the forearm. The radiograph showed erosive defects on the radius and ulna on the lines of attachment of the interosseous ligament. There was no apparent neurovascular deficit. Fibrosarcoma was diagnosed and permission obtained to amputate the arm, should the operative findings support the diagnosis.

At operation the tumour was fleshy and fixed, having all the appearances of a sarcoma, except that the median and ulnar nerves passed through the tumour, being closely embedded within it. Because it had been previously noted that their function was not grossly impaired, the tumour was assumed to be benign and subsequent histological examination strongly supported this.

These tumours are readily mistaken for sarcomas and it is likely that some children who have lost limbs for 'fibrosarcoma' owe their survival more to the nature of the tumour than to the treatment.

Desmoid tumours

Desmoid tumours are non-metastasizing but infiltrating fibromas. In two of our patients they were first noticed at about 6 years of age as painless swellings in the calf which were excised locally, only to recur more proximally and be removed again on several occasions. At about 15 years of age they had infiltrated the hamstrings and were adherent to the pelvis. Operation disclosed a white scirrhous tumour investing nerves and vessels so closely that total excision was not possible without sacrificing the limb. In neither patient was there evidence of vascular or nervous insufficiency.

These tumours spread in the long axis of the limb in the line of the muscles originally involved and should, on diagnosis, be treated by total excision of the muscle or muscles concerned.

Fibrosarcoma

It is believed that neither fibroblastic nor desmoid tumours naturally undergo malignant metaplasia, but there is evidence (including a personal case) that radiotherapy, which is neither necessary nor helpful, may stimulate this.

There is no difficulty in accepting that fibrosarcoma arose *de novo* when an older child has a painful, rapidly growing and very malignant tumour. When, however, a recurring fibrous tumour seems to vary in its histological appearance on succeeding local excisions, until finally a diagnosis of fibrosarcoma is unequivocal, one may wonder whether there was, throughout, a slowly growing fibrosarcoma within a fibrous tumour from which the sections available showed only

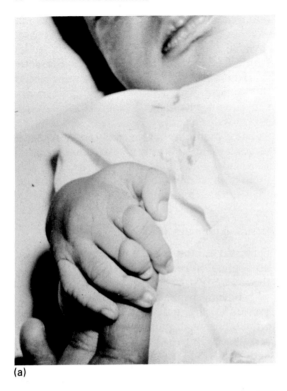

(a)

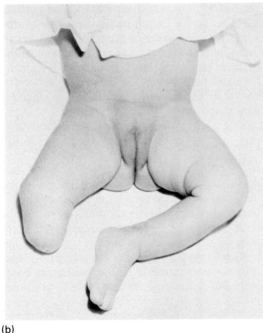

(b)

Figure 8.7 (a) Constriction rings on the index and middle fingers of the right hand. (b) The same child with congenital below-knee amputation by a constriction ring of the right leg. Note the scar of surgery on the left lower leg, to release the constriction ring above the left ankle

benign features. One such baby had evidence of increasing anaplasia, culminating in unquestionable fibrosarcoma for which a forequarter amputation was performed at the age of 3 years, but he died with multiple metastases a year later (Stout and Lattes, 1967).

Synovial tumours

Benign synovial tumours which include intra-articular polyps and synovial osteochondromatosis are very rare. Synovial sarcoma, although rare, is unfortunately more common. In one patient treated by amputation when there was no evidence of distant spread there has been no further recurrence of the tumour. Willis (1962) reported three cases of pigmented villonodular synovitis in finger joints.

Constriction rings

Constriction rings (Figure 8.7) may be superficial or deep, and although not invariably, usually encircle the limb distal to the elbow and knee. Their cause is unknown. When superficial, the problem is purely cosmetic and is dealt with accordingly. When deep and extending to deep fascia, or even bone, they are responsible for serious consequences.

Congenital amputation, with a tapering bony and soft tissue stump without rudimentary digits is usually due to tight rings. Such amputations may occur *in utero* and the newly delivered child may rarely be followed by a mummified limb. In others it is seen to occur during the neonatal period.

When associated with other deformities, notably club feet, there is an adverse effect on prognosis. Gross oedema distal to a ring should be relieved promptly by surgery before it becomes established, as in other forms of chronic lymphoedema. Lastly, they frequently appear in association with compound syndactyly but oedema seems to improve when the fingers are separated (Pillay and Hesketh, 1965).

References

Annotation (1985) Histiocytosis X – current controversies. *Archs. Dis. Childh.* **60**, 605

Arden, G. P. and Ansell, B. M. (1978) *The Surgical Management of Juvenile Chronic Polyarthritis*. London: Academic Press; New York: Grune & Stratton

Baldursson, H., Burke Evans, E., Dodge, W. F. and Jackson, W. T. (1969) Tumoral calcinosis with hyperphosphatemia. *J. Bone Jt. Surg.* **51A**, 913

Beighton, P. and Horan, F. (1969) Orthopaedic aspects of Ehlers-Danlos syndrome. *J. Bone Jt. Surg.* **51B**, 444

Bennett, G. C., Rang, M., Raye, D. P. and Aprin, H. (1982) Dislocation of the Hip in Trisomy 21. *J. Bone Jt. Surg.* **64B**, 289–294

Caffey, J. (1967) In *Pediatric X-ray Diagnosis*. Chicago: Year Book Medical Publishers

Caffey, J. (1946) Multiple fractures in the long bones of infants suffering from chronic subdural haematoma. *Am. J. Roentgenol* **56**, 163

Carter, C. and Sweetnam, R. (1958) Familial joint laxity and recurrent dislocation of the patella. *J. Bone Jt. Surg.* **40B**, 664

Carter, C. and Wilkinson, J. (1964) Persistent joint laxity and congenital dislocation of the hip. *J. Bone Jt. Surg.* **46B**, 40

Darlington, D. and Hawkins, C. F. (1967) Nail–patella syndrome with iliac horns and hereditary neuropathy. *J. Bone Jt. Surg.* **49B**, 164

Devas, M. B. (1963) Stress fractures in children. *J. Bone Jt. Surg.* **45B**, 528

Friedlander, H. L., Westin, G. W. and Wood, W. L. Jr (1968) Arthrogryposis multiplex congenita (a review of 45 cases). *J. Bone Jt. Surg.* **50A**, 89

Fripp, A. T. (1958) Vertebra plana. *J. Bone Jt. Surg.* **40B**, 378

Graf, R. (1983) New possibilities for the diagnosis of congenital hip joint dislocation by ultrasonography *J. Ped. Orthop.* **3**, 354–359

Griffiths, M. J. (1976) Slipping of the capital femoral epiphysis *Ann. Roy. Coll. Surg. Eng.* **58**, 34–42

Harris, N. H. (1961) Myositis ossificans progressiva. *Proc. R. Soc. Med.* **54**, 70

Kempe, H., Silverman, S. N., Steel, D. S. *et al* (1962) The battered child syndrome. *J. Am. Med. Ass.* **181**, 17.

Lloyd-Roberts, G. C. (1968) Diagnosis of injury to bones and joints of young babies. *Proc. R. Soc. Med.* **61**, 1299

Lloyd-Roberts, G. C. and Lettin, A. W. F. (1970) Arthrogryposis multiplex congenita. *J. Bone Jt. Surg.* **52B**, 494

McCarroll, H. R. (1950) Clinical manifestations of congenital neurofibromatosis. *J. Bone Jt. Surg.* **32A**, 601

McCarroll, H. R. (1956) Soft-tissue neoplasms associated with congenital neurofibromatosis. *J. Bone Jt. Surg.* **38A**, 717

McGavran, M. H. and Spady, H. A. (1960) Eosinophilic granuloma of bone. *J. Bone Jt. Surg.* **42A**, 979

Mead, N. G., Lithgow, W. C. and Sweeney, H. J. (1958) Arthrogryposis multiplex congenita. *J. Bone Jt. Surg.* **40A**, 1285

Murray, R. O., Jacobson, H. G. (1971) *The Radiology of Skeletal Disorders*. Edinburgh: Churchill Livingstone

Pillay, V. K. and Hesketh, K. T. (1965) Intra-uterine amputations and annular defects in Singapore. *J. Bone Jt. Surg.* **47B**, 514

Scaglietti, O., Marchetti, P. G. and Bartolozzi, P. (1979) Effects of methylprednisolone acetate in the treatment of bone cysts. *J. Bone Jt. Surg.* **61B**, 200

Sillence, D. O., Senn, A. S. and Danks, D. (1979) Genetic heterogeneity in osteogenesis imperfecta. *J. Med. Genet.* **16**, 101–000

Staheli, L. T., Chew, D. E., Elliott, J. S. and Mosca, V. S. (1987) Management of hip dislocations in children with arthrogryposis. *J. Ped. Orthop.* **7**, 681–685

Stout, A. P. and Lattes, R. (1967) *Tumors of Soft Tissues*, fascicle 1. Washington DC: Armed Forces Institute of Pathology

Williams, P. (1978) The management of arthrogryposis *Orthop. Clin. N. Am.* **9**, 67–88

Willis, R. A. (1962) *Pathology of Tumours in Children*. London: Oliver & Boyd

Writing Group of the Histiocyte Society: Chu, T., D'Angio, G. J., Favara, B., Ladisch, S., Nesbit, M. and Pritchard, J. (1987) Histiocytosis syndromes in children. *Lancet,* **1**, 208

Wynne-Davies, R., Williams, P. F. and O'Connor, J. C. B. (1981) The 1960s epidemic of arthrogryposis multiplex congenita. *J. Bone Jt. Surg.* **63B**, 76

Further reading

Arden, G. P. and Ansell, B. M. (1978) *Surgical Management of Juvenile Chronic Polyarthritis*. London: Academic Press; New York: Grune & Stratton

Akbarnia, B., Torg, J. S., Kilpatrick, J. (1944) Manifestations of the battered child syndrome *J. Bone Jt. Surg.* **56A**, 1159

King, J., Diefendors, S. D., Apthorp, J., Negrete, V. S. and Carlson, M. (1988) Analysis of 429 fractures in 189 battered children *J. Ped. Orthop.* **8**, 585–589

9

The neck

The atlanto-occipital region

Disorders of the atlanto-occipital region may be divided into stable and unstable, the latter having the capacity to damage the spinal cord.

Stable lesions

Stable lesions include absence in whole or part of the posterior arch of the atlas, and congenital fusion of the atlanto-occipital and atlantoaxial joints. These fusions are capable of restricting neck rotation but to a lesser extent than one would expect. This is doubtless due to compensatory hypermobility at a lower level in the cervical spine. This may expose the cord to damage at the level of abnormal movement. Anomalies of this type may also occur with posterior fossa disorders and compression of the brain stem at the foramen magnum.

In the young child with immature bone, atlanto-occipital fusion is difficult to detect radiologically but it is important as a cause of unexplained torticollis in which lack of rotation is more conspicuous than loss of lateral flexion.

The physiological variations of atlantoaxial movement should be recognized lest instability be wrongly suspected. The anterior arch of the atlas may override the odontoid in extension, and there may be widening of the gap between the odontoid and body of the atlas in flexion in 20% of normal children between 1 and 7 years of age (Cattell, 1965).

Unstable lesions

Absence or dysplasia of the odontoid is dangerous, for the cord is exposed to damage

from either injury of modest severity or the cumulative effects of the intermittent pressure of recurrent subluxation. Cord effects are more common in adult life but this in no way alleviates anxiety when this anomaly is found in a child.

The lesion is discovered either by change or because a minor injury has caused a stiff neck. Flexion and extension radiographs confirm instability (Figure 9.1). The dens is either absent or dysplastic as in os odontoideum, when there is a small ossicle separated by a gap from a short odontoid peg in the normal position. This is easily distinguished from an old fracture which involves the root of the peg or the epiphysis, which lies below the superior border of the axis and may be visible up to the age of 11 years (Wollin, 1963).

Surgical stabilization is obviously desirable in one so patently at risk but unfortunately this is very difficult to achieve in young children. One problem is that the posterior arch of the atlas is attenuated, so a stabilizing wire tends to cut through and there is a very inadequate bed for grafts. Furthermore, the juvenile skull is poor material for successful occipitocervical fusion (Newman and Sweetman, 1969). Wiring through the occiput and down to C3 can give improved fixation in these cases. Immobilization postoperatively, using a halo attached to a thoracic jacket or cast, provides good fixation while waiting for the bone grafts to fuse. We have not tried the anterior approach through the pharynx as recommended by Andrade and Macnab (1969).

Infective atlantoaxial subluxation is due to hyperaemic decalcification of the body of the atlas, which affects and loosens the attach-

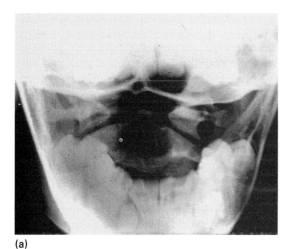

(a)

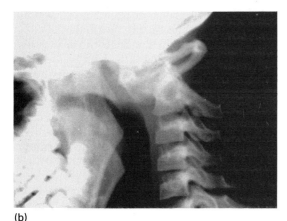

(b)

Figure 9.1 Absent odontoid. (a) Anteroposterior, open-mouth view; (b) lateral view, showing marked instability in flexion

ments of the transverse ligament of the dens upon which stability depends (Watson-Jones, 1932). It should be emphasized that only severe pharyngeal infections, such as retropharyngeal abscesses or post-tonsillectomy infected haematomas, are likely to be responsible.

A child with such a history suddenly develops a stiff neck with some torticollis, and the radiograph is diagnostic. Most stabilize if rested in bed for 3 weeks followed by the use of a Minerva plaster or collar, but this can fail (Werne, 1957). Stabilization is then indicated because of the hazard of cord compression when forward subluxation occurs around an intact dens. Unlike congenital subluxation, the anatomy is normal and successful fusion is probable (Garber, 1964).

Rotary subluxations

In rotary subluxations, one facet joint of either the C1/2 or the C2/3 level subluxates following a mild injury. Stiffness is more conspicuous than pain, and rotation deformity more than lateral tilting. Movement is free towards the deformities but painful away from them. A radiograph through the open mouth may disclose the subluxation, but more commonly a loss of the normal vertical midline alignment of the chin, the odontoid and the spine of the axis is disclosed (Stimson and Svenson, 1935). In the lateral view the neural canal of the atlas is visible, whereas that of the axis is not. Gentle traction with exaggeration of the deformity followed by its correction usually reduces the subluxation and relieves the symptoms dramatically. However, cases of irreducible rotatory subluxation do occur. The diagnosis is frequently missed and should be considered in all patients who have persistent torticollis. The neck X-rays may be difficult to interpret, but tomograms and CT scanning can be helpful (Fielding and Hawkins, 1977; Fielding *et al*, 1978).

Physiological variations in movement of cervical vertebrae

A knowledge of the range of normal movement, and in particular the significance of cervical vertebral subluxations, is of great importance. A child may be seen following a minor injury, with a radiograph which on lateral projection in flexion discloses a degree of subluxation between either C1 and 2 or C2, 3 or 4, which in an adult would be abnormal and alarming but which in childhood is a normal variation.

Cattell (1965) studied these pseudosubluxations and made the following observations. Of children between 1 and 7 years of age, 20% display 'abnormal' forward subluxation between either C2 and 3 or C3 and 4. In a similar proportion the gap between the atlas and the odontoid is increased on flexion, and on extension the arch of the atlas overrides the top of the odontoid. The 'normal' cervical lordosis is absent in 15 per cent but separate ossification centres at the tip of the spinous processes, simulating fractures, are rare.

These observations are important and very

helpful, but, if there is doubt, clinical assessment after a day or two in bed will usually be reassuring. If the displacement is physiological there will be neither pain nor tenderness nor lack of movement.

The Klippel–Feil deformity

A pedantic definition describes the Klippel–Feil deformity as a syndrome with a short, straight neck with limited movement, a low hair-line behind and webbing of the skin of the neck. The radiograph should show absence of one or more cervical vertebrae and congenital fusion. In practice the definition is extended to include all varieties of cervical spine muddle with or without thoracocervical scoliosis, spina bifida, congenital elevation of the scapula and malformation of the uppermost ribs.

In the event, they fall into three categories: the short straight neck with webbing (resembling Turner's syndrome), a short neck with scoliosis and torticollis (Figure 9.2) and cervical kyphosis.

Treatment depends not so much upon the severity of deformity as on its practicability and the neurological complications. Although plastic correction of skin webbing and removal of the prominence of an elevated scapula has some effect, the result is usually disappointing. Upper thoracic thoracoplasty is a tempting approach, but in one patient widening of the root of the neck largely neutralized the improvement.

Spinal cord involvement is uncommon, but may arise when there is cervical kyphosis or the syndrome is associated with a high congenital thoracocervical scoliosis. It is important to realize, however, that compression is as likely to involve the brain stem as the cervical cord, for dermoid cysts of the posterior fossa are recognized concomitants (Logue and Till, 1952). The orthopaedic surgeon should remember the association with deafness, renal anomalies and congenital heart disease (Hensinger *et al*, 1974).

Torticollis (wry neck)

The established deformity consists of a tilt of the head to one side and rotation of the chin to the other, frequently with some asymmetry of the face which is larger on the convex side – the side facing the sun – and most evident when eye levels are compared (Figure 9.3). Hulbert (1950) reviewed 100 patients who attended The Hospital for Sick Children during 7 years; there are also reviews by Coventry and Harris (1959), Macdonald (1969) and Lee, Kang and Bose (1986).

The newborn baby seems normal, although head moulding (not asymmetry) may appear rapidly. A hard fusiform tumour may be felt in the sternomastoid at the level of the angle of the jaw at any time after birth, but is usually noted between the third week and the second month, disappearing between the third and the eleventh month. It is most evident when the baby cries. The true incidence of the tumour is uncertain, for in the short thick neck of a baby a small one may be readily overlooked.

There may be no structural torticollis during the time that the tumour is evident, and indeed only about 1 in 7 develops the deformity later. Alternatively, one may say that only 1 in 5 of those presenting with a structural torticollis has a previous history of tumour. The deformity, if present, seldom becomes conspicuous before 3 years of age, when the neck begins to lengthen.

Great controversy and much speculation have been expended on the nature of this fascinating self-limited tumour. These include familial defects, infections, ischaemia and hamartoma of the muscle. Two theories deserve further consideration: firstly, that it is due to pressure on the neck from intrauterine malposition causing local ischaemia (Chandler and Altenberg, 1944; Chandler, 1948; Dunn, 1973) and, secondly, injury during delivery (Sanerkin and Edwards, 1966). Both have appeal, and are supported by the high incidence of obstetrical abnormality, particularly breech presentation, and of head moulding which is double the normal. Furthermore, Lloyd-Roberts and Pilcher (1965) observed the tumour several times in patients with idiopathic resolving scoliosis of infancy. Sanerkin and Edwards (1966) were fortunate in finding a tumour at autopsy on a baby, born by the breech, who died at 2 days. They described haemorrhage, fragmentation and necrosis of muscle, and emphasized the disruption of endomysial sheaths, which in experimental animals is followed by a proliferative fibroblastic reaction.

Diagnosis is not always easy. Head mould-

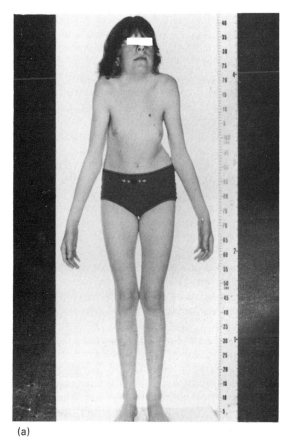

(a)

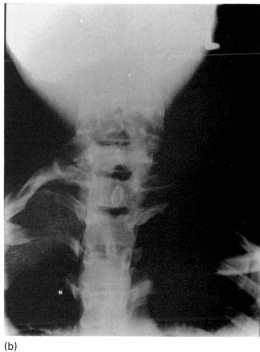

(b)

(c)

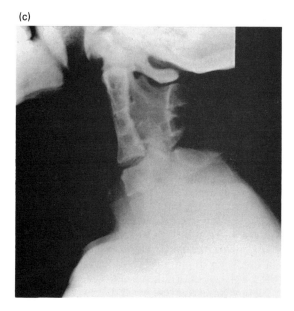

Figure 9.2 Klippel–Feil deformity. (a) A typical case. Note the short neck and elevated shoulders. (b) Anteroposterior X-ray. Note how difficult it is to see the cervical vertebrae because of the short neck. (c) Lateral X-ray. Note the multiple congenital fusion of C2 to C5

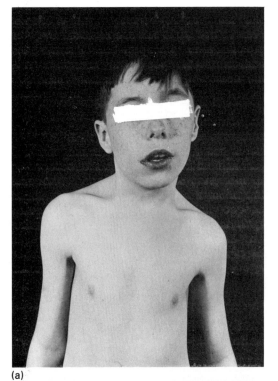

(a)

(b)

Figure 9.3 Right torticollis. (a) Note how the shoulder is elevated on the right, and the facial asymmetry. (b) Posterior view of the same patient

ing, when seen with scoliosis of infancy, may be distinguished by involvement of the occiput since in torticollis this is confined to the frontal zone. Klippel–Feil deformity and atlanto-occipital fusion must be excluded. Acute torticollis is due to sepsis (deep glands or atlantoaxial dislocation), injury, or a common or garden stiff neck. Tumours of the cervical spine should be remembered. In ocular torticollis the head is tilted to balance the eyes and counteract diplopia due to squints which may be seen if the head is placed in the neutral position.

Treatment is governed by prognosis. The favourable outcome in most patients with known tumours contraindicates early operation and implies that stretching exercises are of uncertain value. When the deformity is established it is best to operate at between 3 and 4 years of age, for by then the neck is longer and dissection easier. The essential postoperative physiotherapy and exercises are also better understood by the child and easier to carry out. The presence of facial asymmetry should not be a deterrent, for, if the contracture is released, it tends to improve at any time before maturity. It is wise, however, to demonstrate asymmetry to the parents before operation. Beyond maturity, improvement in the appearance of the neck is still possible, although some secondary skeletal deformity may have developed by then.

Our preference is for supraclavicular division of tight structures under vision, not forgetting the tight anomalous bands that may cross the posterior triangle and the possibility of contracture of the scaleni and deep investing fascia. We do not personally recommend subcutaneous tenotomy, and have no experience of detachment from the mastoid process. Operation must be followed by corrective stretching exercises, which may have to be continued for a considerable period of time.

Congenital pseudarthrosis of the clavicle

A congenital pseudarthrosis of the clavicle (Figure 9.4) is a curious condition, whose cause is unknown. It is nearly always on the right side but has been described on the left in a patient with dextrocardia (Gibson and Carroll, 1970).

Lloyd-Roberts, Apley and Owen (1975)

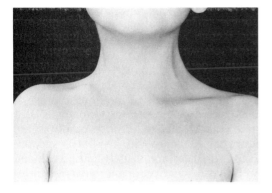

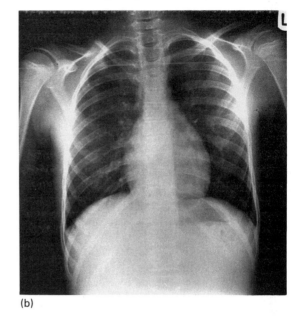

(b)

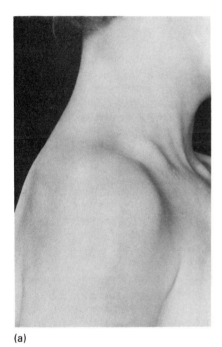

(a)

Figure 9.4 (a) Anteroposterior and lateral views of right pseudarthrosis of the clavicle. (b) Chest X-ray showing right pseudarthrosis of the clavicle

postulated that the lesion may be due to pressure upon the developing clavicle by the subclavian artery which is normally at a higher level on the right side except in dextrocardia when the relative positions of the subclavian arteries are reversed. There is no relationship with neurofibromatosis or obstetrical injury. It is interesting that in cleidocraniodysostosis, where there is also a defect in the clavicle, the first ribs are abnormally elevated and this could also produce pressure from the subclavian artery. The clavicle is no longer thought to develop in membrane but there is some debate as to whether it develops from one or two primary centres of endochondral ossification. Alldred (1963) suggested that failure of the two centres of endochondral ossification to fuse was the cause of the lesion.

There is no tendency to spontaneous healing, so operation is indicated (preferably at about the age of 4 years) to prevent shortening and drooping of the shoulder, and consequent difficulty with braces or brassiere.

Union is readily obtained if the fragments are transfixed with a Kirschner wire and surrounded by bone grafts. Alldred (1963) suggested that union was obtained more easily under the age of 8 years.

Obstetrical paralysis of the brachial plexus

Improvements in the standards of obstetrics are, fortunately, reducing the number of babies presenting with birth palsy due to brachial plexus injury (Figure 9.5). Nevertheless, they still occur, particularly when delivery is rapid and unexpected, and in large babies presenting by the breech or with an abnormal lie in which for one reason or another caesarian section is not performed.

At birth the arm lies immobile by the side, and there may be an associated fracture of the humerus or clavicle. Swelling and bruising may be seen in the neck. There is usually little doubt about the diagnosis, but fractures alone and the flaccid stage of spastic cerebral palsy or athetosis should be considered, although not necessarily to the exclusion of plexus injury, for the precipitating circumstances may be common to both.

Initially there may be some uncertainty about the degree and pattern of paralysis and the extent to which it will take place. In the past, exploration of the plexus has been unrewarding. At present, however, both in adults and in children with brachial plexus injuries a more aggressive policy of exploration and, if possible, repair of the injured brachial plexus is being advised in some specialist centres; the results of these procedures are encouraging. Traditionally a splint is applied, but this is unnecessary, usually ineffectual, and may do harm by encouraging posterior dislocation of the radial head (Aitken, 1952). At this age a mother will be devoting much of her time to the baby, and should be taught to put all the joints of the arm through a full range of movement twice a day, paying particular attention to external rotation of the shoulder (*see* below). The physiotherapist gives periodic supervision and encouragement, and tries to assess the amount of the damage and the progress of recovery. Recovery is sometimes rapid and often near perfect, as in half of Aitken's patients with upper arm paralysis.

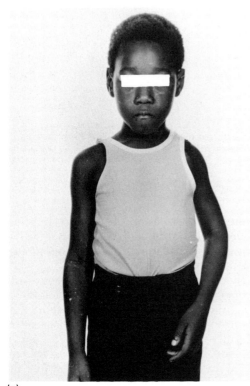

(a)

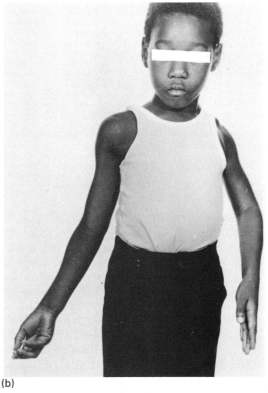

(b)

Figure 9.5 Left Erb's palsy. (a) In neutral position. (b) Same patient, trying to externally rotate the arms at the shoulders; note the inability to do this on the left

Full assessment is usually possible at 1 year, by which time the majority of the spontaneous recovery will have taken place although further recovery can take place up to 2–3 years of age. Sensory loss is less than the motor involvement would suggest, and Horner's syndrome is rare. The distribution of residual paralysis is around the shoulder (C5, C6) in two-thirds of the patients. One-tenth are localized to the hand and forearm (C8, T1 – Klumpke's paralysis) and the remainder have mixed or total paralysis (Wickstrom, Haslam and Hutchinson, 1955).

Operation is contemplated at about 4 to 5 years of age, when the common clinical patterns are established and the child can co-operate.

Residual paralysis of external rotation only

If there is no deformity and only residual paralysis of external rotation, disability is negligible, for the hand reaches the mouth with only slight abduction of the shoulder. If an internal rotation deformity has developed, abduction must approach 90 degrees when eating. We prefer rotation osteotomy (Goddard and Fixsen, 1984) to release of the subscapularis and pectoralis major (the method used by Sever) because this encourages anterior subluxation of the shoulder joint when the arm is laterally rotated. We personally rarely use the transfer of the latissimus dorsi and teres major described by L'Episcopo (1934) and advocated by Wickstrom, Haslam and Hutchinson in 1955.

Residual paralysis of abductors and external rotators

Residual paralysis of abductors and external rotators is much less common, and is probably best treated by arthrodesis of the shoulder at maturity – a decision encouraged by the secondary changes which often occur in the shoulder later.

Claw hand with paralysis of intrinsics, long flexors and partial sensory loss

Claw hand with paralysis of intrinsics, long flexors and partial sensory loss lends itself no more to surgical correction than does total arm paralysis.

Mixed paralysis or Erb's palsy which fails to recover

Mixed paralysis or Erb's palsy which fails to recover is treated on the lines developed for the treatment of similar situations in poliomyelitis. Two special problems merit emphasis: first, paralysis of elbow flexion which is correctable by pectoral transplantation (Brooks and Seddon, 1959); and, second, disabling fixed supination by rotation osteotomy of the radius (Zaoussis, 1963).

Skeletal deformities may develop with time, and include dislocation of the radial head with ulnar bowing, shortening of the humerus, lengthening of the acromion and coracoid processes, elevation of the scapula, and deformity and dislocation of the humeral head, first described from The Hospitals for Sick Children by Fairbank in 1913.

Miscellaneous conditions of the neck

Cervical meningoceles usually have a good prognosis. Cervical ribs seldom cause symptoms in childhood, but, if so, the signs tend to be vascular (for example, one blue arm) rather than neurological. Rheumatoid arthritis is sometimes heralded by a stiff neck, and the neck may ankylose, thus exposing the child to grave danger from injury. Myositis ossificans progressiva (page 85) frequently begins in this area. Congenital nuchal rigidity (Sutra and Mishkin, 1952) should not be diagnosed unless arthritis, myositis and congenital vertebral anomalies have been excluded. Kyphosis causing cord compression is not uncommon after cervical laminectomy, and was first discussed by Cattell and Clark (1967). In Turner's syndrome, webbing of the neck, by itself or in conjunction with other deformities, may occur.

References

Aitken, J. (1952) Deformity of the elbow joint as a sequel to Erb's obstetrical palsy. *J. Bone Jt. Surg.* **34B**, 352

Alldred, A. J. (1963) Congenital pseudarthrosis of the clavicle. *J. Bone Jt. Surg.* **45B**, 312

de Andrade, J. R. and Macnab, I. (1969) Anterior occipito-cervical fusion using an extra-pharyngeal exposure. *J. Bone Jt. Surg.* **51A**, 1621

Brooks, D. M. and Seddon, H. J. (1959) Pectoral transplantation for paralysis of the flexors of the elbow. *J. Bone Jt. Surg.* **41B**, 36

Cattell, H. S. (1965) Pseudosubluxation and other normal variations in the cervical spine in children. *J. Bone Jt. Surg.* **47A**, 1295

Cattell, H. S. and Clark, G. L. (1967) Cervical kyphosis and instability following muliple laminectomies in children. *J. Bone Jt. Surg.* **49A**, 713

Chandler, F. A. (1948) Muscular torticollis. *J. Bone Jt. Surg.* **30A**, 566

Chandler. F. A. and Altenberg, A. (1944) 'Congenital' muscular torticollis. *J. Am. Med. Ass.* **125**, 476

Coventry, M. B. and Harris, L. E. (1959) Congenital muscular torticollis in infancy. *J. Bone Jt. Surg.* **41A**, 815

Dunn, P. N. (1973) Congenital sternomastoid torticollis: an intra-uterine postural deformity. *J. Bone Jt. Surg.* **55B**, 877

Fairbank, H. A. T. (1913) Birth palsy. Subluxation of the shoulder joint in infants and very young children. *Lancet.* **1**, 1217

Fielding J. W. and Hawkins, R. J. (1977) Atlanto-axial rotatory fixation. *J. Bone Jt. Surg.* **59A**, 37

Fielding, J. W., Stillwell, W. T. York Chynn, K. and Spyropoulos, E. C. (1978) Use of computed tomography for the diagnosis of atlanto-axial rotatory fixation. *J. Bone Jt. Surg.* **60A**, 1102

Garber, J. N. (1964) Abnormalities of the atlas and axis vertebrae – congenital and traumatic. *J. Bone Jt. Surg.* **46A**, 1782

Gibson, D. A. and Carroll, N. (1970) Congenital pseudarthrosis of the clavicle. *J. Bone Jt. Surg.* **52B**, 629

Goddard, N. J. and Fixsen, J. A. (1984) Rotation osteotomy of the humerus for birth injuries of the brachial plexus. *J. Bone Jt. Surg.* **66B**, 257

Hensinger, R. N., Lang, J. E. and MacEwen, G. D. (1974) Klippel–Feil syndrome. *J. Bone Jt. Surg.* **56A**, 1246–1253

Hulbert, J. K. (1950) Congenital torticollis. *J. Bone Jt. Surg.* **32B**, 50

Lee, E. H., Kang, Y. K. and Bose, K. (1986) Surgical correction of muscular torticollis in the older child. *J. Pediat. Orthop.* **6**, 585

L'Episcopo, J. B. (1934) Tendon transplantation in obstetrical paralysis. *Am. J. Surg.* **24**, 122

Lloyd-Roberts, G. C. and Pilcher, M. F. (1965) Structural idiopathic scoliosis in infancy. *J. Bone Jt. Surg.* **47B**, 520

Lloyd-Roberts, G. C., Apley, A. G. and Owen, R. (1975) Reflections upon the aetiology of congenital pseudarthrosis of the clavicle. *J. Bone Jt. Surg.* **57B**, 24

Logue, V. and Till, K. (1952) Posterior fossa dermoid cysts, with special reference to intracranial infection. *J. Neurol. Neurosurg. Psychiat.* **15**, 1

Macdonald, D. (1969) Sternomastoid tumour and muscular torticollis. *J. Bone Jt. Surg.* **51B**, 432

Sanerkin, N. G. and Edwards, P. (1966) Birth injury to the sternomastoid muscle. *J. Bone Jt. Surg.* **48B**, 441

Stimson, B. B. and Swenson, P. C. (1935) Unilateral subluxations of cervical vertebrae without associated fractures. *J. Am. Med. Ass.* **104**, 1578

Sutro, C. J. and Mishkin, R. D. (1952) Familial nuchal rigidity. *Bull. Hosp. Jt. Dis., NY* **13**, 155

Watson-Jones, R. (1932) Spontaneous hyperaemic dislocation of the atlas. *Proc. R. Soc. Med.* **25**, 586

Werne, S. (1957) Studies in spontaneous atlas dislocation. *Acta Orthop. Scand.* suppl. 23, pp. 1–150

Wickstrom, J., Haslam, E. T. and Hutchinson, R. H. (1955) Surgical management of residual deformities of the shoulder following birth injuries of the brachial plexus. *J. Bone Jt. Surg.* **37A**, 27

Wollin, D. G. (1963) Os odontoideum. *J. Bone Jt. Surg.* **45A**, 1459

Zaoussis, A. L. (1963) Osteotomy of the proximal end of the radius for paralytic supination deformity in children. *J. Bone Jt. Surg.* **45B**, 523

10

The shoulder and elbow

The clavicle (page 94) and obstetrical paralysis (page 96) have already been considered.

The shoulder joint

Congenital anomalies

Congenital anomalies are infrequent, but reversal of the joint – that is, the glenoid becomes the ball and the humerus the socket – and idiopathic enlargement of the coracoid and acromion processes may occasionally occur although they are usually symptom free. Coracoid and acromion enlargement occur more frequently following Erb's palsy. Acromionectomy may be of value when trying to mobilize the shoulder in this condition.

Dislocation of the shoulder

Dislocation of the shoulder may happen by obstetrical mishap, with or without an associated fracture. If not recognized immediately, this may become irreducible and require open reduction. Anterior or posterior instability may be present in patients with extreme joint laxity (Carter and Sweetnam, 1960) and probably is best left alone. It can also occur as a late complication of Erb's palsy when the head of the humerus may lie below the glenoid. A similar appearance is seen with Sprengel's shoulder.

Humerus varus

In humerus varus, the normal neck shaft angle is reduced in varying degree, and the tuberosity enlarges to lessen the distance between it and the acromion. Abduction may therefore be limited, but not below 90 degrees so the disability is slight. The associated shortening of the humerus together with the deformity suggest that an injury to the proximal humeral growth plate is the cause. This may be traumatic or infective. If traumatic, it may be part of the battered baby, or non-accidental injury syndrome, and this seems a satisfactory explanation for the development in some patients of this otherwise puzzling condition (Lloyd-Roberts, 1968).

Treatment is rarely indicated, but, if there is pain or if restoration of full abduction seems to be desirable, this may be achieved by either abduction osteotomy of the humerus (Lucas and Gill, 1947) or acromionectomy (Lloyd-Roberts, 1953). Of the alternatives, osteotomy is preferable because acromionectomy carries its own peculiar complications.

Abduction contracture

In abduction contracture the intermediate third of the deltoid is fibrotic and adduction ceases at about 30 degrees from the trunk. If further adduction is attempted the skin may be indrawn over the contracted muscle. Excision of the fibrotic muscle restores full movement (Bhattacharyya, 1966).

The condition seems analogous to quadriceps contracture following injections (*see* page 175), and is sometimes seen in association with a vaccination scar. Hill and colleagues (1967) reported a patient who was premature by 30 days and had multiple injections in the 3 months during which he was isolated. Unfortunately there was no record of the injection sites, but, since he also developed a quadriceps contracture, the implication seems clear.

Congenital elevation of the scapula (Sprengel's shoulder)

In Sprengel's shoulder, the scapula is small and high, protruding into the base of the neck to a variable extent (Figure 10.1). It is seldom an isolated deformity, usually being accompanied by cervical or upper thoracic vertebral anomalies or abnormal ribs. The deformity produced is thus commonly as much the result of other anomalies as of scapular displacement. Although most cases are unilateral some are bilateral, especially if the cervical spine is conspicuously faulty.

The disability is cosmetic rather than physical. That part of the scapula above the spinous process is in the posterior triangle, and the contour of the neck is asymmetrical. Furthermore, the supraspinous portion curves sharply forward, and its superior and medial promontory enlarges to become a conspicuous hook bulging anteriorly. Function is only mildly impaired because abduction of the shoulder, although restricted, is not less than 90 degrees. If an omovertebral bone is present in the plane of the levator scapulae and pinning the scapula to the cervical spine (1 case in 3), this limitation is explicable, even when the abnormal bone articulates at both ends. When it is absent, however, the same restriction remains.

Treatment is dictated by cosmetic considerations and so varies with the degree of the blemish. Mild displacements may be ignored, but in other instances only operation is helpful. Many operations have been described. These resolve themselves into partial or complete excisions *in situ* (with or without the periosteum), and attempts to reposition the whole bone by either detaching muscles from the scapula and securing it lower down by internal fixation and even traction, or detaching them from the vertebrae and transferring these to a lower level after mobilizing the scapula (Woodward, 1961).

Moderate deformity is probably best treated later in childhood, by subperiosteal excision of that part of the scapula above and including the spinous process, being careful to remove the superomedial angle. The residual periosteal lined cavity is obliterated by sutures. Function

is uninfluenced. In the past we have used Woodward's operation for more severe deformities in children under the age of 5. It can achieve correction of the greater part of the deformity, which may later be completed by excision of the upper scapula. There is, however, some danger to the brachial plexus if either displacement is overenthusiastic or, when dissecting the muscles from the superior margin, the surgeon forgets the propinquity of the plexus and the probability of muscle and nerve anomalies when the skeletal elements of the same myotome are abnormal. Improvement in abduction is an incidental bonus. Wilkinson and Campbell (1980) have described a vertical displacement osteotomy of the medial border of the scapula with division of the fibrous attachments and excision of the superomedial angle, with encouraging cosmetic and functional results.

The humerus

Phocomelia

In phocomelia the humerus is replaced by a rudimentary arm and incomplete hand. This term, which means a seal flipper, is an apt description of the commonest type, but of course the possible variations in longitudinal and transverse deficiency are almost infinite. Surgery has little to offer these children but good management of both parents and child is vital.

Decisions must be adapted to the total disability of the child. Thus, if one arm is normal, the dysplastic limb may be more valuable as it is as a holder, and steadier than any contemporary prosthesis. Indeed, function following one congenital above-elbow amputation is likely to be well-nigh full, and with a phocomelic limb it may be even better. Unfortunately, however, phocomelia is usually bilateral; but even then we should remember the adaptive capacity of the legs if they are normal. There is a woman with no arms and only one leg who has married and brought up a family. She is a heavy smoker, and apparently her only serious problem is removing the nicotine stains from between her big and second toes.

Developments in prosthetics are now so rapid that these children should be referred to special centres within the first 3 months, for if

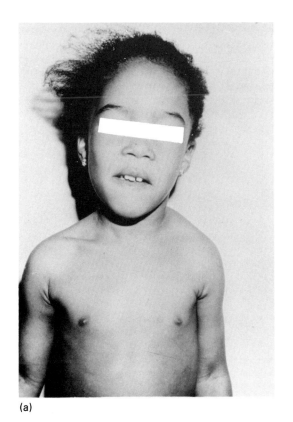
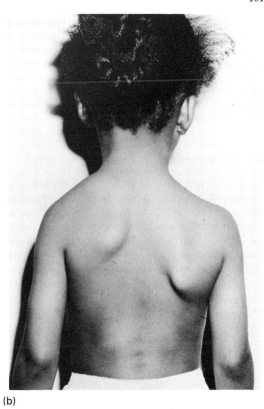

(a)   (b)

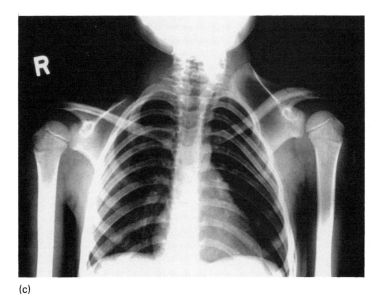

(c)

Figure 10.1 Congenital elevation of the left shoulder (Sprengel's shoulder). (a) Anterior view. (b) Posterior view of the same patient. Note how the lower pole of the left scapula is not only high but also nearer the midline to the rotation of the scapula. (c) Anteroposterior X-ray of left congenital elevation of the scapula

it is decided to use artificial arms those responsible prefer to begin at an early age.

Power-operated prostheses and mechanisms for initiating their movements are becoming progressively more sophisticated. A recent development is the use of myoelectric prostheses in the upper limb (Hubbard, Galway and Milner, 1985).

Supracondylar spur

Supracondylar spur is a palpable, bony semicircle which is continued as a fibrous band to surround the median nerve and brachial artery a short distance above the elbow on the medial side (Figure 10.2). The spur is atavistic, for it is a constant feature in some climbing animals. Both vascular and median compression syndromes are seen. Children are not immune, so this anomaly should be thought of when a child complains of symptoms suggestive of carpal tunnel compression of the median nerve, for this is extremely rare in the young (Kessel and Rang, 1966).

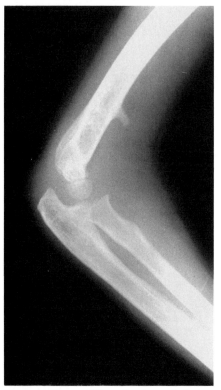

Figure 10.2 Lateral X-ray showing typical supracondylar or humeral spur. This patient presented with symptoms of median nerve compression

The elbow joint

Congenital dislocation of the radial head

The characteristics of congenital dislocation of the radial head (Figure 10.3) have been described by McFarland (1936). Dislocation

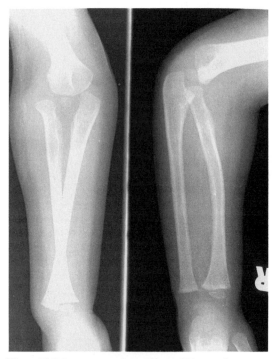

Figure 10.3 Anteroposterior and lateral X-rays of congenital dislocation (lateral) of the radial head

may be anterior, posterior or lateral. The displaced radial head is palpable. Movement is either full or mildly limited. There is relative stability, so the wrist joint rarely subluxates.

Radiologically the radius seems too long for the ulna, which is slightly bowed anteriorly in its proximal third. Secondary changes include a misshapen radial head which is conical, and dysplasia of the capitellum which is deprived of its contact.

The changes are very similar to those one would expect following a Monteggia fracture, if the ulna has a greenstick fracture only and the radial head remains uncorrected. Although it is possible to reduce the head of the radius by shortening the shaft and holding it with a Kirschner wire to the humerus, there is difficulty in obtaining stability of the radial head and a risk of sacrificing some rotary movement. As the functional disability is

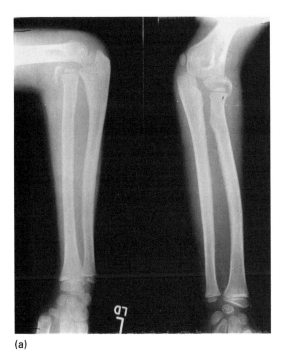

(a)

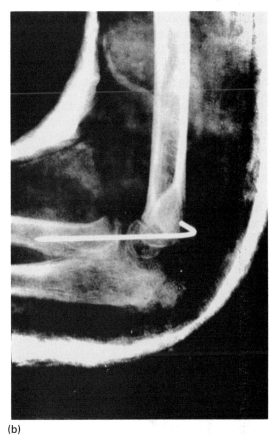

(b)

Figure 10.4 (a) Anteroposterior and lateral X-rays of post-traumatic (acquired) dislocation of the radial head. Note the calcification in the fibrous tissue in relation to the displaced radial head. (b) Postoperative lateral X-ray showing the radial head replaced and held with Kirschner wire

usually negligible, it is best to accept the dislocation.

In the nail–patella syndrome (page 83) the radial head may be displaced backwards and limit extension, and in congenital absence of the ulna the radial head will in time lose contact with the humerus.

Acquired dislocation of the radial head

Acquired dislocation of the radial head (Figure 10.4) develops in Erb's palsy when supination fails to recover, or following prolonged splinting in supination (page 97). Recurrent dislocation is very rare and associated with congenital joint laxity, which predisposes to the first traumatic dislocation in a manner similar to recurrent dislocation of the patella. Any condition in which the ulna shortens or becomes bowed will tend, with growth, to cause displacement of the radial head, even if

(as in a Monteggia fracture) the dislocation is not part of the initial injury. Thus in fibrous dysplasia of the ulna with fracture and some loss of length during healing, eventual dislocation is probable. In these dislocations the radial head is likely to be widely displaced posteriorly and laterally, and, if obstructing movement, it may be removed without anxiety about wrist joint subluxation, for the radius has by now lost contact with the humerus and no longer stabilizes the distal joint. Recently lengthening of the ulna has been described with some success in replacing the subluxing radial head (Pritchett, 1986).

When, however, post-traumatic dislocation occurs alone or in association with a Monteggia fracture, and secondary changes have not developed, open reduction of the head with reconstruction of the annular ligaments, and straightening of the ulna if necessary, is justified to prevent further displacement of elbow and wrist and to improve function (Bell, 1965; Lloyd-Roberts and Bucknill, 1977).

Pulled elbow (subluxation head of radius)

Pulled elbow is an alarming syndrome. The distracted, trailing child is urged forwards by a smart tug on the hand with the elbow extended. There is a scream and the arm lies limp at the side as if the brachial plexus has been injured. Pain is negligible but 'paralysis' persists. Supination of the elbow is limited. The radiograph shows no bony injury or displacement, although occasionally an air arthrogram of the elbow joint may have been produced. A sharp supination movement with the elbow flexed is accompanied by a click, a howl and dramatic recovery, for the child will immediately reach out for the rewarding sweet. The episode is usually not repeated but we have seen recurrences which finally ceased spontaneously.

Pulled elbow is believed to be due to partial displacement of the head of the radius so that it becomes fixed within the grip of the annular ligament. McRae and Freeman (1965) reproduced this by pulling on the straight elbow in the line of the arm in anatomical preparations. They found that impaction was perpetuated in pronation and released by supination.

Recurrent dislocation of the elbow

Recurrent dislocation of the elbow is rare, but sometimes follows a traumatic dislocation in a loose-jointed child. The dislocation is posterior and veers to the lateral rather than the medial side.

The stability of the elbow depends largely on the hinge joint between the ulna and humerus, and so instability has been ascribed to dysplasia of the coronoid process or the capitulum. These abnormalities are certainly common, but it is uncertain whether they are primary or secondary. We are familiar with the humeral head defect due to osteochondral fracture in recurrent dislocation of the shoulder, and it is probable that a similar injury occurs here. Flattening of the capitulum, shallowness at the coronoid notch and reduction in the height of the upper radial epiphysis are all seen, and may all be secondary effects of osteochondral injury.

However, why some traumatic dislocations become recurrent if the articular surfaces are initially normal has still to be explained. Osborne and Cotterill (1966) advanced a most persuasive hypothesis. The first injury tears the humeral attachment of the lateral collateral ligament, and this either fails to reunite with the bone or does so lower down, thus causing an effective lengthening of the ligament. This theory is supported radiographically by the frequency with which avulsion chip fractures are seen in this area. Lateral instability coupled with the lateral inclination of the lower humerus (to provide the carrying angle) allow the coronoid to rotate beneath the trochlea when a moderate force is applied. Osborne and Cotterill reinforced their argument by showing that further dislocation may be prevented by reattaching the lateral ligament in its correct position.

Recurrent dislocation does not inevitably require operation, for there is a tendency for stability to be restored spontaneously, especially if there is general joint laxity. Sometimes, however, dislocation is not only repetitive but requires reduction under anaesthesia, and in these cases (in which secondary changes are usually present) operation is indicated.

The senior author has used Kapel's operation (1951) with success but this is difficult, for its purpose is to construct cruciate ligaments across the joint from the biceps and triceps tendons. The alternative method of reconstructing the lateral ligament is obviously simpler and in no way prejudices a second, more radical, procedure.

Osteochondritis of the elbow

Generalized osteochondritis of the elbow may affect either the radial head or the capitulum (Panner's disease) (Figure 10.5). The changes are similar to those in Perthes' disease, for density merges into fragmentation and healing, with permanent flattening in some. The head of the radius may become enlarged.

In both, aching is associated with some limitation of extension and pain on stress. At first, symptoms may indicate a short period in plaster, but this is purely symptomatic because the ultimate prognosis is good (Trias and Ray, 1963; Smith, 1963).

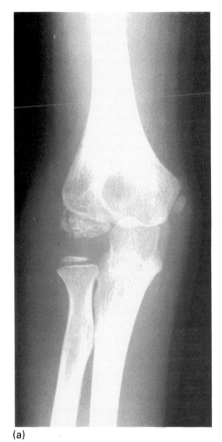
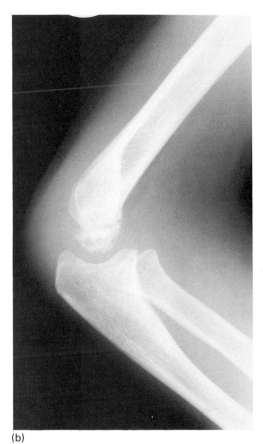

(a)   (b)

Figure 10.5 (a) Anteroposterior and (b) lateral X-rays of osteochondritis of the capitulum (Panner's disease)

Osteochondritis dissecans of the elbow

The symptoms of osteochondritis dissecans of the elbow are similar to those of osteochondritis and, as in the knee, the condition is very rare before the age of 12 years. It occurs predominantly in boys, and separation of a loose body is unusual in childhood. The capitulum and radial head are the areas affected.

The capitulum may show subchondral rarefaction below its convex surface, which later becomes cystic and finally demarcated as a dense semilunar segment. In the radius the medial side of the head is the usual site for similar changes and the epiphysis as a whole may become enlarged.

In children the rarity with which a loose body separates encourages an expectant attitude. Temporary protection in plaster may be necessary if the joint is more painful and irritable than usual but observations and warnings about rough play are generally all that is needed until healing is advanced (Roberts and Hughes, 1950; Osborne, 1967).

Cubitus varus

The normal carrying angle (cubitus valgus) in children is about 5 degrees and when this is lost, or the forearm lies medially angulated in relation to the arm, cubitus varus deformity is present. It is invariably due to malunion of a supracondylar fracture (Figure 10.6).

The malalignment is in two planes: medial inclination and medial rotation (French, 1959) of the lower fragment. The second rotary element is not always appreciated if it is not noted that the characteristic anterior spike of the proximal fragment, seen in the lateral projection, is in fact in the anteroposterior plane but rotated outwards with the major fragment. The use of a sling in medial rotation ensures that the lower fragment becomes even

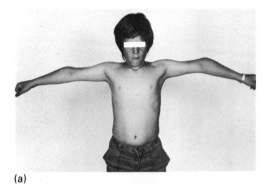

(a)

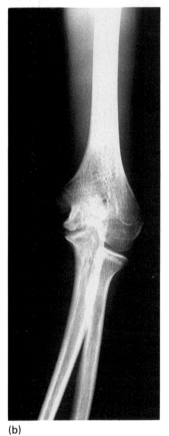

(b)

Figure 10.6 (a) Left cubitus varus following an old supracondylar fracture. (b) X-ray of cubitus varus or gunstock deformity of the left elbow following supracondylar fracture

more rotated inwards in relation to the upper fragment. Soon after the fracture is healed, comparing rotation between the two shoulders with the forearm at 90 degrees to the arm will demonstrate the axial malrotation.

Although posterior displacement tends to mould away with growth and the lack of elbow

flexion recovers as the anterior buttress absorbs, medial rotation and angulation usually persist. However, the fracture is well above the growth plate and the elbow is stable, so there is no tendency for the deformity to increase with growth. Consequently, a decision for or against correction may be taken as soon as elbow movements are restored.

There is no functional disability and no risk of late complications, but the appearance may be most displeasing when the elbow is straight or the arm abducted. When the elbow is flexed the deformity is masked. If it is decided to interfere, a valgus osteotomy with internal fixation above the level of the healed fracture is appropriate. It is advisable to apply the plaster initially in full extension, which enables the surgeon to confirm that correction is satisfactory. With the elbow flexed this is often difficult to judge and it is very easy to undercorrect the deformity. The purist will wish to overcome medial rotation as well but this adds to the difficulty at operation, and in practice seems unnecessary.

Cubitus valgus

Cubitus valgus is an increase in the carrying angle of the elbow and is again usually the result of malunion of a fracture, but may occasionally be seen in Turner's syndrome (page 83) and the nail–patella syndrome (page 83).

As in cubitus varus, function is good but here the resemblance ends, for the deformity is progressive and there is the late complication of ulnar nerve paralysis due to stretching around the convexity of the deformity.

The original injury is a displaced fracture running obliquely from the lateral metaphysis (to transect the outer part of the trochlea) which inevitably crosses the epiphyseal growth plate. Failure of accurate reduction may be followed by non-union or growth plate arrest on the lateral side. Progressive deformity is the quotient of continuing medial growth, failure of lateral growth and upward displacement of the head of the radius due to instability of the capitulum.

Non-union and its accompanying displacement should be corrected regardless of the state of the growth plate, in order to give some support to the head of the radius (Jeffrey, 1958). Cosmetic considerations may indicate wedge osteotomy later, when the opportunity is taken to transpose the ulnar nerve forward to reduce the risk of tardy paralysis.

Miscellaneous conditions of shoulder and elbow

Deformities of the elbow are features of Turner's syndrome and nail–patella syndrome (page 83). In the 'battered baby' syndrome (page 81) displacements of the metaphyses at both ends of the humerus are common. At the lower end dislocation of the elbow is closely simulated. Myositis ossificans following injury (page 85) and tumoral calcinosis (page 80) are seen most frequently here, as is small pox arthritis. Rheumatoid arthritis (page 80) often affects the elbow and suppurative arthritis of infancy the shoulder. Congenital skin webbing, with restriction of elbow extension, may expose the median nerve to surgical hazard during correction. The upper humerus is a common site for simple bone cysts (page 29) and monostotic fibrous dysplasia (page 29).

References

Bell Tawse, A. J. S. (1965) The treatment of malunited anterior fractures in childen. *J. Bone Jt. Surg.* **47B**, 718

Bhattacharyya, D. (1966) Abduction contracture of the shoulder from contracture of the intermediate part of the deltoid. *J. Bone Jt. Surg.* **48B**, 127

Carter, C. and Sweetnam, R. (1960) Recurrent dislocation of the patella and of the shoulder: their association with familial joint laxity. *J. Bone Jt. Surg.* **42B**, 721

French, P. R. (1959) Varus deformity of the elbow following supracondylar fractures of the humerus in children. *Lancet.* **2**, 439

Fulford, G. E. and Hall, M. J. (1968) *Amputation and Prostheses*. Bristol: Wright

Hill, N. A., Leibler, W. A., Wilson, H. J. and Rosenthal, E. (1967) Abduction contractures of both glenohumeral joints and extension contracture of one knee secondary to partial muscle fibrosis. *J. Bone Jt. Surg.* **49A**, 961

Hubbard, S., Galway, H. R. and Milner, M. (1985) Myoelectric training methods for the preschool child with congenital below-elbow amputation. *J. Bone Jt. Surg.* **67B**, 273

Jeffrey, C. C. (1958) Non-union of the epiphysis of the lateral condyle of the humerus. *J. Bone Jt. Surg.* **40B**, 396

Kapel, O. (1951) Operation for habitual dislocation of the elbow. *J. Bone Jt. Surg.* **33A**, 707

Kessel, L. and Rang, M. (1966) Supracondylar spur of the humerus. *J. Bone Jt. Surg.* **48B**, 765

Lloyd-Roberts, G. C. (1953) Humerus varus: report of a case treated by excision of the acromion. *J. Bone Jt. Surg.* **35B**, 268

Lloyd-Roberts, G. C. (1968) The diagnosis of injury of bones and joints in young babies. *Proc. R. Soc. Med.* **61**, 1299

Lloyd-Roberts, G. C. and Bucknill, T. M. (1977) Anterior dislocation of the radial head in children. *J. Bone Jt. Surg.* **59B**, 402

Lucas, L. S. and Gill, J. H. (1947) Humerus varus following birth injury to the proximal humeral epiphysis. *J. Bone Jt. Surg.* **29**, 367

McFarland, B. L. (1936) Congenital dislocation of the head of radius. *Br. J. Surg.* **24**, 41

McRae, R. K. and Freeman, P. A. (1965) The lesions in pulled elbow. *J. Bone Jt. Surg.* **47B**, 808 [summary]

Osborne, G. (1967) The elbow and forearm. In *Clinical Surgery*, vol. 13, *Orthopaedics*. London: Butterworths

Osborne, G. and Cotterill, P. (1966) Recurrent dislocation of the elbow. *J. Bone Jt. Surg.* **48B**, 340

Pritchett, J. W. (1986) Lengthening the ulna in patients with hereditary multiple exostoses. *J. Bone Jt. Surg.* **68-B**, 561–565

Roberts, N. and Hughes, R. (1950) Osteochondritis dissecans of the elbow joint. *J. Bone Jt. Surg.* **32B**, 348

Smith, M. G. H. (1964) Osteochondritis of the humeral capitulum. *J. Bone Jt. Surg.* **46B**, 50

Trias, A. and Ray, R. D. (1963) Juvenile osteochondritis of the radial head. *J. Bone Jt. Surg.* **45A**, 576

Wilkinson, J. A. and Campbell, D. (1980) Scapular osteotomy for Sprengel's shoulder. *J. Bone Jt. Surg.* **62B**, 486

Woodward, J. W. (1961) Congenital elevation of the scapula. *J. Bone Jt. Surg.* **43A**, 219

Further reading

Rang, M. (1983) *Children's Fractures,* 2nd edn. Philadelphia, Toronto: J. B. Lippincott

Wadsworth, T. G. (1982) *The Elbow.* Edinburgh, London, New York: Churchill Livingstone

11

The forearm and hand

General considerations

With the exception of radioulnar synostosis, congenital disorders of the forearm have an effect on the function of the hand and, often, on its structure. The interrelationship between the two bones during growth has been mentioned because it affects the elbow joint. Discrepancy in length or alignment may also affect the wrist, when lower radioulnar subluxation is caused thereby. Similarly, soft tissue abnormalities, especially contractures, are important because of their influence distally; for example, Volkmann's ischaemic contracture. Although this chapter is divided into two parts – first, disorders of the forearm and, second, disorders primarily in the hand – this is largely an artificial distinction.

One must never consider abnormalities of the forearm and hand without paying frequent attention to the other arm. Congenital anomalies are frequently bilateral but are by no means always mirror images. Hands work as pairs and their efficiency is mutual.

Inheritance is not unusual in deformities of the hand, and it is wise not to pronounce on prognosis while the father's hands remain in his pockets.

Lastly, nowhere is the adaptability of young children in overcoming apparently disabling situations more dramatic than in the hand. For example, bilateral congenital absence of the thumbs is compatible with full function for, if normal, the index fingers will develop the property of pinch. Widening of the web space and medial rotation of the metacarpal occurs spontaneously. It is wise not to be hasty in deciding upon treatment (except in the pre-

sence of the most obvious indications) until a few years have passed. This allows time for structure and function to adapt themselves as best they may, and this is often surprisingly effective.

The forearm

Radioulnar synostosis

In radioulnar synostosis (Figure 11.1) the bones are joined at, or just below, the superior radioulnar joint on one or both sides. The position of the forearm is fixed at a point from which no rotation is possible. Fortunately, this is usually in full pronation or slightly supinated – a position in which function is virtually full, especially when there is an adaptive increase in shoulder rotation.

There are three basic types of radioulnar synostosis. One is the headless type in which the radius springs from the ulna which is solidly fused and there is no vestige of a radial head. The second type is where the radial head is present but frequently deformed; the radius and ulna are clearly fused by bone just distal to the radial head. Finally, there is the type where there is no obvious bony fusion between the radius and the ulna but the clinical signs of loss of rotation of the forearm are present; in these the radial head lies behind the ulna in a partially dislocated position and the ulna may be somewhat bowed.

Function is so good that it may not be noticed for many years. One boy, a keen cricketer, was known to be unsafe as a boundary fielder because he could not catch high balls. In these circumstances treatment

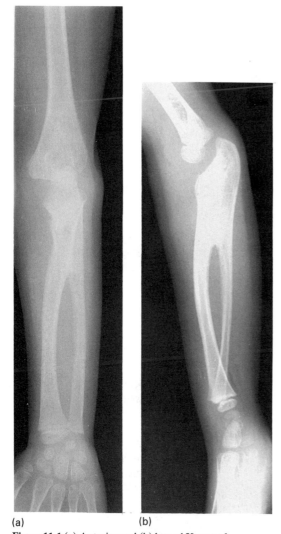

(a)   (b)

Figure 11.1 (a) Anterior and (b) lateral X-rays of radioulnar synostosis

Congenital amputation

The forearm is a common site for congenital amputation (Figure 11.2). The level is usually just below the elbow leaving enough forearm to act as an activated hook. If, as is usual, the amputation is unilateral, function will be near perfect, for the stump will be a valuable aid as a holder and steadier to assist the normal hand. Most prosthetic surgeons feel that a dress arm should be introduced, if possible, in the first year of life so that the child becomes used to wearing a prosthesis even though, for function, the unencumbered limb is likely to be used as it possesses normal sensation. The myoelectric arm is becoming of increasing value, but still suffers from the problem of lack of sensation.

When the amputation is bilateral and the stump is of adequate length, Krukenberg's operation merits consideration (Swanson, 1964) as an alternative to a powered prosthesis. By dividing one forearm bone from the other,

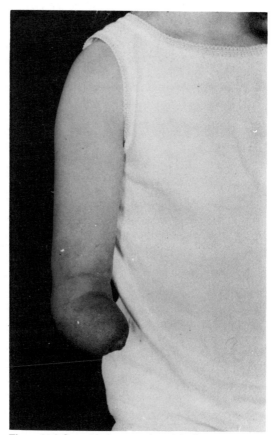

Figure 11.2 Congenital amputation of the forearm

seems superfluous, particularly as the operation required is moderately formidable and the results of doubtful virtue. Simple excision of a uniting bar fails because there is no active supination available and cross-union recurs. The ingenious swivel (Kelikian and Doumanian, 1957) has met with some success in old post-traumatic synostosis for which it was designed, but is rarely if ever successful in congenital cases. Osteotomy to place the hand in a more functional position is sometimes indicated.

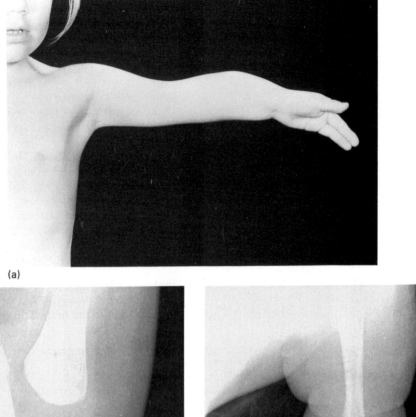

(a)

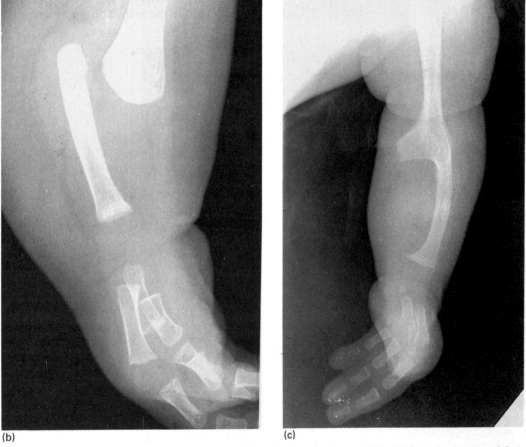

(b)　　　　　　　　　　　　　　　　　　　　(c)

Figure 11.3 (a) Congenital absence of the ulna (ulnar club hand). Note the absence of the little and ring fingers and the short forearm. (b) X-ray of congenital absence of the ulna. (c) Congenital absence of the ulna with congenital fusion of the elbow

this operation aims to construct a pincer grip on one side. Swanson pointed out that a dress prosthesis can always be worn over the pincer, thus answering the criticism of offensive ugliness. The child can at least feed himself with chopsticks in addition to establishing other skills to ensure his independence.

Absence and duplication of ulna

Absence

Abnormalities of the ulnar component are much less common than those of the radial (*see* below). If the radius is relatively normal the wrist is stable and loss of one or more ulnar digits does not seriously interfere with the function of the hand which merely deviates ulnarwards on gripping and pinching.

As on the radial side, the abnormality may involve any part of the arm, but predominantly its post-axial side. Thus the humerus may be short, the elbow fused, the radius short and curved or, at the other extreme, the ulna may be present but dysplastic and the hand lack its ulnar fingers and associated carpal bones (Figures 11.3 and 11.4).

When localized to the forearm and hand the main problem is instability of the elbow, for the radius soon loses contact with the humerus. Fortunately, the proximal end of the ulna with its olecranon is frequently present, and then fusion of proximal ulna to distal radius in mid-pronation, with excision of the displaced radius, resolves the difficulty (Figure 11.4b). Otherwise there seems no alternative to elbow arthrodesis postponed until maturity. Sometimes it may also be necessary to treat the wrist in a similar fashion.

Duplication

Duplication is even less common. The arm and forearm are short and there may be other abnormalities in the limb. The elbow and wrist

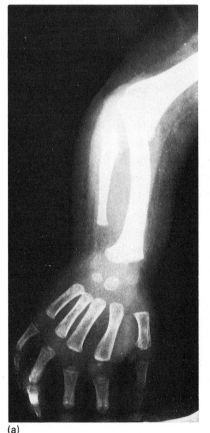
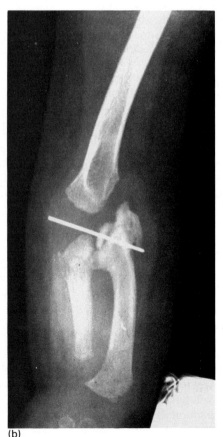

(a) (b)

Figure 11.4 (a) Partial absence of the ulna. (b) Operation to free the radius from the ulna, to preserve elbow stability

are stable but the hand is double (mirror hand) and lacks thumbs, being an eight-fingered assembly with a good grip but little pinch. Reduction by partial amputation is the obvious solution but this should be delayed until the function of individual fingers can be assessed, for this is variable and operation must obviously be planned to preserve the more useful digits (Harrison, Pearson and Roaf, 1960).

Madelung's deformity

In Madelung's deformity (Figure 11.5) there is posterior dislocation of the ulna at the lower radioulnar joint, and the articular surface of the radius is inclined towards the ulnar side. The deformity seems due to premature epiphyseal arrest of the anterior and medial quadrant of the radial plate, which causes both forward and medial inclination and some shortening of the radius. The unimpaired ulna impinges on the carpus, deviates the wrist radially and finally dislocates backwards.

The cause in most cases is unknown but a minor, forgotten, injury crossing the growth plate rather than passing through the metaphysis or the proximal layers of the plate is an obvious theoretical explanation.

In childhood, the parents will notice the prominent ulna, but symptoms are unlikely to develop before maturity. Later there may be aching in the wrist, weakness of grip and deformity, coupled with limitation of pronation and dorsiflexion.

When seen before symptoms develop it is difficult to decide what to do, for growth is likely to be continuing. Excision of the prominent ulna may encourage bowing of the radius, thus adding to the deformity of the wrist. This may be ameliorated to some extent by shortening the ulna and performing a lateral wedge osteotomy of the radius, but ulnar instability and deformity remain and further growth encourages recurrence. Reconstruction of the lower radioulnar joint may still further reduce forearm rotation.

Dissatisfaction with the outcome of surgery during growth has persuaded us that, in the majority of cases, it is better to wait until maturity and then to deal with the problem symptomatically. Many will have no significant disability, cosmetic or functional, and so need no treatment. Deformity alone may be treated by removal of the lower ulna, provided that the

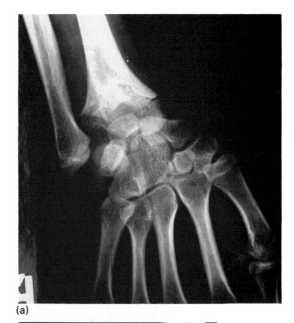

(a)

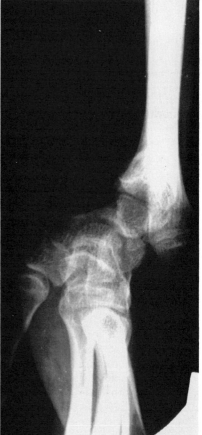

(b)

Figure 11.5 Severe Madelung's deformity. (a) Anterior view. (b) Lateral view

lower radial obliquity is not excessive in which case the wrist will deviate considerably. Radial osteotomy and shortening of the ulnar now seem rational (Dwyer, 1955). When pain is present one should try to distinguish between that arising in the radioulnar-lunate complex and that arising from the wrist joint. In the former, excision of the ulna is helpful, but otherwise arthrodesis of the wrist is necessary (Henry and Thorburn, 1967).

Madelung's deformity is found in association with Turner's syndrome (*see* Chapter 8); it is also seen in diaphyseal aclasis and in dyschondrosteosis, a rare disorder in which there is some shortness of stature, shortening of the forearm bones and shortening of the tibia and fibula (Dawe *et al*, 1982).

Radial club hand and abnormalities of the radial component

There are wide variations in deformity and disability within this syndrome, which may involve both arms to a variable extent in about half the patients affected. Although this was specially associated with thalidomide poisoning, it was seen before and is still being seen years after withdrawal of the drug, and in some there is an obvious factor of inheritance. It is chastening to reflect upon our comments at that time. We noted a marked increase in this somewhat rare 'congenital' disorder, but failed to appreciate the implications. It is to be hoped that this lesson may compensate in some way for the tragedies of this episode, and alert us to investigate urgently any similar change in the incidence of other deformities in the future.

Radial club hand is the common manifestation (Figure 11.6): the abnormality may extend beyond this into the arm or be restricted to the hand alone. Thus we may find that the shoulder joint is dysplastic, the humerus short and the elbow ankylosed in extension. At the other extreme the radius is present, though often dysplastic, but the radial carpal bones are small and the thenar muscles absent.

In radial club hand the radius is either absent or shortened, thin and useless. The ulna, which is short, is bowed so that its distal end is inclined to the radial side and, although rotation is lost, the forearm is usually fixed in the mid-position. The elbow is stable but frequently lacks extension or flexion to a variable degree. The wrist is unstable and the hand lies in fixed radial deviation and palmar flexion. The thumb is absent or rudimentary, and there is fixed flexion deformity and stiffness of the proximal interphalangeal finger joints, which is most marked on the radial side but often negligible on the ulnar side. Finger power is very variable.

Confronted by so grave and apparently so disabling a deformity one's natural reaction is to try to improve matters, but one should first consider very carefully the advisability of interfering at all. One should approach this problem from both the functional and the cosmetic aspects.

There are two main schools of thought about the management of this deformity. The conservative school points out the excellent function shown by many patients who have no treatment in the way of surgery or splintage. Certainly it is vital not to sacrifice function for cosmesis. In those patients with persistent stiffness or ankylosis of the elbow in extension the radially deviated position of the hand allows the fingers to be brought to the mouth. Similarly, in those patients in whom the thumb is absent and the index and middle fingers are stiff and hyperplastic, the ulnar two fingers are by far the most functional. These fingers can function much better, particularly in relation to the mouth, if the hand is left is its radially deviated position.

At the other end of the scale there are those surgeons who agree with Riordan (1965) and Buck-Gramcko (1971) and urge very early operation by centralization and pollicization in the first year of life.

Lamb (1977) has made an extensive study of this condition. He stresses the paramount importance of making an accurate functional assessment of both upper limbs before coming to a decision about surgery. He advises splintage from birth, which is continued only at night once the child starts to use its hand so that it does not interfere with the normal use of the hands during the day. If there is limitation of elbow flexion but no bony ankylosis the elbow should be mobilized as soon as possible. At the age of 3–4 years centralization of hand on the ulna is undertaken. A Kirschner wire is used for internal fixation and external splintage maintained at least at night for 6 months.

Lamb points out the dangers of the centralization operation due to the abnormal anatomy on the radial side; for example, the median

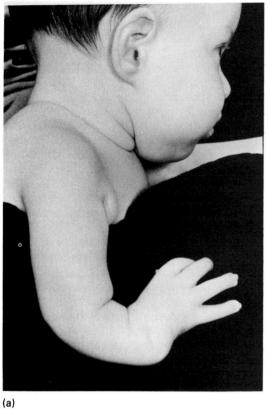

(a)

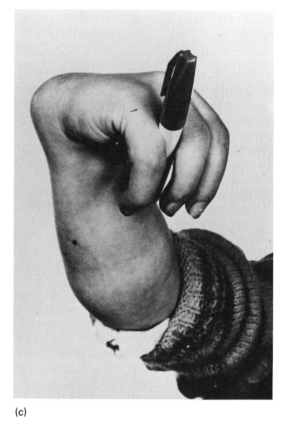

(c)

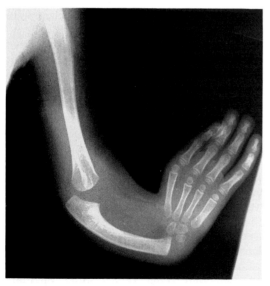

(b)

Figure 11.6 (a) Right radial club hand. Note the absence of the thumb. (b) X-ray of the same patient, showing complete radial absence and the absent thumb. (c) Radial club hand in use. Note how the ulnar fingers are used for pushing and holding the pen

nerve may be immediately under the skin on the radial side. The lower end of the ulna must be slotted deeply into the carpus if the centralization is to remain stable.

Following centralization the child will again be observed carefully; if it can be shown that pollicization would improve function then this can be considered. Clearly this is not a field for the surgeon who treats only the occasional patient, and a more detailed account of the management of this and other congenital hand anomalies is given by Flatt (1977).

Ischaemic contracture (Volkmann's contracture)

Fractures around the elbow in children are prone to cause vascular occlusion, reflex spasm of the brachial artery (Griffiths, 1940) and a forearm compartment syndrome. This is the commonest cause of muscle ischaemia, infarction and contracture in the forearm. Rarely, this may follow severe crushing injuries. Better primary treatment of fractures particularly susceptible to this complication and an aggressive approach to incipient ischaemia, measurement of compartment pressure and early fasciotomy are responsible for a great reduction in the number of affected hands.

The effects of vascular insufficiency will depend upon its degree and duration, so it is not surprising that the lesion which follows is of varying severity. At worst there is total necrosis of muscle and irremediable ischaemic neuritis causing permanent paralysis, deformity and loss of sensibility. At best the nerves are normal and there is little or no permanent weakness but some contracture is demonstrable when the wrist is dorsiflexed, for then the proximal interphalangeal joints will flex – the 'constant length phenomenon'.

Ischaemia shows a predilection for the deep flexor muscles – flexor digitorum profundus and pollicis longus – but sparing the flexor digitorum sublimis. The median nerve, by virtue of its course, is more likely to become ischaemic than the ulnar nerve. The infarct is oval in the longitudinal plane and the effect varies from total muscle necrosis to minor fibrosis, and between gliosis of a nerve for several inches and slight swelling with or without transitory disturbance of conduction.

The disability in established deformity will be the quotient of contracture, weakness (myogenic and neurogenic) and anaesthesia. Excluding the neural element, there are two common patterns of presentation and these may overlap. Firstly, deep flexor contracture, which is demonstrated by the constant length phenomenon. When the wrist is dorsiflexed the interphalangeal joints flex, but when it is palmar flexed they can be passively extended, provided that secondary joint flexion contractures have not developed. Secondly (less common in children), the interossei are contracted, so the interphalangeal joints cannot be flexed if the metacarpophalangeal joints are extended ('intrinsic plus') (Parkes, 1945; Bunnell, 1948).

Early treatment is governed by the need to prevent unnecessary fibrosis and, so, contracture in affected muscles at a time when the extent to which power will be retained and nerve recovery will advance is uncertain.

In children, corrective splinting is certainly of benefit. The wrist is held in slight dorsiflexion and the fingers and thumb are stretched continuously by some form of lively splinting. At between 6 and 9 months following the ischaemic episode the extent of the permanent muscular and nervous deficit will be apparent.

The rarity of this condition today and the complexity of the techniques which successful repair demands should prompt most of us to refer these patients to surgeons with a special interest in this problem.

The hand

Congenital abnormality in the hand is common and protean, and only those patterns which are seen relatively frequently will be discussed. Patterson (1959) studied the case notes of 600 children with such deformities attending The Hospital for Sick Children. From among these he selected 200 for review. Other surveys have been written by Barsky (1958), Buchan (1966), Stelling (1968) and Flatt (1977). The role of the plastic surgeon and the orthopaedic surgeon frequently overlap in the management of these deformities, the more complex of which should be referred to the specialist hand surgeon.

Disorders of the carpal area

Minor anomalies of carpal bones are frequently seen, and often reflect more proximal abnormality. Congenital amputation is usually at the carpometacarpal level and thus provides a useful hook. Rudimentary fingers with nails may need excision. Median nerve compression is exceedingly rare (Lettin, 1965) but we have seen compression of the ulnar nerve by ganglia and by an enlarged pisiform bone. Osteochondritis of the lunate (Kienbock's disease) is rare below 12 years of age.

The thumb

Absent thumb

Absent thumb is usually a *forme fruste* of radial club hand but may occur independently, and in these the index finger is likely to be normal. Two lines of treatment are possible. One is to allow the index finger to autopollicize itself because a pinch will develop between the index and middle fingers, and as a result the gap between them enlarges and the index rotates to face the middle finger. The second approach is to formally pollicize the index finger, if this does not appear to be occurring spontaneously, and to improve cosmesis.

Floating thumb

In cases of floating thumb, the first metacarpal is absent and a small but well formed thumb, attached by a slender pedicle to the base of the index or thereabouts, is completely unstable. Tendons are usually absent and reconstruction by a graft to replace the metacarpal and tendon transfer are not greatly favoured. Amputation is probably the best policy, followed in some cases by pollicization of the index finger.

Short thumb

In cases of short thumb, the long flexor and extensor tendons are often present but the thenar muscles are absent. Function, however, is good.

Five-finger hand

In cases of five-finger hand, the thumb is replaced by an extra digit, thus offering a good opportunity for pollicization.

Duplication of thumb

Duplication of the thumb presents in various ways. Small tags with a narrow pedicle are simple to treat. Projections containing cartil-

age are small and flat. They must be dissected out completely or the cartilage will continue to grow. A fused distal component with two phalanges articulating with the proximal phalanx is more difficult. The abnormal segment is usually on the radial side and small, and this is excised. Unfortunately, however, the remaining ulnar segment deviates from the midline and this deformity may increase with growth, despite careful removal of the abnormal proximal epiphysis. This has led some surgeons to treat this by wedge resection of the central area of soft tissue, leaving the bones intact.

The duplication may be more proximal, arising from the metacarpophalangeal joint. Sometimes there is real difficulty in deciding which to remove, and careful exploration may be necessary. Again the radial thumb is generally the abnormal component. Progressive deformity after excision is common and this may need osteotomy for its correction.

A similar progressive deformity is seen when the supernumerary digit is represented only by an epiphysis which lies on the radial side or, more rarely, in the presence of a delta phalanx. This is a complex anomaly of the epiphysis of the proximal phalanx in which the epiphyses are bracketed so that progressive deformity occurs. Flatt (1977) has described an osteotomy in which the bracketed epiphysis is divided and open wedge osteotomy performed.

Thumb in palm

Thumb in palm is normal in infancy, but when it persists unduly and is accompanied by shortening of the first web space, cerebral palsy should be suspected as the most likely cause.

Less frequently there is hypoplasia of the extensor tendons. This is difficult to treat, for the web space is markedly reduced and the volar surface of the thumb is contracted. Extensive release with the addition of skin to fill the defect must be perpetuated by the introduction of a new motor using either a superficial finger flexor or extensor carpi radialis prolonged by a free graft (Crawford, Horton and Adamson, 1966).

Trigger thumb

This is the most common abnormality of the hand seen in childhood, and most patients are

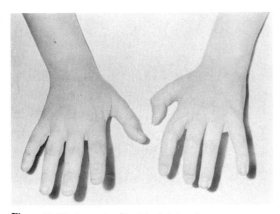

Figure 11.7 Trigger thumb of the left hand

under 2 years of age (Figure 11.7). The term is a misnomer, for there is no snapping as seen in the fingers but a fixed flexion deformity of the interphalangeal joint. The condition is misdiagnosed with regularity, usually as a dislocation of the thumb, because the thickened sheath and the nodule on the enclosed tendon which is felt at the level of the proximal volar crease are mistaken for the displaced metacarpal head.

Many recover spontaneously (Dinham and Meggitt, 1974) so, in those under the age of 3, it is worth waiting at least a year after diagnosis for spontaneous recovery before dividing the tendon sheath. There seems to be no risk of a fixed deformity developing.

The fingers

Flexion deformities

It is not unusual to see a baby with one or more flexed fingers with some fixed deformity at the proximal interphalangeal joints.

The little finger and sometimes its neighbour are involved most frequently (camptodactyly, congenital contracture of the little finger). The metacarpophalangeal joint is extended and the proximal interphalangeal is flexed. The condition is frequently present in one or other parent with whom the need for treatment may be discussed. They will have found that it causes no significant disability, although there may be slight difficulty in putting on a glove and it may cause embarrassment on shaking hands. Surgery is largely unrewarding. Flatt (1977) recommends bony correction by osteotomy only as a last resort.

The remaining fingers may be individually or collectively flexed. This may be due to bony or sound fibrous ankylosis, but is more commonly the result of tendon anomalies. Contracture of flexor sublimis is usually responsible and the effect is therefore mainly on the proximal interphalangeal joints, which may or may not have a fixed flexion deformity. Regular stretching with splinting in infancy will improve most of these significantly, but not necessarily correct them fully. Some residual deformity is no disability and we have not been persuaded that lengthening of the sublimis tendons at the wrist is necessary. The third variety is due to hypoplasia of the extensor tendons similar to that already described in the thumb and managed in the same fashion.

Similar deformities are seen following birth injuries to the brachial plexus of the lower arm type (page 96), ischaemic contracture (page 115), arthrogryposis multiplex (page 85) and leprosy (Brand, 1966).

Syndactyly

Syndactyly is a common congenital abnormality within the province of the plastic surgeon. When the fingers appear otherwise normal, their separation is usually postponed until about 4 years of age. However, when there is undue discrepancy in length between two joined fingers, operation should be undertaken as soon as possible lest secondary deformity develop in the longer digit.

Polydactyly

Most commonly seen on the ulnar border of the hand, these supernumerary digits are usually hypoplastic and there is little difficulty in deciding which to remove. As in the thumb, well formed digits may articulate with an epiphyseal plate of the neighbouring normal finger and care must be taken to remove them entirely so as to prevent progressive deformity. Duplications of the central fingers are rare but when present are frequently associated with complex syndactyly or abnormalities elsewhere in the arm, such as a double ulna.

Brachydactyly

There are two types of brachydactyly. In the first, all elements of the fingers are present but in abbreviated form, and in the second there is absence of one phalanx or fusion of one interphalangeal joint. Function is good.

Macrodactyly

In macrodactyly one finger is involved and it outstrips its fellows in girth and length. It is also deformed, more particularly distally, but movement is usually preserved. This anomaly may be isolated or seen in association with more proximal abnormality. In neurofibromatosis and haemangiomatous malformations of the arm it is not uncommon to find such an abnormality of a finger, and this has led to the belief that these conditions are the usual cause of enlargements confined to the fingers. This is in fact not so, for although there is some increase in fibrofatty subcutaneous tissue, the remaining structures within the finger are microscopically normal, merely being enlarged for no apparent reason.

It is possible to control the growth in length by epiphysiodesis of the involved bone when it reaches what is deemed to be adult size. However, reduction in size of the soft tissues is very difficult, and frequently unsatisfactory. Amputation is often the most successful treatment, particularly if the increased size inhibits hand function.

The single-finger hand

Provided that the digit is mobile, it can usually be opposed to some other part of the hand and function is good. It is in these cases that the building of a post or transfer of a toe against which the finger can be more readily opposed finds its greatest application. When the single digit is stiff the situation is analogous to a congenital amputation at the metacarpophalangeal level.

Lobster claw hand

In lobster claw hand, the hand is divided by a central cleft resulting in a pincer-like deformity with near-normal function but unpleasing appearance (Figure 11.8). There is considerable variation between the different types, but in general two patterns emerge.

In the first pattern the peripheral fingers are normal but the middle is absent or hypoplastic, although the metacarpal may be present.

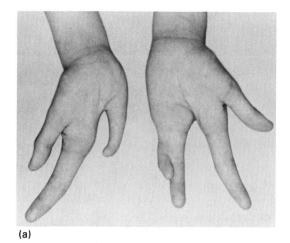

(a)

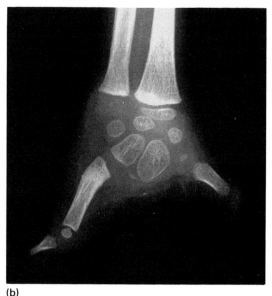

(b)

Figure 11.8 (a) Bilateral lobster claw hands. (b) X-ray of a lobster claw hand

These are frequently familial and there may be similar deformities in the feet. Excision of the abnormal central ray and closure of the remaining defect improves the appearance considerably without disturbing dexterity.

The second variety is more complex. The peripheral fingers are often fused together and the central cleft is an amalgam of rudimentary fingers which reduce its depth and thus the grasping ability of the hand. In these cases, removal of the rudiments and deepening of the cleft is more likely to be called for (Flatt, 1977).

Tumours of the hand

Anomalous muscles may simulate tumours very closely. Thus prolongation of the muscle belly of palmaris longus into the hand resembles a compound palmar ganglion. The latter is a chronic tenosynovitis around the flexor tendons above and below the carpal tunnel, which was once a common manifestation of tuberculosis. This is not an uncommon site for a cavernous haemangioma, but other soft tissue tumours including ganglia are very rare.

Chondromas may be single or multiple (dyschondroplasia). Solitary tumours are treated by curettage and cancellous bone grafting, but multiple tumours are likely to be associated with severe deformity. Osteochondromas are similarly single or multiple (diaphyseal aclasis). Both may interfere with hand function and require excision. A solitary osteochondroma may simulate a bone cyst if not seen in profile.

Dactylitis is infection of a phalanx or metacarpal and is characterized by central radiolucency surrounded by layers of periosteal new bone so that there is palpable thickening. Once a feature of tuberculosis, this is now almost exclusively due to subacute osteomyelitis.

Sucking finger

Persistent finger and thumb sucking in the early years may produce a deformity. This is usually angulation of the digit at an interphalangeal joint but when the index finger is rotated in the mouth a rotary deformity may be produced. In severe examples the finger will flex towards the radial side, when it may be a handicap to a typist or musician (Figure 11.9). Rotation osteotomy at the neck of the metacarpal resolves the problem. The orthodontist is likely to be involved because of the associated abnormal dentition.

Flaccid paralysis

Surgery of the hand was once a most important aspect of the management of poliomyelitis and accordingly considerable knowledge has accumulated on this subject. Today its application is relatively rare in the developed world but the same principles apply to reconstructive operations in peripheral neuritis, in obstetric and other injuries to the brachial plexus and the peripheral nerves and in leprosy (Brand, 1966; Brooks, 1966).

Miscellaneous conditions in the forearm and hand

Diaphyseal aclasis (page 11) has a special predilection for the radius and is associated with premature lower ulnar epiphyseal fusion, which also occurs in Turner's syndrome. Neurofibromatosis (page 83) produces destructive effects in the lower ulna, and haemangiomatosis (page 15) may have a similar effect. Desmoid tumours (page 87) are seen in front of the wrist and forearm, and Caffey's infantile cortical hyperostosis (page 82) may involve both bones – as may Englemann's disease. The hand is rarely affected in juvenile chronic arthritis (page 80). Ellis–Van Creveld syndrome (page 7) and polydactyly may be associated with congenital heart lesions, as may the long thin hands of arachnodactyly (page 6). Melorheostosis (page 14) may involve one border of the hand. The nail–patella syndrome (page 83) is characterized by dysplasic nails, and myositis ossificans progressiva (page 85) by short thumbs. Many of the more florid general disorders are mirrored in the hand – for instance, trident hand in achondroplasia (page 6), bunch of grapes in dyschondroplasia (page 7), and so on. Skeletal age is usually calculated on carpal development, which is retarded in disorders such as cretinism.

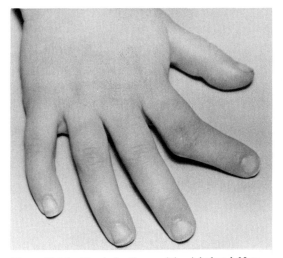

Figure 11.9 Sucking index finger of the right hand. Note the elevation and rotation towards the radial side

References

Barsky, A. J. (1958) *Congenital Anomalies of the Hand.* Springfield, Ill: Charles C.Thomas

Blundell Jones, G. (1964) Delta phalanx. *J. Bone Jt. Surg.* **46B**, 226

Brand, P. W. (1966) The hand in leprosy. In *Clinical Surgery*, vol. 7, *The Hand*. London: Butterworths

Brooks, D. (1966) Treatment of the paralytic hand. In *Clinical Surgery,* vol. 7, *The Hand*. London: Butterworths

Buchan, A. C. (1966) Congenital malformations of the hand. In *Clinical Surgery*, vol. 7, *The Hand*. London: Butterworths

Buck-Bramcko, D. (1971) Pollicization of the index finger. *J. Bone Jt. Surg.* **53A**, 1605

Bunnell, S. , Doherty, E. W. and Curtis, R. M. (1948) Ischaemic contracture, local, in the hand. *Plast. Reconstruct. Surg.* **3**, 424

Crawford, H. H., Horton, C. E. and Adamson, J. E. (1966) Congenital aplasia or hypoplasia of the thumb and finger extensor tendons. *J. Bone Jt. Surg.* **48A**, 82

Dawe, C., Wynne-Davies, R. and Fulford, G. E. (1982) Clinical variation in dyschondrosteosis. *J. Bone Jt. Surg.* **64B**, 377–381

Dinham, J. M. and Meggit, B. F. (1974) Trigger thumbs in children. *J. Bone Jt. Surg.* **56B**, 153

Dwyer, F. C. (1955) Treatment of traumatic Madelung's deformity by shortening the ulna. *Proc. R. Soc. Med.* **48**, 100

Flatt, A. E. (1977) *The Care of Congenital Hand Anomalies*. St Louis, Mo: C. V. Mosby

Griffiths, D. L. (1940) Volkmann's ischaemic contracture. *Br. J. Surg.* **28**, 239

Harrison, R. G., Pearson, M. A. and Roaf, R. (1960) Ulna dimelia. *J. Bone Jt. Surg.* **42B**, 549

Henry, A. and Thorburn, M. J. (1967) Madelung's deformity. *J. Bone Jt. Surg.* **49B**, 66

Kelikian, H. and Doumanian, A. (1957) Swivel for proximal radioulnar synostosis. *J. Bone Jt. Surg.* **39A**, 945

Lamb, D. W. (1977) Radial club hand. *J. Bone Jt. Surg.* **59A**, 1

Lettin, A. W. (1965) Carpal tunnel syndrome in children. *J. Bone Jt. Surg.* **47B**, 556

Parkes, A. (1945) Traumatic ischaemia of peripheral nerves, with some observations on Volkmann's ischaemic contracture. *Br. J. Surg.* **32**, 403

Parkes, A. (1966) Ischaemic contracture. In *Clinical Surgery*, vol. 7, *The Hand*. London: Butterworths

Patterson, T. J. S. (1959) Congenital deformities of the hand. *Ann. R. Coll. Surg.* **25**, 306

Riordan, D. C. (1965) Congenital absence of the radius: a 15-year follow-up. *J. Bone Jt. Surg.* **45A**, 1783 [report]

Swanson, A. B. (1964) The Kruckenberg procedure in the juvenile amputatee. *J. Bone Jt. Surg.* **46A**, 1540

Further reading

Flatt, A. E. (1977) *The Care of Congenital Hand Anomalies*. St Louis, Mo: C. V. Mosby

12

The spine and trunk

Peter J. Webb

The treatment of spinal deformity still presents a considerable challenge in spite of the advances of surgical methods during the last decade. Furthermore, the aetiology of the largest group of deformities remains unknown.

Definition and terminology

The term *scoliosis* is often used as if it were a diagnostic entity implying knowledge of the causative agent; it is, however, only a description of the deformity and implies a lateral curvature of the spine (coronal). *Kyphosis* is a forward angulation (sagittal). Both may exist together. *Lordosis* is a posterior angulation in the sagittal plane.

Kyphosis and lordosis are present in the normal spine and are abnormal only if there is either an increase in their extent or loss of flexibility. Scoliosis is never part of the normal spinal shape and must always be considered as potentially serious.

Perhaps the most important observation that needs to be made is whether the deformity has normal or restricted mobility. *Postural* or *compensatory* deformities exist but the segment of the spine involved retains normal flexibility. A *structural* curve, however, is considered to be present in a segment of spine that does not have normal flexibility. A compensatory curve exists above or below a structural one in order to maintain body symmetry. Compensatory curves may remain non-structural, but over the course of time the soft tissues tend to become fixed and the bony shape adapted so that stiffness increases and the curve becomes structural. It is thus not true

that compensatory deformities retain their flexibility. The term *postural scoliosis* has long been in use and implies that there are no fixed anatomical changes. The term is confusing because flexible curves may exist secondary to a short leg or a structural curve as defined above, or because there is a tendency for the person to adopt a posture outside the expected normal range (e.g. in cerebral palsy). In these cases the observed deformity is secondary to another cause.

Classification

Spinal deformity (scoliosis) may be (1) congenital, (2) neuromuscular or (3) idiopathic, or it may (4) occur in association with other known conditions.

Congenital

In congenital deformity (Figure 12.1) a structural abnormality exists in one or more vertebrae at birth. There may be failure of formation (*type I*), failure of segmentation (*type II*) or a mixture (*type III*). The abnormalities may be single or multiple. If single, there is no reported risk to subsequent siblings. If multiple or if associated with spina bifida, there may be a hereditary tendency (Wynne-Davies, 1975a).

Congenital deformities are not always isolated to one structure, and the spine is no exception. Abnormalities of the ribs are commonly seen, which might be expected from a consideration of the development. Of far greater importance is the possibility that neurological anomalies may ˙coexist (spinal

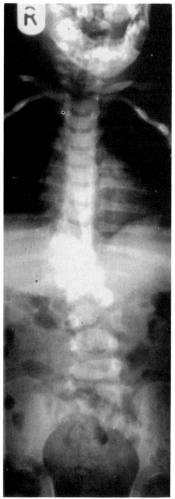

Figure 12.1 Congenital abnormalities can be seen (hemivertebrae T9, T12, L2)

dysraphism). Clinical assessment can give a clue to the existence of such abnormalities; care should be taken to examine the posterior aspect of the trunk for minor anomalies of skin pigmentation, texture or tufts of hair – not forgetting the possibility of distal neurological change, which may be represented in an alteration of foot size with no other evidence of abnormality.

There are important associations with thoracic or abdominal malformations. The radiological features of spinal dysraphism may be obvious if there is gross abnormality but the changes may be as minor as slight widening of the interpeduncular distance.

Diastematomyelia

There is a central spur of bone or soft tissue within the neural canal dividing the neural elements, which may be responsible for a deterioration of neurological function during growth. There is a difference of opinion about the need for excision of such a spur. If correction of the deformity is planned, full radiographic examination is prudent and great care necessary with any correction undertaken.

Spina bifida

The most dramatic and challenging anomaly is that present in association with spina bifida, which may be as diverse as a minor anomaly of ossification of the neural arch, present as a radiological feature only, or as a major anomaly with no cord function and hydrocephalus, at the other extreme. Scoliosis is only one of the possible deformities which may be present. A severe kyphosis often exists, which increases from birth onwards. This presents a formidable challenge to the skill and ingenuity of the surgeon and is associated with complications in nearly every case.

Posterior hemivertebrae

This anomaly deserves particular mention because it is associated with potential for neurological abnormality. Early recognition of the problem with surgical stabilization anteriorly and posteriorly will prevent neurological involvement and allow preservation of spinal column function. The author's personal preference is to undertake a short segment fusion when the angle of kyphus is approximately 40 degrees (however young the patient may be). Reduction of growth has often been raised as a major disadvantage to early fusion, but the anomalous segment does not have normal potential and, in addition, such growth may be associated with increased deformity. The fusion therefore cannot be held responsible for increased deformity, but rather the initial abnormality.

Neuromuscular

There are a large number of conditions which may be associated with a progressive spinal deformity secondary to muscle weakness. The normal shape of the spine is maintained by the anatomy of the joints and its associated ligaments, together with the muscle pull which is altered by these disorders. Even though the condition itself may not be progressive (i.e. poliomyelitis) the resulting curve may be. Spinal deformity related to progressive conditions should be assumed to be progressive. There may be reduction in respiratory function or an associated mental subnormality. If the paralysis is symmetrical, 'collapsing' deformities may occur (Figure 12.2).

Neuromuscular disorders present a challenge to the surgeon and the anaesthetist if a spinal fusion has to be undertaken. The deformities are best treated early in the natural history of the condition, certainly if the child is wheelchair-bound, since the surgery is less demanding of the patient or surgeon and the results are more acceptable. Prolonged bed rest after a fusion is no longer required if adequate internal fixation is undertaken, particularly if each segment of the spine is instrumented. The natural fear that the condi-

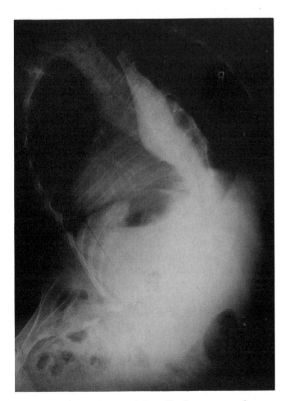

Figure 12.2 Scoliosis secondary to Duchenne muscular dystrophy

tion will be allowed to deteriorate by the bed rest is therefore, to a large extent, a thing of the past.

Idiopathic scoliosis

Idiopathic scoliosis is by far the commonest type and is identified by exclusion of other causes. Although, as its name implies, the aetiology is unknown, there are, nevertheless, consistent patterns of presentation.

Infantile

James (1951) reported a small series of patients with scoliosis who had presented under the age of 3 years. Lloyd-Roberts and Pilcher (1965) reported 100 cases of infantile curves; spontaneous resolution occurred in 92. Infantile curves are typically present in males, convex to the left in the dorsal region and associated with ipsilateral anterior plagiocephaly. Other features of moulding may be associated torticollis, pelvic obliquity and calcaneovalgus feet. Mehta (1972) reported 361 patients. X-ray analysis of the curve pattern revealed that the prognosis for progression could be established by comparing the relationship between the rib and vertebra on the two sides (rib vertebral difference).

This pattern of scoliosis is rarely seen in North America and is thought to be in part related to the sleeping position; that is, children nursed prone are less likely to develop infantile scoliosis, although there is likely to be a genetic as well as an environmental factor (Wynne-Davies, 1975b). Early treatment with spinal plaster jackets may prevent severe deformity later in the child's life.

Adolescent

The adolescent pattern of scoliosis (Figure 12.3) contrasts directly with the infantile, being commoner in females than in males, present most often convex to the right in the mid-dorsal region and commonly progressive with growth. It presents in association with the pubertal growth spurt. The prevalence of this condition has been variously reported from 13.5% (Brooks, 1975) to 0.1% (Hensinger *et*

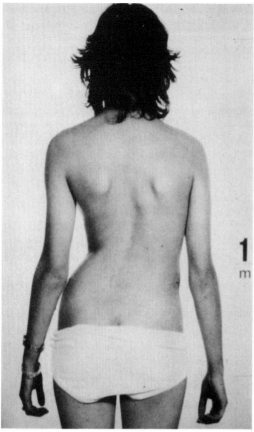

(a)

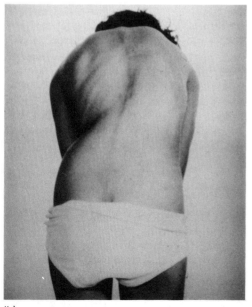

(b)

Figure 12.3 (a) and (b) Adolescent idiopathic scoliosis in a female aged 15 years

al, 1975). The true incidence in the population is difficult to determine accurately and the natural history of the majority of the curves is unknown since only the more significant present to clinical studies. School screening programmes, started in the USA, have suggested an incidence of around 3%, of whom only 0.3% may require treatment.

Juvenile

The juvenile presentation of scoliosis is almost certainly a mixture of late presenting infantile and early onset adolescent pattern, and is equally distributed in males and females and in side. The prognosis for progression, however, may be worse than the adolescent because a longer period of growth remains to be completed.

Aetiology

The aetiology of idiopathic scoliosis has been investigated by a large variety of techniques. Two fields of study have produced more positive results than others.

First, the biomechanical/growth theories publicized by Dickson and colleagues (1983) suggest that a median plane asymmetry (flattening or, more usually, reversal of the normal thoracic kyphosis at the apex of the curve) superimposed during growth is responsible for anterior overgrowth of the vertebrae (in contradistinction to Scheuermann's) which predisposes to a progressive scoliosis, the site of which is determined by other biomechanical factors.

Secondly, the neuromuscular theories (Lloyd-Roberts *et al*, 1978) accumulated evidence. Pincott divided the dorsal roots of *Cynomolgus* monkeys and found that a scoliosis reliably developed convex to the side of section, the severity of the curve being proportional to the number of roots divided. He suggested that a neurosensory imbalance may be associated with the development of the scoliosis.

A structural scoliosis is almost invariably associated with rotation of the vertebrae at the apex, such that the vertebral body is rotated to the side of the convexity. Whether this rotation is previously related to myoneuronal causes, themselves generated by a peripheral or perhaps central lesion in the nervous system or to growth disturbance, has not yet been determined. However, it is likely that there are a variety of possible primary events disturbing the delicate balance of spinal posture which, when altered, generates the conditions under which progressive change may occur which, when initiated, becomes the final common pathway leading to a severe spinal deformity.

Scoliosis in association with other conditions

There are a large number of conditions which may be associated directly or indirectly with spinal deformity.

Neurofibromatosis

The primary defect of tissue in neurofibromatosis is tumour formation on both peripheral and central nerves, associated with cafe au lait spots in the skin. The spinal deformity which characteristically occurs is that of a 'sharp C' pattern, distinguishable from the 'long C' curve of other neurological scolioses. Furthermore, the vertebrae themselves and the associated ribs may have abnormal shape. The presence of kyphosis is a sign of potential for the development of severe disabling deformity and an indication to consider anterior and posterior spinal fusion.

This condition is transmitted as an autosomal dominant with variable penetrance.

Bone dysplasia

Spinal deformity occurs in a variety of conditions having abnormal bone texture – mucopolysaccharidoses, achondroplasia, spondyloepiphyseal dysplasia, diastrophic dwarfism and osteogenesis imperfecta, to name but a few. The pattern of abnormality in these types may be different but they are usually more rigid than the neuromuscular or idiopathic types and should each be considered in their own right. Particular attention should be paid to the cervical spine in the infant, since there may be sufficient abnormality to generate instability. X-ray of the whole spine is mandatory when one of these conditions is suspected.

Spinal tumours

Tumours of the neural or bony elements of the spine should be suspected whenever pain is a presenting feature in association with the deformity. Osteoid osteoma, for example, presents with a characteristic spinal deformity, concave to the side of the tumour which is often placed in the laminae at the apex of the curve (Mehta, 1978; Kirwan, 1984). When the tumour is removed, resolution of the deformity may be complete if no secondary changes occur.

No child with a painful back should be ignored without an attempted explanation. Bone scans allow a variety of conditions to be excluded without requiring a large dose of radiation. Standard radiographs may show a widening of the interpeduncular distance or scalloping of the posterior aspect of the vertebral body. Neurological signs require neurological explanation, and radiculography or magnetic resonance imaging (MRI) may be necessary to exclude pathology.

It should not be forgotten that tuberculosis can cause deformity and neurological dysfunction, and still presents to spinal clinics in spite of available treatment.

Irritative conditions

Irritation of nerve roots in an adult may present as a painful scoliosis characterized by stiffness and associated with limitation of straight leg raising and neurological signs, but juvenile or adolescent prolapsed intervertebral discs may present with stiffness alone in spite of the presence of a large disc protrusion.

Destructive lesions

Destruction of the vertebral body, or disc space, secondary to tumour, although rarely seen, may present as a spinal deformity. Spinal deformity may occur after radiotherapy given for a Wilms' tumour or neuroblastoma in the early years of infancy. These deformities are secondary to growth disturbance and, as a rule, are very rigid. Altered radiotherapeutic techniques have markedly reduced the incidence.

In association with other dysmorphic
conditions or syndromes

Spinal deformity, usually scoliosis, may be a
recognized part of an association of abnormalities, such as the VATER association of
anomalies, or part of a recognized syndrome
(i.e. Marfan's, Prader–Willi, Freeman–Sheldon, Coffin–Lowry, prune belly or Larsen's)
as a frequent finding. The association between
cardiac abnormalities and scoliosis has given
rise to the term 'cardiac scoliosis'; although
there is no direct link, it is not surprising to find
abnormalities arising in embryologically closely associated structures. The cardiac scoliosis
presents with an idiopathic pattern but is more
likely to be stable. It is sometimes difficult to
define the part played in the diagnosis of the
deformity by the corrective surgery that many
of these patients have undergone.

Kyphosis

Kyphosis may be associated with many of the
conditions mentioned above but other possibilities deserve special mention.

Developmental kyphosis

The natural position for a fetus to adopt is a
long C kyphus involving the whole spine.
When head control is developed, a cervical
lordosis develops. When the child begins to sit,
the spine changes shape to allow a lordosis to
develop in the lumbar region which is completed when the child walks. If, for one reason
or another, development is delayed, so will be
the development of spinal posture. This is
particularly likely if there is hypotonia in
association with global retardation. If the
kyphus is allowed to become stiff, a particularly taxing problem will develop. Great care
should be taken, therefore, to maintain a full
range of joint motion at each segment,
concentrating particularly on extension. The
early provision of a 'sitting' orthosis may be
helpful; 'buggies' which do not control the
lordosis may be particularly harmful.

Juvenile kyphosis (Scheuermann's disease)

Poor posture is often said to be the cause of an
upper dorsal kyphosis, which it may be.
Postural deformity, however, remains mobile

or perhaps with an associated tightness of the
hamstrings. The postural round back deformity
is best treated with hyperextension exercises.
Care, however, should be taken to distinguish
the more rigid deformity secondary to vertebral osteochondritis – that is, a wedging of the
vertebrae in association with abnormal radiological appearances of the ring apophyses.
Scheuermann (1920) described this abnormality and suggested that avascular necrosis of the
ring apophyses might be responsible. More
recent suggestions have been herniation of the
nucleus pulposus into the growth plate, repeated mechanical trauma or persistence of the
vascular ring. Scheuermann's original series
suggested an increased incidence in young men
involved in heavy work. The condition, however, can occur in otherwise normal healthy
adolescents.

If the condition progresses, treatment may
be indicated: initially hyperextension exercises, or a brace, or, on occasions, anterior and
posterior fusion may be required.

Typically the patient is male, in the early
teenage years and presents with a painless
kyphosis, radiological features of which are
wedging of three to five adjacent vertebrae
with anterior irregular apophyses. Scoliosis
may also be present but is usually non-
progressive, and may be present in a section of
the spine distal to the kyphotic segment.

Kyphus may also be associated with any
osteoporotic condition; that is, osteogenesis
imperfecta, bony dysplasia or idiopathic
osteoporosis.

Prognosis of spinal deformity (indications for treatment)

If the causative pathology is itself progressive,
the spinal deformity should also be considered
progressive. Each of the conditions described
above has its own potential or otherwise for
progression. Risser (1958) observed that completion of ossification of the superior iliac
apophyses coincided with cessation of spinal
growth and that deterioration in the curve was
unlikely after that event. This observation has,
in association with others, contributed to the
belief that all spinal deformity stops progressing after growth ceases. However, Collins and
Ponseti (1969) and Nachemson (1968) reported
progression after skeletal maturity in some

patients with larger curves. There seems to be general agreement now that curves of 40 degrees are likely to be stable but curves of 60 degrees are likely to be progressive. Edgar (1980) reported long-term follow-up of patients and showed progression of deformity related to the extent of the curve and Cobb angle; furthermore, patients who had received spinal fusions had less back pain. It is not true that idiopathic scoliosis is a benign condition. Paediatricians have learned to recognize the condition but often fail to appreciate its significance. The referral pattern of spinal deformity patients to a scoliosis clinic is often such that the deformity has already reached the point where spinal fusion may be the only feasible means of treatment (Figures 12.4 and 12.5).

If observation or assessment of a spinal deformity allows the conclusion that stability will be lost by the time growth has ceased (or has already been lost), treatment should be considered. If the stability has been lost, attempts should be made to regenerate it. Mehta and Morel (1979) reported a series of 21 patients with progressive infantile idiopathic scoliosis treated by early intervention in serial plaster of Paris jackets applied in the position of maximum correction. Although only 16 of the patients had completed treatment by the time of the report, they concluded that resolution of spinal deformity can be induced by conservative treatment and that this was most likely to succeed if started early. As a general rule, prognosis is related to the age of onset and the apical level of the curve. The

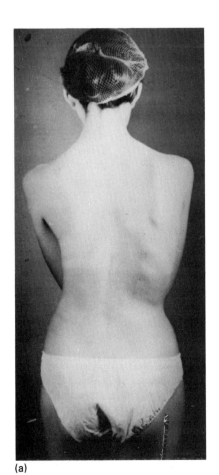

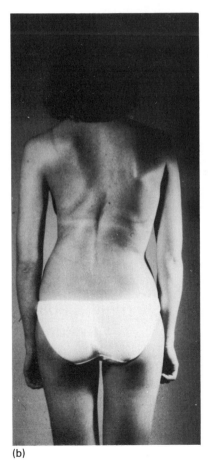

(a)   (b)

Figure 12.4 (a) Adolescent idiopathic scoliosis in a female aged 16 years. (b) The same patient aged 26 years

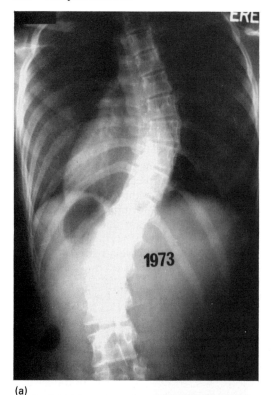

(a)

(b)

Figure 12.5 (a) X-ray of the patient shown in Figure 12.4a.
(b) X-ray of the patient shown in Figure 12.4b

younger the patient and the higher the level, the worse it is likely to be.

Congenital scoliotic deformities have a more predictable prognosis, being related to the balance of growth between the two sides of the spine. If there is extra growth potential on one side, progression is likely; if this can be predicted from either serial radiographs or a knowledge of the individual condition then treatment to maintain balance, or to create it if it is lost, is justified at whatever age this conclusion is reached. A posteriorly placed hemivertebra has a particularly bad prognosis. The author believes that spinal fusion is justified if the angle of kyphus approaches 40 degrees because stability of the spine can be achieved with less risk of major neurological complications either at the time of surgery or as a result of progressive deformity later in life.

The overall aim of treatment for any spinal deformity must be to prepare the child or adolescent for adult life with a stable spine by protecting *the child* against the development of a deformity which has been untreated during the growing years and to prevent the secondary physiological events consequent upon spinal deformity which may not appear until the fourth decade.

Management of spinal deformity

If spinal deformity is detected before it has become severe or fixed, non-operative treatment is often successful. However, severe deformity still may occur, and then operative treatment has to be recommended.

Non-operative methods

Observation

Observation of an established curve is mandatory until it can be clearly seen that no potential for further progression exists. Congenital scoliosis frequently does not need either non-operative or operative treatment, but there is always room for doubt. Far too little is known about the natural history of the commonest (idiopathic) group for even the most experienced to be complacent.

Physiotherapy

It is right to maintain that physiotherapeutic techniques, exercises or manipulation have not been shown to prevent deformity progressing when the curve has been established at 30–40 degrees. However, particularly in the delayed developmental group, careful attention to the maintenance of a full range of movement can make subsequent development of spinal deformity less likely. The spine has potential for three-dimensional movement at each segment, which allows significant deformity to be unnoticed because of the possible compensatory changes. In just the same way as with single plane joints such as the knee, fixed deformity should not be tolerated, certainly if it has the potential for progression or limits function.

Plaster of Paris techniques

Risser (1955) described the localizer cast which, in modified form, is still used in the treatment of the younger child or of the mildest curves in older children. Cotrel and D'Amore (1966) described a modification to this cast by using traction (elongation), derotation and flexion of the lumbar spine (EDF) (Figure 12.6). These principles of application are now used in most centres.

The indication for cast treatment is in a mobile but progressive curve to provide support to the growing spine to prevent further deformity or, on occasions, in the much younger child, to maximize the potential for spontaneous correction (Mehta and Morel, 1979). Casts may also be used preoperatively to assess the capability of the severely mentally retarded patient to co-operate in the uncommon event of a spinal fusion being required.

The casts are for the most part applied after the patient has been placed on a special plaster table which allows the corrective forces to be applied. Younger children need to be given an anaesthetic for the task to be conducted satisfactorily.

Casts are used prior to the application of a brace in the younger patient because they can be changed regularly to accommodate either the effect of growth on body size or improved posture. A significant number of parents find a localizer cast easier to handle than the more complicated application of a brace.

Brace support

Blount (1958) described the Milwaukee brace which, with few modifications, is still in use, having particular value in the scoliotic curves whose apex is T8 or above (Figure 12.7). Watts, Hall and Stanish (1977) described the Boston modular brace which is cosmetically more acceptable, being for the most part under the arm (Figure 12.8). However, if the apex of the curve is above T9 then a superstructure may need to be added.

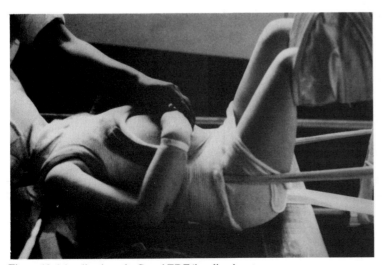

Figure 12.6 Application of a Cotrel EDF 'localizer' cast

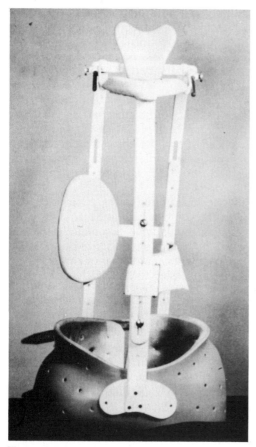

Figure 12.7 The Milwaukee brace

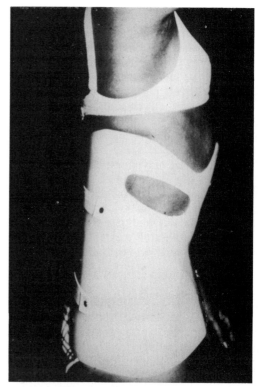

Figure 12.8 The Boston brace

Electrospinal stimulation

Bobechko (1975) described the use of internal electrodes, and Axelgaard, McNeal and Brown (1978) the use of external electrodes, placed usually over the convexity of the scoliosis to stimulate corrective muscular activity. As yet this has not become an established technique for treatment. O'Donnell *et al* (1988) followed up 62 patients for an average of 3.2 years who were being treated by electrical stimulation, and concluded that the curve progression paralleled that found in natural history studies.

Non-operative treatment is used when a significant curve has been diagnosed but has not progressed to the point that surgical treatment has to be considered. Commonly 20 degrees is given as the point to start treatment, although in the known progressive neuromuscular conditions the author's practice is to start earlier in order to prevent further deformity.

Treatment must be continued until potential for·progression has ceased.

Brace wearing can be expected to maintain the curve in the position in which it was initially applied. It is an unreasonable expectation to believe that the often dramatic correction seen when the brace is first applied will be maintained (Mellencamp, Blount and Anderson, 1977).

The individual choice of brace is dependent upon the diagnosis, the age of the patient and the flexibility of the curve. The Boston modular brace imposes a flexion on the lumbar spine as part of the attempt to derotate the spine at that level. The patient's own muscle power is required to auto-correct posture above the brace. In muscle-weakening conditions this cannot be relied upon and a more supportive brace (spinal holding jacket) may be needed.

Operative methods

When a segment of spine lacks stability, as evidenced by progressive or painful deformation, spinal fusion may be required if the age and condition of the patient allow it. The aim of fusion is to provide a biologically stable spine – that is, a spine which will withstand the stress placed upon it without progressive deformation or pain.

Fusion implies loss of movement; it is thus a price that may need to be paid to provide the advantages of stability. However, fusion is also associated with cessation of growth over the area fused, which has disadvantages in the young child. Fusion is therefore delayed for as long as is safely possible. It may be suggested for patients with progressive muscle weakness when it is clear that external support is either no longer acceptable to the patient or unlikely to succeed in the long term. In practice, this decision can be taken when the curve is around 40 degrees and the patient already confined to a wheelchair. Under these circumstances the natural history of the condition and the

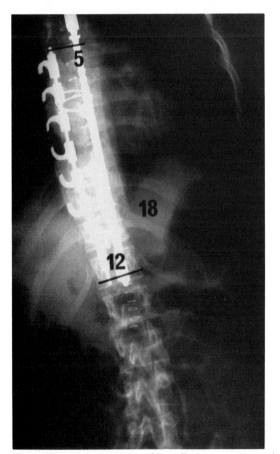

Figure 12.9 Adolescent idiopathic scoliosis treated by Harrington compression and distraction

patient's present and future fitness to withstand the surgical trauma must be taken into account.

Posterior spinal fusion

Posterior fusion with the use of Harrington distraction rods is still the most common form of fusion undertaken (Figure 12.9). Correction is achieved by distraction over the concavity of the curve. Recently other implants have been designed which allow a combination of distraction and compression forces to be applied segmentally to achieve a better correction mechanically.

The choice of implant to be used will depend on the type of curve, the size and age of the patient and the experience of the surgeon. Implant design has been refined considerably since the days of Harrington: Cotrel and Dubousset (1984) have designed a system of implants for use posteriorly which allows a significantly better hold to be achieved on the vertebral column. A sound biological fusion must still be the primary aim, but thorough excision of the posterior intervertebral joints and complete decortication with autogenous graft from the iliac crest is necessary to provide the conditions under which successful fusion can occur.

Segmental spinal instrumentation

Luque (1982) has described the technique of passing wires under each lamina and attaching them to rods placed alongside the spinous processes (Figure 12.10). Although this method allows considerable correction together with great mechanical strength, such that postoperative protection in a brace is seldom required, the joints cannot be excised as completely or the spine decorticated so thoroughly without removing some of the mechanical strength of the bone under which the wires are placed. Nevertheless, this method is particularly useful for the muscular dystrophy patient. Immobilization by external support is not required, reducing the risk of further neurological or myological deterioration because the patient can be mobilized early. The need to pass the wires under the laminae, however, increases the risk of neurological damage.

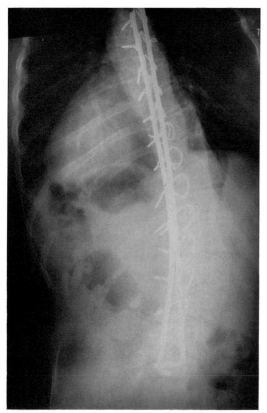

Figure 12.10 Scoliosis secondary to Duchenne muscular dystrophy (see Figure 12.2) treated by the Luque technique

Preoperative correction in a Risser cast was commonly undertaken but is seldom used nowadays; little if any increase of correction was achieved and the intra- and postoperative problems were greatly increased. Lateral bending or maximum dynamic traction films allow a reasonable estimate of the correction to be obtained which can then be safely achieved operatively, particularly if spinal cord monitoring or 'wake up' tests are used to assess cord function.

Correction of deformity is considered particularly risky if there are congenital abnormalities or associated spinal dysraphism because of the possible associated diastematomyelia. If this is suspected, preoperative myelography must be undertaken. Opinion is divided about the wisdom of excising the spur of bone or fibrous band, but certainly great care needs to be taken in such cases.

Anterior spinal fusion

Anterior fusion may be indicated if there is kyphos greater than 60 degrees or specifically to increase bone mass in those patients where the only support may be from the spine itself or where it is placed under unusual stress (e.g. paralytic curves or spina bifida or in some cases of cerebral palsy with athetoid movements). Dwyer (1969) described a technique of anterior fusion using a screw with attached cable to maintain the corrected position (Figure 12.11).

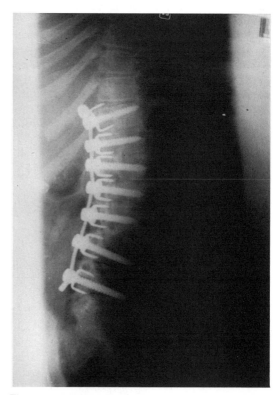

Figure 12.11 Scoliosis secondary to hydrocephalus treated by the Dwyer technique

This method provides great opportunity for correction of rotation and thus may, on occasions, be used to reduce the number of vertebral levels requiring fusion. Its disadvantage, however, is that it cannot be used if a kyphus is present, thus effectively limiting its use to the lumbar and lower thoracic region. However, more recent designs of implants allow them to be used in compression and in distraction, and are thus suitable for treating both scoliosis and kyphosis anteriorly.

Combined anterior and posterior fusion

This may be indicated in heavy paralytic patients or in spina bifida patients to provide the greatest opportunity for correction and the largest amount of bone.

Release or excision of vertebral disc contents can also provide opportunity for postoperative correction of deformity by skeletal traction on some of the more severe curves, the disc space being filled with chip graft often taken from the rib excised during the approach to the spine. The movements of correction through the grafted area during the immediate postoperative period of 2–3 weeks on skeletal traction does not impede eventual solid fusion. Posterior fusion with instrumentation may then be undertaken to further correct and stabilize the spine.

Disc and plate excision may be considered necessary to achieve increased correction of the deformity but also in the author's experience has a place in the younger patient whose subsequent anterior spinal growth after a posterior spinal fusion may result in the return of some of the previously corrected spinal deformity.

Limited spinal fusion

A short segment of spine may be fused in a congenital curve to provide balance of growth by reducing the later growth on the convexity. This method is not a major procedure and, if successful, may allow correction to be achieved safely through the growth process.

Leatherman and Dickson (1979) described 'closing wedge' osteotomy for congenital curves, supplemented by excision of the posterior elements and compression arthrodesis as a second stage.

Complications of surgery

Spinal fusion is achieved in 98% of patients with idiopathic scoliosis if careful attention is paid to the detail, but neurological complications are reported in approximately 1%. Deep

infection or rod/hook failure may require removal of the implants at a later stage.

Almost all spina bifida patients, however, have complications and, although the rewards of successful surgery can be impressive radiologically, the patient may spend long periods of time in hospital. Great care must therefore be taken before deciding to submit the patient to a lengthy surgical programme.

Spondylolisthesis

Forward slipping of one vertebra on the next distal segment occurs most commonly at the lumbosacral junction. The defect that allows this may be associated with congenital abnormalities of the upper sacrum or posterior arch of the fifth lumbar vertebra (dysplasic type) or a lesion in the delicate pars interarticularis (isthmic type) or due to degenerative change in the posterior joints (degenerative) or traumatic as a result of vertebral fracture other than through the pars (traumatic type) or pathological as a result of generalized bone disorder. The first and last of these commonly present with symptoms of pain and/or deformity during the early second decade and may thus present to a paediatric clinic. If the defect is associated with spina bifida, progression of the slip is likely (Velikas and Blackburn, 1981). Occasionally, spinal fusion may be required to prevent further deformity. The simplest approach is to undertake a fusion between the transverse process of the fifth lumbar vertebra and the ala of the sacrum, which can be performed quite easily if there is a 25% slip or less. Occasionally, however, the fourth lumbar transverse process has to be included as well, or, more rarely, anterior interbody fusion between the fifth lumbar vertebra and the sacrum.

Disc space disorders
Non-specific discitis

Non-specific discitis may present any time after the second year of life, commonly in the lumbar spine. There are often no clinical features other than pain in the early stages. X-rays taken early in the condition fail to reveal the pathology although a bone scan may be positive. In the later stages there is tenderness to local pressure, limitation of movement and the disc height may be reduced and the adjacent end plates appear irregular. The erythrocyte sedimentation rate may be increased. Bacterial culture of the blood rarely reveals a pathogen although antibiotics often relieve the symptoms quite dramatically, together with bed rest. The condition may result in fusion of the two vertebrae involved, but commonly completely resolves.

Acute calcific discitis

This presents dramatically with severe pain associated with a limitation of movement and calcification of the intervertebral disc shown on plain radiographs. The condition is, fortunately, self-limiting and rare, although one recent patient has had two episodes. Disc calcification may also occur without symptoms. The cervical spine is most often affected and up to eight discs may be involved (Melnick and Silverman, 1963). After the symptoms resolve, resorption of the calcified material may take months or years to complete. Later follow-up reveals loss of disc height but increased height of adjacent vertebrae (Ozonoff, 1979).

References

Axelgaard, J., McNeal, D. R. and Brown, J. C. (1978) Lateral electrical surface stimulation for the treatment of progressive scoliosis. In *External Control of Human Extremities*, Proceedings of 6th International Symposium, Dubrovnik Yugoslavia, p. 63

Blount, W. P. (1958) Scoliosis and the Milwaukee brace. *Bull. Hosp. Joint Dis.* **19**, 152

Bobechko, U. P. (1975) Electrospinal stimulation. *J. Bone Jt. Surg.* **58A**, 156

Brooks, H. L., Azen, S. P., Gerberg, M. E., Brooks, R. and Chan, L. (1975) Scoliosis: a prospective epidemiological study. *J. Bone Jt. Surg.* **57A**, 968–977

Collins, D. K. and Ponseti, I. V. (1969) Long term follow up of patients with idiopathic scoliosis not treated surgically. *J. Bone Jt. Surg.* **51A**, 425–445

Cotrel, Y. and D'Amore, M. (1966) Spinal traction in scoliosis. In *Proceedings of a Second symposium on Scoliosis*. Ed. by P. A. Zorab. Edinburgh: Livingstone pp. 37–43

Cotrel, Y. and Dubousset, J. (1984) Nouvelle technique d'osteosynthese rachidienne segmentaire par voit posterieure. *Rev. Chir. Orthop.* **70**, 489

Dickson, R. A., Lawton, S. O., Archer, I. A. and Butt, W. P. (1983) The pathogenesis of idiopathic scoliosis. *J. Bone Jt. Surg.* **66B**, 8–15

Dwyer, A. F. (1969) Experience of anterior correction of scoliosis. *Clin. Orthop.* **62**, 192

Edgar, M. A. (1980) Long term review of fused and unfused patients with adolescent idiopathic scoliosis. In *Scoliosis 1979*. Ed. by P. A. Zorab and D. Siegler. London, New York: Academic Press, pp. 181–193

Hensinger, R. N., Cowell, H. R., MacEwan, G. D., Shands, A. R. and Cronis, S. (1975) Orthopaedic screening of school age children – review of ten year experience. *Orthop. Rev.* **4**, 23–38

James, J. I. P. (1951) Two curve patterns in idiopathic structural scoliosis. *J. Bone Jt. Surg.* **33B**, 339–406

Kirwan, E. O'G., Hutton, P. A. N., Pozo, J. L. and Ransford, A. O. (1984) Osteoid osteoma and benign osteoblastoma of the spine. *J. Bone Jt. Surg.*. **66B**, 21–60

Leatherman, K. E. and Dickson, R. A. (1979) Two-stage corrective surgery for congenital deformities of the spine. *J. Bone Jt. Surg.* **61B**, 324–328

Lloyd-Roberts, C. G. and Pilcher, M. F. (1965) Structural idiopathic scoliosis in infancy: a study of the natural history of one hundred patients. *J. Bone Jt. Surg.* **47B**, 520–523

Lloyd-Roberts, G. C., Pincott, J. R., McMeniman, P., Bayley, J. I. L. and Kendall, B. (1978) Progression in idiopathic scoliosis. *J. Bone Jt. Surg.* **60B**, 451–460

Luque, E. R. (1982) The anatomic basis and development of segmental spinal instrumentation. *Spine.* **7**, 256–259

Mehta, M. H. (1972) The rib vertebral angle in the early diagnosis of idiopathic scoliosis and its implication in patient treatment. *J. Bone Jt. Surg.* **54B**, 230–243

Mehta, M. H. (1978) Pain evoked scoliosis: observations on the evolution of the deformity. *Clin. Orthop.* **135**, 58–65

Mehta, M. H. and Morel, G. (1980) The non-operative treatment of infantile idiopathic scoliosis. In *Scoliosis 1979*. Ed. by P. A. Zorab and D. Siegler. London, New York, Toronto, Sydney: Academic Press, pp. 71–84

Mellencamp, P. D., Blount, W. P. and Anderson, A. J. (1977) Milwaukee brace treatment of idiopathic scoliosis: late results. *Clin. Orthop. Related Res.* **126**, 45–57

Melnick, J. O. and Silverman, F. P. (1963) Intervertebral disc calcification in childhood. *Radiology.* **80**, 399

Nachemson, A. (1968) A long-term follow-up study of non-treated scoliosis. *Acta Orthop. Scand.* **39**, 466–476

O'Donnell, C. S., Bunnell, W. P., Betz, R. R., Bowen, J. R. and Tipping, R. T. (1988) Electrical stimulation in the treatment of idiopathic scoliosis. *Clin. Orthop.* **229**, 107

Ozonoff, M. B. (1979) *Pediatric Orthopedic Radiology*. Philadelphia, London, Toronto: W. B. Saunders, p. 59

Risser, J. O. (1955) The application of body casts for the correction of scoliosis. *AAOS Instruct. Course Lect.* **12**, 255

Risser, J. O. (1958) The iliac apophysis: an invaluable sign in the management of scoliosis. *Clin. Orthop.* **11**, 111

Scheuermann, H. W. (1920) Kyphosis juvenilis. *Ugeskr. Laeg.* **82**, 385

Velikas, E. P. and Blackburn, J. S. (1981) Surgical treatment of spondylolisthesis in children and adolescents. *J. Bone Jt. Surg.* **63B**, 67–70

Watts, H. C., Hall, J. E. and Stanish, W. (1977) The Boston brace system for the treatment of low thoracic and lumbar scoliosis by the use of a girdle without superstructure. *Clin. Orthop. Related Res.* **126**, 87

Wynne-Davies, R. (1975a) Congenital vertebral anomalies: aetiology and relationship to spina bifida cystica. *J. Med. Genet.* **12**, 280– 288

Wynne-Davies, R. (1975b) Infantile idiopathic scoliosis – causative factors. *J. Bone Jt. Surg.* **57B**, 138–141

13

The hip and thigh

Congenital dislocation of the hip and its variants

The basic facts of congential dislocation of the hip (CDH) are well known: girls are affected more than boys (6:1); there are more unilateral cases than bilateral (2:1); winter births are more affected than summer births (1.5:1); incidence varies between races (Bantu, 0; northwest Europe, 1.5 true dislocations per 1000 births); and the first-born of the family predominates.

Familial influences are well recognized. the risk may be expressed in terms of that to succeeding siblings of affected children. According to Wynne-Davies (1970), in Edinburgh the risk varies from 6%, when the parents are normal, to 36% when one parent has a dislocated hip. The influence of familial joint laxity is also an important factor (Wilkinson, 1963), especially in boys (Carter and Wilkinson, 1964).

Environmental factors are also important. there is a high incidence of CDH in breech deliveries and late versions. There is an increased incidence in babies born by caesarian section, which are frequently performed for abnormal lie *in utero*, and in association with calcaneovalgus, talipes equinovarus and other foot deformities. Finally, some of the most severe forms of congenital dislocation can be seen in severe oligohydramnios. All this suggests that the intrauterine environment as well as inherited factors are important in the development of congenital dislocation of the hip and its variants.

Anatomy

The primary fault is still uncertain because those operated upon are likely to demonstrate only the secondary effects of the dislocation, which obscure the initial anomaly. To be sure, even dissection of a dislocated hip in a newborn may be misleading, for even then there is ignorance of the time it has been displaced. It is probable that deformity of the femoral head, imperfect articular cartilage, false acetabulum, anteversion (increased forward inclination of the femoral neck beyond the normal 20 degrees at birth), acetabular deficiency or malposition, infolding or adherence of capsule, shortening of some muscles such as psoas, adductors and hamstrings, and inversion of the acetabular labrum (limbus) and so on, are all secondary to, rather than the cause of, dislocation.

McKibbin (1970) dissected with great thoroughness the dislocated hip of a baby born by the breech who *in utero* had extended legs. The baby died at 2 days from cerebral haemorrhage due to the application of forceps to a tardy aftercoming head. He was otherwise normal. The only significant abnormalities were capsular redundancy and elongation of the ligamentum teres. McKibbin paid special attention to the inclination of the femoral neck and acetabulum – both were normal (compared with controls) in this and all other respects.

Ogden and Moss (1978) have published their extensive studies of a number of neonatal hips and have suggested three types.

Type 1 (which probably makes up 80–90% of all CDH) may be called positionally unstable. These usually show mild lateral and marginal changes in the acetabulum with an anteverted femoral head. This is associated with mild adduction and flexion contractures which, if left untreated, may progress to a more severe deformity, becoming subluxated or even dislocated.

Type 2 There is loss of sphericity of the femoral head as well as anteversion. The acetabulum becomes shallower and the labrum everted. In association with this the acetabular roof fails to ossify laterally and, in time, inversion of the labrum develops.

Type 3 There is significant deformation of the acetabular margin and the femoral head with posterosuperior displacement of the head to form a false acetabulum. This is associated with inversion hypertrophy of the fibrocartilage to form the limbus.

Although the essential lesion is as yet uncertain, its secondary effects are of great moment in treatment. These features (which are listed above) are all significant, varying only in degree and relative importance from patient to patient and from infancy to childhood. Thus extension in the newborn is avoided lest the shortened psoas lever out the unstable hip, and the tendon is divided during operative reduction for the same reason, thus reducing tension in the restored joint. Similarly, anteversion is neutralized by flexing and abducting the hip in the very young, but corrected by operation when the leg must be extended for walking and it remains as a cause of instability.

The acetabular labrum (limbus) has evoked controversy and interest elucidated further by Ogden (1978). In McKibbin's patient the labrum was normal, as described in Ogden and Moss's type 1 patients. The limbus may be pressed against the acetabular rim in partial upward displacement (subluxation; Ogden and Moss type 2) or inverted within the socket with its attached superior capsule (Ogden and Moss type 3). There is no doubt that the limbus may return to its normal position with conservative treatment and we therefore take issue with Somerville (1967) that, if demonstrated on arthrography, it should necessarily be removed, and that at operation it is commonly the only barrier to reduction.

Variations on the theme of congenital dislocation, their diagnosis and management

The variations are seldom static, for with growth and secondary adaptive changes there is a trend towards deterioration from the mild to the severe derangements.

Instability in the newborn

Great impetus was given to programmes of elimination of dislocation by the detection of instability at birth and its prompt treatment. This notion was initiated in Italy, and a particular debt is owed to Ortolani and Putti.

Diagnosis

Unstable hips are detected by clinical examination. Radiography is, in our opinion, less helpful or even misleading, in spite of special techniques. Ultrasound in experienced hands is the most accurate method of assessment (Graf, 1983; Clarke *et al*, 1985). Barlow's two-stage manoeuvre (1962) is one of many methods of clinical examination.

Stage 1

With the hips and knees flexed, the hips are abducted while pressure is applied forwards from behind the greater trochanter. When positive, there is a 'clunk' or jerk (not a click), which is palpable and often visible and audible as the femoral head snaps over the posterior acetabular rim into the socket.

Stage 2

The hips are flexed and slightly abducted while pressure is applied to the upper medial thigh. A clunk indicates that the hip can be dislocated backwards.

These clunks are very common. Barlow found them in the ratio 1:67 births, Von Rosen (1968) in the ratio of 1:77 and Smaill (1968) in the ratio of 1:120. The incidence of hip dislocation in the countries concerned is between 1 and 1.5:1000 births, so clearly a state of instability is being seen, which in most cases corrects itself. Thus, in Barlow's series based on 9000 births there were 159 clunking hips, whereas it may be calculated that 14 cases at the most would have persisted as dislocations in later childhood – about 9%.

These are, of course, extreme figures, and are used only to emphasize the high rate of spontaneous 'cure' – the assumption being that most were never abnormal, or at least were within the physiological deviations of normal. Barlow noted a rapid and spontaneous disappearance of the clunk in a high proportion of patients. Nelson (1966) found clunking hips in 16% of a group of babies at birth; at 1 week the incidence was 7% and at 3 weeks less than 0.5% (1:290).

There is, of course, no direct evidence that unstable hips become dislocated hips; but the circumstantial evidence is strong, for in communities in which every newborn baby can be skilfully examined and (if 'abnormal') treated, established dislocation has been reduced to a very low level – 0.07 per 1000 live births (Fredensborg, 1976). Ultrasound can demonstrate relative anatomical immaturity of the hip which may progress with time to dysplasia and frank dislocation.

Management

What, then, should be done when a clunk is detected? The empiricist will treat them all by some form of abduction splint (Von Rosen's or Barlow's) for 3 months. They will justifiably argue that at this age to treat 9 out of 10 cases unnecessarily is both harmless and acceptable as a policy, because the 1 in 10 who might otherwise dislocate (having perhaps failed to attend for supervision in the early months) do well. Unfortunately, in all large series of abduction splintage there is a small but definite incidence of damage to the capital femoral epiphysis, leading to avascular necrosis (AVN, epiphysitis). Mild forms of this condition will recover completely, but severe forms can damage the hip irrevocably and so splintage cannot now be considered entirely harmless (Kalamchi and MacEwen, 1980).

The eclectic, on the other hand, will prefer to discriminate between the many patients with a probable favourable outcome and the few at significant risk. Our policy is to distinguish between Barlow's two tests. If stage 1 is positive we regard the hip as habitually dislocated, but capable of reduction when fully abducted. Consequently these are treated in abduction, our preference being for an irremovable 'mother-proof' splint, such as the von Rosen or the Denis Browne hip harness (*see* page 143). The Pavlik harness has recently become very popular, as it appears to be associated with a low incidence of AVN, although it is not without its problems (Mubarak *et al*, 1981). If stage 2 is positive the hip is habitually intact, but capable of being dislocated. Provided that the instability (clunk) has disappeared in 2 weeks, no treatment is advised but a precautionary radiograph is taken at about 4 months, when the femoral head is usually sufficiently ossified for its congruity to be assesssed. The distinction between these two types was well described by Finlay, Maudsley and Busfield (1967). The use of ultrasound scanning both of neonatal hips and hip development in the first 6–9 months of life is adding a new dimension to our knowledge and management of hip instability.

Comment and criticism

There is no doubt that in relatively small well controlled centres such as Malmö and Edinburgh, screening of all newborn babies by skilled examiners can virtually eradicate congenital dislocation. This is only possible when all births (or at least all primigravidae) or those with obstetric abnormalities are delivered at hospitals where the staff are not only familiar with, but also practiced in, the screening test. Frequently, succeeding obstetric or paediatric house physicians become disillusioned and lose heart when they have examined perhaps 100 normal hips without avail. It would be only natural if the next 100 received less careful attention. The obstetric or paediatric house physician may possibly meet his first 'clunk' just before he hands over to his successor, who then goes through the same process of keenness, disillusion and complacency.

At The Hospitals for Sick Children in London almost as many dislocations requiring admission are being seen as were encountered 5–10 years ago, and a brief survey does not suggest that they are largely in babies born at home. Prevention demands that a senior, experienced, permanent and dedicated doctor be allocated to this tedious but important task – an ideal which is too rarely practicable.

Lastly, and most important, there are two types of patient who may elude detection by eliciting the 'clunk' sign of instability. First, those who have irreducible dislocations at birth cannot by definition be reduced and so have no clunk. Abduction in flexion (*see* below) is limited and should therefore be tested for in screening. Second, those with excessive joint laxity can flop in and out without a significant clunk or, if irreducible, are difficult to recognize by the abduction/flexion test, but declare themselves when walking begins. Again ultrasound has been able to detect hip abnormality in the absence of clinical signs.

Acetabular dysplasia and the uncovered femoral head

The word 'dysplasia' is often used loosely and applied to all the variants. It means that there is no upward (as opposed to lateral) displacement of the hip joint, but the acetabulum provides an inadequate cover for the head. This situation may present early or late in the evolution of the deformity.

Early acetabular dysplasia

At any time after infancy but usually within the first year the mother notices a lack of symmetry, including crease differences between the hips or difficulty in abducting one or both. On applying the comprehensive hip test abnormal signs are found. In this test, the hips and knees are first flexed so that the knees are in contact with the feet, parallel and touching both the table and each other. This means that the hips are flexed about 70 degrees and the knees beyond 90 degrees. If one hip is at fault the knee on that side will be lower than, or proximal to, its fellow. On abducting the legs in the same position, the abnormal hip will have a more limited range than the other.

This test is fundamental in the diagnosis of all varieties of hip disorders. Thus it is positive in coxa vara, Perthes' disease and when hips are involved in myelomeningocele and cerebral palsy. There is no difficulty when the disorder is unilateral, but when both hips are symmetrically involved, diagnosis depends on good fortune, experience, a high index of suspicion and a request for a radiograph. Unfortunately, there is no normal range for abduction in flexion, which may vary from 45 to 90 degrees, but other signs – such as prominence or upward displacement of the greater trochanter – should be sought.

In acetabular dysplasia the femoral head will appear to be somewhat lying away in propor-

tion to the degree of its ossification (which is often delayed on the side under suspicion). In addition, the acetabular roof will be inclined more vertically. Wynne-Davies (1970) found that the femoral head ossific nucleus is visible at 6 months in 78% of normal hips, in an investigation which concluded (on the basis of a study of genetic and other aetiological factors) that there are significant differences between neonatal hip instability and primary acetabular dysplasia.

Differential diagnosis

Identical signs are found when the hip is normal but the pelvis oblique because of scoliosis (usually resolving in infancy – the moulded baby syndrome – Lloyd-Roberts and Pilcher, 1965), with or without contracture of the adductors. In both there will be apparent shortening and limited abduction, but in pelvic obliquity careful scrutiny of the radiograph detects a difference. In pelvic obliquity (Figure 13.1) the acetabulum appears shallow but this is an artefact reflected in the narrowing of the wing of the ilium above. It is important to correct the contracture of the adductors or true subluxation may develop. Stretching is usually enough, and there is no tendency to recur once the pelvis is seen to be level on the radiograph (Heikala, Ryoppy and Louhimo, 1985). Manipulation under anaesthesia or wide abduction splintage should be avoided because of the serious risk of avascular necrosis (AVN).

Management

In true acetabular dysplasia, the diagnosis should be confirmed by examination under anaesthetic, arthrogram and adductor tenotomy if necessary, followed by a frog plaster in the modern position for 6 weeks and then Denis Browne's harness (*see* page 143) applied until the acetabulum is similar to its fellow – which usually requires about 4–6 months.

Late acetabular dysplasia

Late acetabular dysplasia represents acetabular growth failure and may follow either non-operative or operative treatment for dislocation or subluxation. It is discussed later.

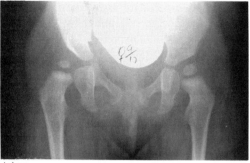

(a)

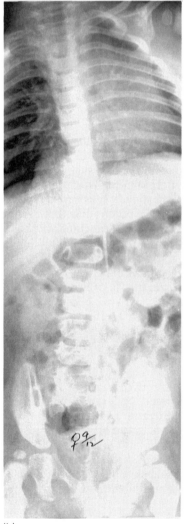

(b)

Figure 13.1 Pelvic obliquity. (a) Anteroposterior X-ray at age 9 months. Note the apparent sloping of the right acetabulum, the tilt of the pelvis up on the right and the apparent narrowing of the right ilium compared with the left. (b) The same patient, showing curvature of the spine and rotation of the pelvis, causing the asymmetry

Dislocation and subluxation

The comprehensive sign of dislocation and subluxation is positive, as in acetabular dysplasia, but more conspicuously, since the femoral head moves upwards. Displacement of the trochanters, too, is easier to feel.

The signs of neglected dislocation in the older child, such as telescoping, Trendelenburg gait and so on, are well known and need not concern us, but three aspects of diagnosis merit emphasis.

Firstly, joint laxity (a factor in aetiology) may allow almost full abduction in flexion with only slight contrast in symmetry in the fully abducted position (Figure 13.2), although of course shortening is detectable. Those who pontificate about delay in diagnosis in older children are likely to have either a limited experience or a limited memory for they would otherwise have failed, on some occasion, to detect a dislocated hip in a lax child.

Secondly, on first walking normal children are unstable and if they walked Trendelenburg fashion they would be falling constantly. To avoid this, the foot on the dislocated side is placed flat on the floor and the shortening is compensated for by flexing the opposite knee. This sign is pathognomonic of hip instability and shortening in young children, because when shortening alone is present they compensate by equinus of the ankle on the shorter side. Undue delay in walking is rare in congenital dislocation.

Thirdly, conspicuous abnormality of one hip should alert the surgeon to the possibility of an abnormality of lesser degree being present in the other. Furthermore, this anxiety should continue throughout growth, for acetabular dysplasia may not declare itself until adolescence is reached.

The management of dislocation and primary subluxation

The methods we will describe are those that are used at The Hospitals for Sick Children. They are a distillate of the work of our predecessors and contemporaries and it must be emphasized that this is the practice of one hospital only, and that there are certainly satisfactory alternatives to most of the recommendations that will be made. Our principles have been described elsewhere (Lloyd-Roberts

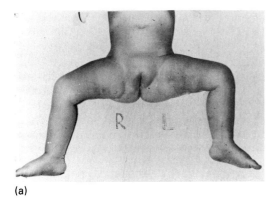

(a)

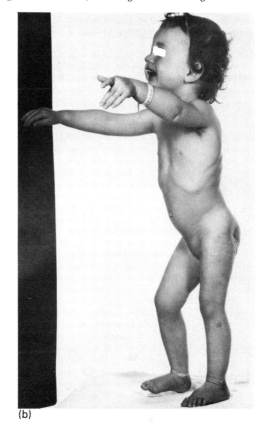

(b)

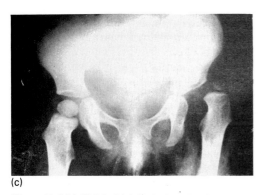

(c)

Figure 13.2 (a) Child with joint laxity, showing almost full abduction on the dislocated left side. (b) Characteristic stance of a walking child with left congenital dislocation of the hip. Note the flexion of the right leg and the dimple in the left buttock. (c) X-ray of the same patient, showing lateral and upward displacement of the hip

and Swann, 1966) and we apply them to any child from infancy to about 6 years of age in whom the radiograph discloses true dislocation or subluxation with limitation of abduction.

Reduction by non-operative means

A choice must be made between manipulation under anaesthesia, manipulation following a period of traction, and traction alone. We use traction alone to the exclusion of manipulation, for although manipulation following traction may be less noxious than primary manipulation, we avoid both because the evidence against is formidable (Scott, 1953, Somerville and Scott, 1957). Wilkinson and Carter (1960) were able to contrast the outcome in patients treated at The Hospital for Sick Children by two former surgeons, neither of whom practiced operative reduction. One

relied on traction exclusively and one on manipulation. The concentric reduction rate was the same, but, whereas the traction series (92 hips) showed no evidence of vascular disturbance in the femoral head, there were 38 examples among 99 manipulated hips. The disturbance is assumed to be vascular. Some may have unusually prolonged delay in ossification and others ossify irregularly. Notwithstanding this, the final results in the two series reflected these changes because, although the reduction rate was the same, the final head shape in those manipulated was significantly worse. Indeed the outcome differed at the expense of the manipulation series in direct relationship to this feature. It is difficult to accept this disturbance in the very young to be innocuous, as is sometimes asserted, for it seems likely that softening of the head allows deformity to develop which mirrors the shape of the mould – which in this case is a dysplastic acetabulum – thereby favouring subluxation later.

We use traction in the form of a hoop erected above the ordinary cot in such a way that the child can be suspended from it (using fixed traction) in the manner of Bryant's method for a femoral fracture (Figure 13.3). Although there is no fracture and so the risk of ischaemia to the limb should be less, it is

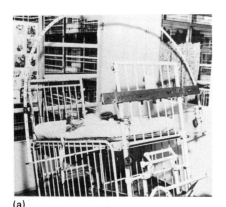

(a)

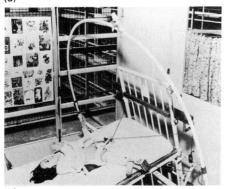

(b)

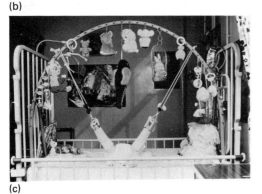

(c)

Figure 13.3 (a) Hoop traction, old style, with 90 degree abduction which is not now recommended. (b) Hoop traction, old style, showing cross-traction. (c) Modern hoop traction, with abduction of not more than 45 degrees

probably inadvisable to use this method in children weighing more than 10–12 kg. The initial pull is with the hips flexed to 90 degrees, in which position the femoral head is lying somewhat behind the acetabulum and so the force is immediately corrective. This position is maintained for 2–3 days and thereafter the legs are gradually abducted on the hoop until, in 7–10 days, they lie abducted about 40 degrees on each side. Cross traction was used in the past but we rarely if ever use it now. If, at any time during the abduction period, adductor tension develops, it should be relieved by tenotomy of the adductors.

This method has certain advantages over an orthopaedic frame. There is no mystique, no need for special nursing skill or orthopaedic workshop, nor any delay in starting treatment. It has special advantages in the very young for it is easier to maintain cleanliness. Vascular disturbance in the form of AVN is rare, compared with an average of 10% in reported frame series. The concentric reduction rate is comparable at about 50% for both methods. We are of the opinion that the low incidence of vascular change is due to the lack of rigid fixation which allows the child to wriggle somewhat, thus reducing by instinct the tension on his retinacular vessels as the hip abducts.

Traction prolonged for more than 2–3 weeks has no virtue; concentric reduction is now unlikely, and stiffness (Mackenzie, Seddon and Trevor, 1960) or even porosis and premature epiphyseal arrest is possible (Botting and Scrase, 1965).

Preliminary traction is virtually always used in primary hip displacement under the age of 2–2.5 years.

In patients under the age of 3–3.5 years, traction is usually employed unless there has been a previous attempt at reduction by surgical means. Over this age the chance of successful reduction by traction is very rare, and nowadays we tend to release the tight muscles at the time of operation rather than use a period of preliminary traction and immobilization prior to surgery.

The first major decision

The first major decision is now taken for or against operative reduction. If the joint is congruous or still widely displaced there is no problem, for in the first eventuality non-operative treatment continues, and in the second, operation is performed. Difficulty arises when the head is lying away from, but not above, the acetabulum.

There are three possible causes. Firstly, the appearance may be an artefact due to the summation of traction, joint laxity, redundant capsule, retarded ossification in the femoral head and a laterally rotated leg. In the lax patient a similar appearance may be seen in the opposite normal hip in unilateral dislocations. Secondly, the limbus may have failed to evert as the femoral head comes down. Thirdly, there may be one or more insuperable barriers to concentric reduction. It is seldom possible to distinguish between these on plain radiographs, but an arthrogram is very helpful.

The patient is anaesthetized and examination under anaesthetic is performed. This should be combined with screening of the hip and an arthrogram to confirm the quality of reduction of the hip. The patient is then put in the modified frog position in which the hips are abducted no more than 40–50 degrees on each side and are flexed above 90 degrees on each side. This position has been shown to be associated with significantly less incidence of AVN than the traditional frog or the Lorenz position in which the hips were abducted 90 degrees and flexed 90 degrees. The plaster is maintained for 6 weeks and then the second major decision is made.

The second major decision

The second major decision follows after 6 weeks in plaster, when the concentric reduction of the hip is assessed. This assessment is so important that we admit the child routinely to avoid the possibility of a hurried or badly considered decision in the outpatients' department. If the hip is still not congruous, we operate; if congruous, we continue with non-operative treatment as if the original reduction had been entirely satisfactory.

Continuing non-operative treatment

In continuing non-operative treatment, no more plaster is used. Denis Browne's hip harness is applied instead (Figure 13.4). This device is designed as a controlled movement

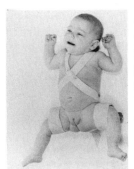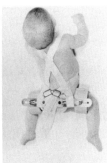

Figure 13.4 Denis Browne hip harness. As in Figure 13.3c, the hips should not be abducted more than 45–50 degrees

splint, permitting full rotation but limiting flexion and extension and abduction and adduction to a range of about 30 degrees in each direction, from the modified frog position of 50 degrees of abduction and above 90 degrees of flexion. The splint is fixed to the child in such a way that unauthorized removal is impossible without the surgeon's knowledge. Essentially, two thigh bands are connected behind by an adjustable bar, the whole being controlled by crossed chest and back straps stitched to each other. The knees are free.

The virtues of this remarkable splint are not recognized as they should be – indeed, we have sometimes wondered if Denis Browne himself appreciated all its admirable qualities! In contrast to plaster, the harness allows crawling and, later, walking. It is easy to keep both it and the child clean, and it may be changed in the outpatients' department without anaesthesia (or the cross-bar adjusted for growth). Furthermore, movement is life not only to the child but also to his articular cartilage (Salter *et al*, 1980). Plaster immobilization of a growing joint denies to articular cartilage that important stimulus of movement with physiological pressure, upon which its health depends. In addition, plaster by fixation may impose an abnormal growth pattern on the femoral head, especially when the joint is not fully congruous. Moreover, muscles – especially the important abductors – develop wonderfully. Lastly (and this is perhaps its most important property), it will not retain an unstable reduction because the hip redislocates. How much better it is to be aware of this situation and deal with it early, than wait for a year or more and have to meet the same problem later, when unsuspected incongruity enforced by plaster fixation may have done irreparable damage to the cartilage and the femoral head.

The harness is usually retained for 4–6 months. During this period the child can crawl or even walk within the limits of his enterprise and seniority.

It may be wondered why plaster is used at all in the early phase instead of a harness. The reason is that plaster seems to be more satisfactory in retaining reduction in the first few weeks after this has been achieved.

The third major decision

When the harness is removed the legs usually adduct to near neutral within 3 weeks. A radiograph must be taken in neutral position at this point to assess the need for osteotomy. If the harness has an imperfection, it is that, by virtue of the free rotation which it permits, there is no opportunity to favour reduction of anteversion by progressive adduction with internal rotation that plaster allegedly achieves. We personally doubt the value of these manoeuvres, and Wilkinson (1963) showed experimentally that internal rotation in fact produces anteversion because the femoral head is pressed against the posterior acetabular wall.

If the joint remains congruous with the legs in the neutral position, no further immediate treatment is needed. However, if it is congruous in internal rotation with 20 degrees of abduction but lies away slightly while in the neutral position (as often occurs), the decision for or against osteotomy is difficult. This may be rendered simple by performing an osteotomy on all such patients and this was our former practice, but we now realize that many of these operations were unnecessary. Correction of the responsible valgus and anteversion sometimes occurs rapidly on normal weight bearing, and we now wait and see for at least 6–12 months. If after this, persistent lying off or lateral displacement is seen, repeat EUA (examination under anaesthesia) screening and arthrography are performed. Based on the radiological appearance of the most congruous position, a femoral or innominate arterotomy is then performed.

Late non-operative treatment

Late non-operative treatment is essentially observation until skeletal maturity, for acetabular failure may develop at any time short of this. We must strive to prevent secondary subluxation (Figure 13.5) by judicious surgical intervention directed against either persisting abnormalities of the femoral head or the acetabular roof, or in both components of the joint. It is during this time that special attention is paid to the opposite 'normal' hip in 'unilateral' dislocations. Regular supervision is the only safeguard, for if subluxation develops in a child over 8 years of age and is not immediately corrected, it rapidly becomes irreducible and the final result is badly compromised.

Commentary on non-operative treatment

When operation was hazardous and seldom performed in the very young, and manipula-

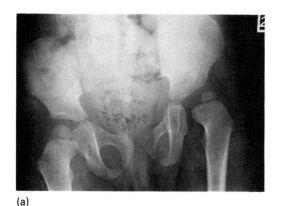
(a)

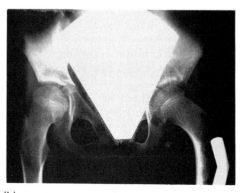
(b)

Figure 13.5 (a) Secondary subluxation following conservative treatment. (b) Ten years after varus rotation osteotomy in the same patient. Note that the acetabulum is developing well

tion under anaesthesia followed by plaster was the rule, the early results were entirely satisfactory in about half the patients treated, but as time passed the proportion of good results decreased. Platt (1953, 1956) wrote about this important aspect of treatment and emphasized the probable significance of deformed femoral heads and imperfect articular cartilage. Both are certainly common findings at operation after prolonged treatment in plaster in a less than congruous position, and may well occur in those who were congruous and in whom no opportunity for seeing the joint is justified.

Conservative treatment initiated by traction and followed by plaster (and in some cases a harness) gives better early results (Wilkinson and Carter, 1960) and it is anticipated that our present regimen will improve on this, especially if treatment based on mobility reduces deformity and articular cartilage damage as it promises to do.

We have discussed non-operative management at some length because today there is a tendency to return to routine operation in most dislocations (Galloway, 1926). Nevertheless, we believe that about half our patients seen after infancy should, with good conservative treatment, be spared operation on the joint itself, although later osteotomy on femur or pelvis will be needed in some of these cases. Furthermore, we believe the best results follow non-operative treatment, provided that no mistakes are made. That these may be the more favourable joints to treat affects the argument in no way.

Operative treatment

We will now consider the various operations from the standpoint of their indications during primary treatment, and for the imperfect results of primary non-operative treatment. In both, the factor of age must be contended with. Techniques are merely touched upon.

Primary treatment from 1 to 5 years of age

Open reduction

Open reduction is needed when closed reduction fails, the hip does not bed down in plaster, or redislocates in the harness – situations already discussed. Although possibly indicated earlier, we personally find it better to postpone

operation until the child is 1 year of age. This is because ischaemic changes, which are less common following open reduction later, seem specially common in infancy. This is possibly due to the pattern of vascular supply. It is seldom, if ever, necessary in primary subluxation at this age. The medial, or Ludloff, approach has been recommended for open reduction in a child under the age of 1 year (Ludloff, 1913; Dwyer *et al*, 1986; Ferguson, 1973).

If reduction seems unsatisfactory in the immediate postoperative radiograph, it should be repeated at once or within a few days. By contrast if unsatisfactory on removing the plaster (before or after osteotomy – *see* below), it should only be repeated after a period of mobilization to restore movement. This no more than reflects the surgical philosophy that an operation, once correctly indicated, is still indicated even if it fails. Following surgical failures the result is likely to be a salvage procedure to gain stability but often at the expense of some stiffness. If the acetabulum has been severely damaged and distorted, Colonna's capsular arthroplasty can still be useful.

For the techniques of open reduction, see Salter (1961), Scaglietti and Calandriello (1962) and Lloyd-Roberts and Swann (1966).

Femoral osteotomy

When open reduction is performed, it will be found that the hip enjoys its greatest congruity when the femur is internally rotated and somewhat abducted. Osteotomy is designed to retain the proximal end of the femur in internal rotation and abduction, while aligning the leg so that it points directly to the ground. Thus the osteotomy must direct the limb towards adduction and external rotation. We favour an osteotomy which compensates for both anteversion (which determines the internal rotation) and valgus (which determines the abduction), for in many both are present. Some surgeons, however, are content with the rotation element only. Harris (1965), working at The Hospitals for Sick Children, made a study of the implications, natural history and effects of both anteversion and valgus.

We rarely omit osteotomy after open reduction. We have already discussed its place at the end of non-operative treatment. It is also frequently indicated in primary subluxation, if a radiograph in about 30 degrees of abduction and full internal rotation shows restored congruity to the hip joint.

The osteotomy may be performed below or between the trochanters, and the higher operation is preferred because this causes less shortening and less obvious deformity – temporary though this may be. The method of internal fixation should avoid interfering with the epiphysis of the greater trochanter, for delay in growth here will encourage valgus deformity to recur. Penrose of Coventry designed an excellent screw and plate for this purpose. Supracondylar osteotomy has disadvantages and should be avoided.

Acetabular reconstruction

By acetabular reconstruction, the acetabulum is either actually deepened, by turning down its still pliable roof and supporting the flap so formed by grafts (ascribed to Parker of Cardiff), or relatively deepened by altering the direction in which it faces in a backward and downward direction (Pemberton, 1958, 1965; Salter, 1961, 1969).

To do either at the time of open reduction implies that the surgeon doubts the capacity of the acetabulum to develop, in spite of congruous reduction. The nub of the matter is acetabular potential and this is difficult to forecast. Wilkinson and Carter (1960) showed that the potential was greater in unilateral dislocation whereas Sallis and Smith (1965), also from this hospital, were unable to find definite factors upon which to base a prognosis, except that congruity of reduction was the common feature in those with good development. According to Harris, Lloyd-Roberts and Gallien (1975), if concentric reduction can be obtained and maintained by the age of 4.5 years, 95% of acetabula will develop satisfactorily without the need for acetabular surgery.

The quandary remains, but before embarking wholesale on acetabuloplasty it is well to recall that Mackenzie, Seddon and Trevor (1960) reported that one in three of those under 3 years of age developed ischaemic changes after Parker's operation. Salter's operation is also prone to this complication and demands rigorous attention to detail and care to avoid tension on the femoral head and the

evil consequences of articular cartilage compression (Salter and Field, 1960; Powell, 1986).

When, then, should it be done? Perhaps always if the acetabulum is anteriorly disposed, inclined and deficient, with an obviously sloping roof. These hips can be recognized at open reduction because in order to maintain stability they have to be flexed as well as abducted and internally rotated. For the rest, the older the child and the more the slope (i.e. the gap between the reduced head and the roof at the free margin), the greater will be the inclination; however, in these cases empiricism governs the decision. Our personal primary acetabuloplasty rate is about 5% – similar to that of Scaglietti, but many surgeons think otherwise and regularly include this procedure with their open reductions (Trevor, 1960; Eyre-Brook, 1966).

Both Pemberton and Salter rotate the socket, and these operations are at present in greatest favour – with justification, for both can achieve most impressive results. An added advantage is that by rotation of the pelvis they may obviate the need for a secondary femoral osteotomy. Recently we have had a number of cases referred to us in which the femoral head has dislocated posteriorly following a Salter osteotomy. This seems to be due to an inadequate capsulorrhaphy such that a redundant pouch of capsule is left posteriorly. This, combined with the relative reduction in the depth of the posterior wall of the acetabulum brought about by the forward and lateral rotation of the acetabulum, allows the head to dislocate posterolaterally. If this is not recognized and corrected, it produces an extremely difficult situation to salvage, frequently associated with severe AVN (Fixsen, 1987).

One contraindication is certain – no form of acetabular reconstruction will compensate for an inadequate open reduction; the surgeon must seek again the obstruction that eludes him.

Primary treatment over 5 years of age

The upper limit for open reduction including capsular arthroplasty is difficult to define. In cases of unilateral dislocation we believe that reduction is justified at any time to restore hip joint anatomy, as an aid to future arthrodesis or definitive arthroplasty. Bilateral dislocations are more difficult, for bilateral capsular

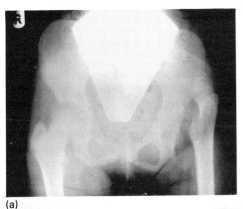

(a)

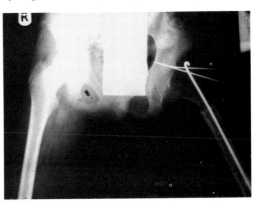

(b)

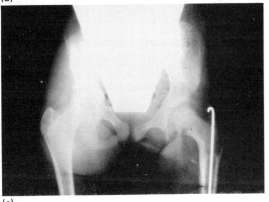

(c)

Figure 13.6 (a) Neglected high congenital dislocation of the hip in an 8-year-old child. No previous treatment. (b) After open reduction and femoral osteotomy with shortening, two Kirschner wires through the greater trochanter into the ilium stabilize the femoral head in the socket. (c) The same patient 2 years later

arthroplasty is less appealing. In general, we regard 7 years of age as being the upper limit, especially if there is an effective false acetabulum (Figure 13.6).

Open reduction

Open reduction is usually technically possible at any age. In the past we used preliminary soft tissue release followed by skeletal traction. However, we now prefer to perform a soft tissue release at the time of open reduction and combine it with femoral shortening. This has allowed high dislocation to be reduced in patients up to the age of 14 without the problems of prolonged traction. Acetabuloplasty may be necessary either at the same time or later if the acetabulum fails to respond to concentric reduction.

Capsular arthroplasty

Hey-Groves of Bristol first described capsular arthroplasty in his Bradshaw Lecture (1927) but it remained in the limbo of the literature until Colonna (1932, 1965) refined and advo-

cated it. The redundant capsule is divided close to the acetabulum and fashioned to enclose the head, which is placed within the acetabulum that is enlarged and deepened to the inner pelvic wall. We regard this as a salvage operation, to be used only in those patients where previously failed surgery has obliterated any reasonable acetabulum.

Osteotomy

Osteotomy is performed for the same reasons as those given under primary treatment in younger children, and for the indications suggested in the following section.

Operations usually performed later for unsatisfactory non-operative or operative treatment

Capsular arthroplasty

Some indications have been mentioned, but in addition capsular arthroplasty may be chosen when there is irreducible subluxation, as an alternative to a superior support.

Osteotomy

If the subluxated hip becomes congruous on abduction and internal rotation, the appropriate osteotomy is indicated.

Acetabular insufficiency or inadequacy

Acetabular reconstruction is combined with osteotomy for the above indication in older children judged to have poor acetabular potential or marked inadequacy. Salter's operation is ideal both in this situation and when the head is poorly covered but not subluxated.

Superior support

If subluxation is irreducible and significantly displaced, and capsular arthroplasty is for some reason rejected, acetabular reconstruction is not suitable. Either a supporting buttress of new bone placed immediately above the head (an augmentation shelf) must be used (Wainwright, 1976; Staheli, 1981), or the pelvis divided at the level of the top of the flattened socket in the coronal plane. The distal fragment, which contains the hip joint including the capsule, is then displaced within and below the proximal, which serves as a wide supporting platform that gradually moulds to conform to the shape of the head (Chiari, 1955). Both may sometimes be combined with osteotomy if some displacement is thereby reduced.

Complications of treatment of dislocation

Complications arising from technical errors and the nature of the disorder have already been described. Sepsis is a disaster, and is likely to proceed to intractable stiffness with deformity, indicating osteotomy or arthrodesis. Stiffness is otherwise usually temporary, but if associated with fixed flexion deformity this should be corrected by traction. Stiffness due to ischaemic change, compression of cartilage or myositis ossificans may, however, be permanent. Fractures (usually supracondylar) are common after operation and immobilization, but these do not affect the issue. Bone plates may loosen, become irremovable or predispose to fractures at the screw holes, and for these reasons their removal is always advised.

Coxa vara

The angle made by the femoral neck and the shaft of the femur is reduced in varying degree from the normal 120 degrees to below 90 degrees in extreme examples. Although this deformity may complicate bone softening (as in rickets or the fractures of fragilitas ossium) and require corrective abduction osteotomies, these will not be considered further. Three varieties will be described: congenital, infantile and adolescent (slipped upper femoral epiphysis).

Congenital coxa vara

Congenital coxa vara (Figure 13.7) must be distinguished from the infantile type, for it is present at birth and associated with early noticeable leg shortening. This will be discussed with the congenital dysplasias of the femur.

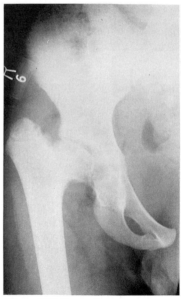

Figure 13.7 Congenital coxa vara. Note the inadequate acetabulum and the small femoral head. Compare with Figure 13.8

Infantile coxa vara

In infantile coxa vara (Figure 13.8) the abnormality is of the proximal femoral epiphyseal growth plate, which is evident on radiographs. The plate is widened, slightly

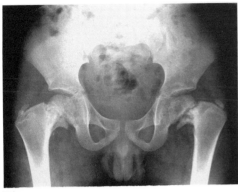

(a)

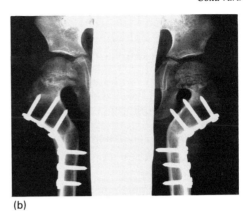

(b)

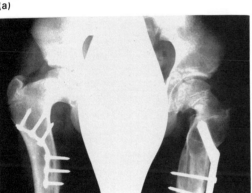

(c)

Figure 13.8 Infantile coxa vara. (a) At diagnosis. (b) After bilateral abduction osteotomies. (c) Seven years later. The osteotomy on the left had to be repeated. Note that the metal should be removed; otherwise it becomes buried, as shown on the right

more vertical than usual, broader and often bifurcating inferiorly to isolate a triangular fragment of bone of which the apex points downwards. The femoral neck is short. The metaphysis has a patchy density and consists of disordered cartilage and new bone (Babb, Ghormley and Chatterton, 1949). Untreated, the head moves downwards on the neck which bends to follow it until finally it points below 90 degrees. Concurrently, the greater trochanter enlarges and may approach the wing of the ilium. The epiphysis closes prematurely. It should be emphasized that all do not behave in this way and spontaneous stabilization is common at some point in development. In fact, shortening rarely exceeds 2.5 cm.

Signs will depend on severity and upon whether it is present on one or both sides. Trendelenburg's lurch or waddle will be seen if varus inhibits the efficiency of the hip abductors. Similarly, limitation of internal rotation and of abduction reflect the degree of posterior displacement and varus present.

The nature is obscure. Some cases are evidently familial for it is often bilateral and

has been reported in identical twins, and an exactly similar deformity is seen in craniocleidodysostosis. Blockey (1969) suggested that some are traumatic, and illustrated his thesis convincingly with radiographs showing normal appearances followed later by those of infantile coxa vara. Unfortunately, the head and proximal neck of the femur are cartilaginous during the early months, so the earliest changes are not visible, but this criticism does not apply to Blockey's patient, whose radiograph was normal much later.

Morgan and Somerville (1960) presented evidence favouring a vascular determinant, which again supports the suggestion that this may be an acquired rather than a congenital lesion.

Treatment aims at increasing abduction, reducing the shortening and varus deformity, directing the growth plate more horizontally and increasing abductor power by widening the distance between their origin and insertion. This is most readily achieved by an abduction osteotomy which is usually of about 60 degrees. The parents should be warned that the operation may need to be repeated if, with further growth, the deformity recurs. To reduce this risk, bone grafting was advocated by Le Mesurier (1948) – a recommendation which he subsequently withdrew – and by Amstutz and Wilson (1962) who combine it with osteotomy. Postponing operation cannot be advised because the deformity may increase rapidly and become irremediable.

Adolescent coxa vara (slipped upper femoral epiphysis)

The synonym is largely a misnomer, for there is no displacement of the head within the acetabulum except somewhat posteriorly, when displacement is considerable. Rather, the deformity is a forward and upward displacement of the femoral neck on the head at the level of the growth plate.

Aetiology and natural history

Most cases are seen between 10 and 16 years of age but the end-point coincides with the closure of the epiphysis. Boys outnumber girls by 3:2 but girls are liable to present earlier and sometimes even below 10 years of age. There is bilateral involvement in 20%. Two physical types predominate: the adiposogenital and the tall, thin, rapidly growing adolescent.

All these features combine to suggest an endocrine basis, and Harris' observations (1950) support this. Harris subjected rabbits' epiphyses to stress on a machine, which indicated the pressure at which they separated from the metaphysis. He found that sex hormones increased the resistance whereas growth hormones decreased it. Their opposing effects were mainly seen in the large cartilage cell layer of the plate which multiplies under the influence of pituitary growth hormone, which is itself inhibited by testosterone.

The fact that spontaneous epiphyseal displacement is confined to this growth plate, whereas the hormonal effects are general, presupposes that some other factors are also involved. Ghormley and Fairchild (1940) observed that during active growth the plane of the growth plate becomes less horizontal and this, combined with cartilage cell hyperplasia, renders the area vulnerable to shearing forces.

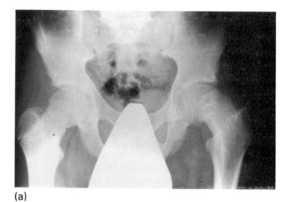

(a)

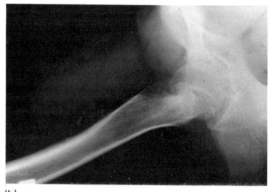

(b)

Figure 13.9 Left adolescent coxa vara (slipped upper femoral epiphysis). (a) Anteroposterior X-ray. (b) Frog lateral of the same patient

Indeed, little more than periosteum binds the proximal and distal segments at this stage. It has been suggested that not only minor direct injury but even habitual sitting habits may initiate the process.

Once started, the course is variable, for in some cases no apparent displacement takes place while in others the neck moves so far forward, hinging on the posterior periosteum, that its posterior border engages with and finally fuses with the anterior and superior quadrant of the head. Unless the onset is very late, epiphyseal fusion is premature and follows on average 18 months later. The inevitable gaps between head and neck in front and behind fill with cartilage and later ossify, following some moulding of the neck in the direction of the head. During this healing process some overgrowth occurs so that exostoses form, especially on the superior surface of the neck where they may obstruct abduction. We have also seen a similar outgrowth anteroinferiorly, acting as a block to adduction. Complications are discussed with treatment.

Clinical features

Unexplained limp is more prominent a presenting symptom than pain, but if either or both develop without obvious cause in the years during which coxa vara occurs, this must be assumed to be the diagnosis until disproved. The limp is of the painful hip variety (quick short step on involved side, long and slow on the other), the leg moving in external rotation. Pain is dull and frequently long standing, but may be exaggerated by trips or stumbles. If dull pain is succeeded by persisting sharp pain it is likely that sudden increased displacement has taken place.

The patient is likely to display one or other of the physical types already mentioned. The leg lies in external rotation. Hip irritability is seldom marked, so limitation of movement is usually governed by the degree of deformity. Thus one may find that only internal rotation is lost in patients with the least slip. This is a very important sign which may precede confident radiological diagnosis. Otherwise, fixed external rotation, lack of abduction, increased extension and shortening will vary with the deformity.

Radiological signs (Figure 13.9)

Displacement of the head is best seen on the lateral projection. A frog lateral is preferable and much easier to take than a 'shoot-through' lateral view. Klein and colleagues (1948) found the lateral view diagnostic in 98% of his patients compared with 68% of the anterior projections, and confirmed the validity of Perkins' sign – that is, a line continuing that of the superior border of the neck no longer cuts across the top of the head. The diagnosis is by no means always easy even with good radiographs and a normal opposite hip. When in doubt, rely on the clinical signs. When healing is complete the head is often bullet shaped.

Signs in the metaphysis are of great importance for they may precede actual displacement. The plate is widened and there is irregularity and patchy porosis on the metaphyseal side. General porosis may be present.

Treatment

Diagnosis demands that the patient be taken off his feet. Conservative treatment which includes traction, bed rest and plaster is of no value, for further displacement may occur, there is no correction of existing deformity and the incidence of late osteoarthritis is high.

When metaphyseal changes are present and are supported by physical signs, and the patient is within the age span of hazard, it is prudent to fix the epiphysis by pinning.

The decision, therefore, concerns only the choice of operation.

There is general agreement that chronic displacement which can be fixed *in situ* should be (Newman, 1960; Durbin, 1960; Dunn, 1964; Fahey and O'Brien, 1965). The amount of deformity deemed suitable for fixation will vary between surgeons, but, in general, if no more than a quarter of the neck is exposed on the lateral projection, this is feasible. Fixation should be by two or three threaded pins or a cannulated screw, and not by a heavy nail which may displace the head or damage the blood supply. Although union may take up to 2 years patients may be allowed to walk at between 6 weeks and 3 months.

Although vascular complications can, and do, occur in the chronic group with minor displacement, they dominate the situation in all others. The vessels feeding the head lie within the synovial reflection and beneath the periosteum behind and below the neck, crossing the periphery of the epiphyseal plate to enter it. Their vulnerability to the displacement or its surgical correction needs no emphasis. Necrotic changes may involve the whole or segments of the head, or the articular cartilage alone (Waldenstrom, 1931).

When it is believed that a sudden increase in displacement has occurred on a background of earlier chronic changes – making pinning impossible – we have often feared to correct this by manipulation because of the alleged danger to the blood supply, and have performed direct corrective surgery (*see* below). Later contributions (Vaughan-Jackson, 1956; Fairbanks, 1969) suggest that we have been overcautious. It now seems proper to treat these by very gentle manipulation and pinning.

If manipulation fails, or chronic displacement has progressed beyond the point when pinning is possible, the choices are to allow fusion to occur spontaneously (with its obvious disadvantages) and then do a femoral osteotomy, to correct the deformity at the neck, or to fuse the epiphysis and remove the exostosis on the neck.

Correction through the neck is performed either by a transcervical cuneiform osteotomy or at the level of the growth plate (Klein and colleagues, 1948). Enthusiasm for these methods has varied with the reported ischaemic necrosis rates, but generally they have not found favour. Dunn (1963) introduced a promising variation. In this operation the retinacular vessels are carefully mobilized by gentle subperiosteal dissection, the neck is shortened (to further reduce tension on the vessels), the epiphysis is obliterated (to encourage the intraosseous circulation) and the head is fixed by threaded pins. In 1975 Angel and Dunn reported the results of 73 operations. Narrowing of the joint space suggesting chrondrolysis occurred in 18%; avascular necrosis occurred in 14%. More recently, Boyer, Mickelson and Ponseti (1981) followed up more than 100 patients for 21–47 years. The results were very good in the majority of the 83 hips where the slip was left unreduced. The results even in moderate and severe slips were better, and with fewer complications, after fixation than after operative and manipulative treatment. Surprisingly few joints suffered degenerative arthritis in the long term.

The alternative, less dramatic but therefore reassuring, operation places a graft across the growth plate without disturbing the position, together with excision of the superior exostosis when this is obstructing movement (Herndon, Heyman and Bell, 1963). Some residual deformity must therefore be accepted, and the method's reputation will ultimately depend on the incidence of degenerative arthritis – as indeed will any method when the danger of ischaemia is past. The intertrochanteric osteotomy described by Griffiths (1976) is a very useful and safe technique for the severe slip.

When the epiphyseal plate is closed, the blood supply to the femoral head becomes largely transcervical and intraosseous, so correction by any form of cervical osteotomy is undesirable. The alternative is femoral osteotomy between or below the trochanters, if the residual deformity seems worthy of correction. Abduction and internal rotation osteotomies have, unfortunately, a poor outlook in

terms of degenerative arthritis and even late ischaemic change (Pearson and Riddell, 1964). The addition of a flexion component to correct hyperextension (Newman, 1960) appears to produce a hip with a functionally satisfactory range of movement, although chondrolysis can occur (Ireland and Newman, 1978). Again, the Griffiths intertrochanteric osteotomy is very useful in this situation.

There remains the problem of ischaemic necrosis developing in a young man. Total and segmental necrosis will be watched with more pessimism than optimism, in the hope that stability and lack of pain will allow prolonged postponement of arthrodesis, in spite of limited movement. Articular cartilage necrosis, which has so many of the clinical features of low-grade infective arthritis, causes stiffness and deformity. In the young patient, arthrodesis is still likely to be the operation of choice in these patients. Total hip replacement in a young, otherwise active, person is likely to fail. Lowe (1970) reported six patients with undoubted cartilage necrosis in whom osteotomy improved movement and satisfactory hips were obtained. This gives credibility to Waldenstrom's original concept of the cause as a failure of synovial fluid secretion rather than avascular necrosis – a proposition supported by Cruess (1963). Sugioka (1984) has reported good results with a trochanteric rotational osteotomy.

Lastly, should the opposite hip be pinned if it is clinically and radiologically normal? This will depend entirely on the surgeon's attitude towards any operation which is unnecessary in 80% of cases but valuable in 20%, the distinction at the time of decision being impossible. If the decision is against operation the patient must be warned to report immediately any symptoms, however mild, in the opposite hip.

The overall results of treatment are not encouraging. In 1957, Hall reviewed results in 173 hips collected at random by a British Orthopaedic Association working party. In total, 23% were classified as fair or poor. Furthermore, the late incidence of osteoarthritis is unknown, but it is certainly high and demands operation much more frequently than the effects of Perthes' disease, though of the two it is much the less common (Lloyd-Roberts, 1955; Boyer, Mickelson and Ponseti, 1981).

Congenital shortening, pseudarthrosis and absence of the femur, proximal focal femoral deficiency (PFFD)

Ring (1959, 1961) reviewed patients from The Hospitals for Sick Children, and Amstutz and Wilson (1962) included some of them in their larger survey and classification. More recently, Hamanishi (1980) and Pappas (1983) have surveyed a large number of patients and stressed the wide spectrum of this disorder.

The possible variations are protean but some definite patterns emerge. The cause is unknown. It is important to appreciate that although the obvious abnormality lies in the femur, the tibia and other parts of the limb may be dysplastic in one form or another, thus adding to the clinical problem.

Simple short femur

The commonest and fortunately the least disabling disorder is simple short femur. Shortening and lateral bowing of the femur is associated with some loss of internal rotation, or fixed external rotation of the leg. Fixed flexion deformity and limited abduction are uncommon. The radiograph discloses some lateral femoral bowing with central sclerosis more marked on the lateral side. The curve may extend into the neck, but there is no true coxa vara.

The leg inequality, which usually does not exceed 6.5 cm unless there is significant tibial growth deficiency, can be managed by femoral lengthening using modern techniques. Ring (1959) observed that the relative discrepancy

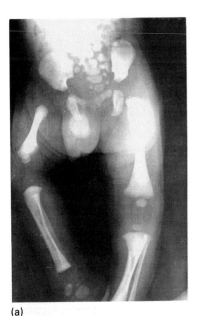

(a)

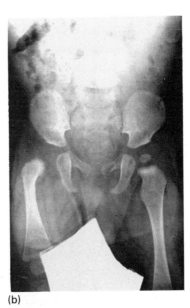

(b)

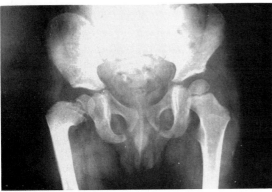

(c)

Figure 13.10 Proximal focal femoral deficiency. (a) At birth. Note the bulbous proximal femoral shaft, which has not migrated proximally and is held away from the ilium by the unossified proximal femoral head and neck. (b) Same patient at 1 year. Note that the femoral neck is ossifying and the head is appearing without any treatment. (c) Same patient at 3.5 years. The femoral head and neck are now ossified but there is some coxa vara and shortening

between the femurs remains constant, so an early and reasonably accurate prognosis is possible.

The condition is sometimes bilateral and symmetrical, thus disposing of both the need for treatment and the suggestion that fractures are responsible.

Short femur with coxa vara

The outlook here is much less favourable, for the ultimate shortening will exceed 7.5 cm and is frequently 15–17.5 cm. The signs are similar to those in simple shortening, but are exaggerated. The coxa vara, as seen on the radiograph, is quite different from the infantile form already described, for although the trochanter may be elongated there are no changes of the growth plate. The neck curves downwards to end in a bullet-shaped head, the epiphysis of which may extend along the superior border of the neck. Furthermore, the acetabulum may be dysplasic.

Shortening dominates the outlook. The coxa vara should be corrected by abduction osteotomy if there is significant abductor insufficiency or adduction deformity. Modern techniques of leg lengthening can be used but the problems with instability both at the hip and at the knee often make it difficult to gain the desired amount of lengthening, in which case disarticulation through the knee or ankle may be indicated, as an alternative to an extension prosthesis, to allow a prosthesis with a good prosthetic knee.

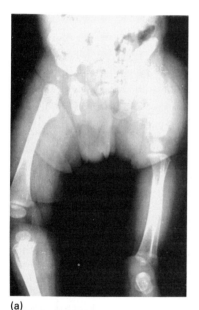

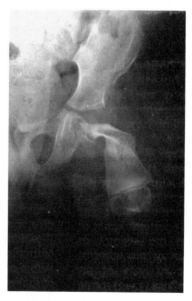

(a)

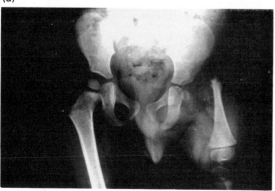

(b)

Figure 13.11 (a) Proximal focal femoral deficiency, unstable type, at 6 months of age. The proximal femur is already migrating upwards and looks irregular. (b) Same patient at 20 months. The femoral head is now ossified but the neck/shaft complex is unstable. (c) Same patient after a King's operation. The femoral head is in severe varus but the neck/shaft complex is now stable

Hypoplasia of the upper third of the femur

In hypoplasia of the upper third of the femur, the femur is narrow and short at birth, often ending in a bulbous proximal extremity. This may be misinterpreted as total absence of the proximal third with instability of the remainder (Figure 13.10). Fixsen and Lloyd-Roberts (1974) pointed out the importance of the appearance of the upper end of the ossified femur in relation to the likely stability of the head and neck. In the bulbous type the cartilage is likely to ossify without a pseudarthrosis. However, some coxa vara may occur and an abduction osteotomy may be necessary. If the proximal end is pointed or tufted, there is nearly always a pseudarthrosis and progressive coxa vara, which should be stabilized by bone grafting or the operation recommended by King (1969) (Figure 13.11). The benefit of this operation is stabilization of the hip to aid the fitting of a prosthesis. If the foot is going to be at approximately the level of the opposite knee, a choice has to be made between amputation of the foot with arthrodesis of the knee to provide a good above-knee stump at maturity (Panting and Williams, 1978) and rotation of the ankle through 180 degrees to produce a knee joint as described by Van Nes in 1950 (reviewed by Kostuik *et al*, 1975).

Absence of the greater part or the entire femur

In the absence of the greater part of or the entire femur, the main issue is whether or not to stabilize the femoral condyles or upper tibia upon the pelvis by arthrodesis, or whether to accept the totally flail assembly. Prostheses are needed in either event, and the decision should be taken with the advice of the prosthetic surgeon as to whether they would prefer a flail limb or an arthrodesis to the pelvis.

Persistent femoral anteversion (fetal alignment)

Some children walk with feet turned in (pigeon toes) and others with medial rotation of the whole leg which is best identified by watching for inward inclination or 'squinting' of the patellae. These will be found to have limited or absent external rotation with the hips extended, but a relatively free range in flexion. These children characteristically sit between the legs in the so-called 'W' or television position. This is one of the commonest causes of intoeing gait.

In describing this, Somerville (1957) pointed out that the femoral neck of the normal fetus at 30 weeks is inclined forwards (anteverted) about 60 degrees, but this angle gradually moulds to the adult value of about 10 degrees during childhood. Failure to mould constitutes persistent femoral anteversion. There is an obvious temptation to include this among the anomalies associated with congenital dislocation.

Provided that some external rotation remains, there is unlikely to be a disability, but otherwise the child's agility may be handicapped and this is exaggerated if a compensating external tibial torsion develops. These cases are not only very clumsy but also very ugly, walking as though knock-kneed, with pronated feet, and running with their legs below the knee flailing laterally. The effects that this malalignment may have on hip or knee joints over the years are still not known.

Clearly, operation is occasionally justified to correct the anteversion and improve the gait, before secondary changes in the tibia, or possibly the hip, develop. Somerville recommended rotation osteotomy if external rotation of the hip was no more than 15 degrees, and in the more severe added a medial rotation osteotomy of the tibia. This is largely a cosmetic operation and should only be undertaken in the most severely affected patients.

McSweeny (1971) suggested that about 13% of the population studied showed intoeing gait associated with persistent femoral anteversion. The majority of these would correct their intoeing by the age of 7 years, although many of them retain some femoral anteversion and correct their intoeing by increasing the external tibial torsion. Only 1 patient out of 174 required femoral osteotomy. Further long-term studies into adult life are necessary to establish whether or not persistent femoral anteversion does predispose to problems in either the hip or the knee in later life. A recent small study (Kitaoka *et al.*, 1989) showed no relation between femoral anteversion and osteoarthritis of the hip.

Femoral retroversion of infancy

Babies are sometimes seen who lie with their legs externally rotated and, on examination, lack internal rotation in extension but not in flexion (Figure 13.12). Harris (1965) showed that these have retroversion of their femoral necks and that many are habitually nursed in the prone position with legs straight and laterally rotated.

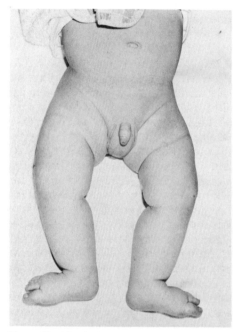

Figure 13.12 Typical clinical appearance of femoral retroversion

Progress towards spontaneous correction is generally very rapid and good, correction usually occurring by the age of 2 years. One problem about this condition is that it can mimic congenital dislocation in the hip in which the leg commonly lies in external rotation, but there should be the other signs of shortening and limitation of abduction unless the condition is bilateral and the child has excessive joint laxity.

Transient synovitis of the hip

'Coxalgia fugax' is a picturesque and descriptive synonym and describes exactly what transient synovitis of the hip is – a fleeting pain in the hip. Another synonym ('irritable hip') describes the physical signs, and a third

('observation hip') reminds us of its earlier significance as a possible presenting feature of tuberculosis (coxalgia).

Today it is the commonest clinical syndrome in the hip joint of children, predominantly affecting boys who are under 10 years of age. There is limp with or without pain, which is usually felt in the knee rather than the hip. Signs are very variable, sometimes no more than limitation at the extremes of all movements. In others there is fixed flexion and greatly restricted movement especially into abduction which, if forced, may stimulate adductor muscle spasm, when if there is fever, an infective arthirtis may be suspected.

The signs are short lived, lasting between a few days and, rarely, 2–3 weeks. Bed rest seems to aid recovery. Occasionally the attack is repeated.

Radiographs of the hip are usually normal, although there is sometimes a suspicion of joint space widening and of capsular thickening or distension, but this may equally be explained by an unusual opacity of the psoas and obturator internus (Adams, 1963). Ultrasound can now be used to identify the presence and size of the effusion.

The cause remains unknown; injury, low-grade local infection and synovial hypersensitivity have all been incriminated, but no hard evidence is forthcoming to support any one candidate (Adams, 1963; Hardinge, 1970).

It is tempting to regard transitory synovitis as a *forme fruste* of Perthes' disease because of their similarity in presentation. This problem is difficult to resolve because a mild pre-existing synovitis may have been ignored and forgotten when Perthes' disease develops later. Adams denied an association, whereas de Valderrama (1963) reckoned 2% to be a low estimate. Jacobs (1960) reported three patients who developed Perthes' disease among 25 with synovitis who were followed up. Kemp's views (1969) are mentioned later.

The significance of transient synovitis lies in the possibility that, in spite of the virtual disappearance of tuberculosis in the western world, it may still be the presenting syndrome of significant disease not yet visible on the radiograph or otherwise not recognized. Thus Perthes' disease, juvenile chronic arthritis, mild low-grade infection and the predisplacement phase of adolescent coxa vara may all, on occasions, pass through a similar initial phase.

The problem is best resolved (except when infection is suspected) either by resting the child in bed at home for a week or in hospital if home conditions do not allow satisfactory bed rest, and re-examining him in 2 weeks. If any signs persist, further investigation should follow; a bone scan can be very useful, particularly in showing a cold spot if early Perthes' disease is suspected.

It is generally believed this synovitis is truly transient and leaves no permanent scars. However, a proportion will later develop Perthes' disease or juvenile chronic arthritis. De Valderrama (1963) followed up 23 patients for an average of 21 years. Two-thirds of the children spent an average of 3.5 months in hospital, which suggests a much more severe disease than the transitory synovitis we know nowadays.

Legg–Calvé–Perthes' disease (coxa plana, osteochondritis juvenalis, pseudocoxalgia)

Perthes' disease is the abbreviated synonym for Legg–Calvé–Perthes' disease in general use, and has the virtue of historical accuracy for Legg and Calvé and Perthes all described the condition independently in 1910, but Perthes published a further, more precise, account in 1913. Waldenstrom is sometimes credited with the original account – one year before, in 1909 – but he forfeits eponymous immortality by regarding it as a variety of tuberculosis and compounding this error in 1910. Furthermore, Perthes recognized the ischaemic nature of the disease.

Aetiology and pathogenesis

Most cases of Perthes' disease arise between 3 and 10 years of age; boys predominate (4:1) and only 10% are bilateral. It is less common than congenital dislocation, but more so than adolescent coxa vara. A full historical, radiological and clinical review is well presented by Catterall (1982).

Disturbance of the blood supply to the epiphysis is accepted as the cause. Having accepted that, one must face the first of the many difficulties in the understanding of the nature of the disease. The known avascular necroses of transcervical fracture, coxa vara,

Gaucher's disease and so on behave in a totally different way, for progressive loss of movement, deformity and even ankylosis follow, whereas in Perthes' disease early limitation of movement usually improves and fixed deformity is transitory, thus more closely resembling vascular disturbance in congenital dislocation.

The relationship to transient synovitis has already been discussed and the late structural effects mentioned. Synovitis may have an obliterative influence on the vessels of the retinaculum, which are at all times vulnerable (*see* 'coxa vara'). If they are obstructed, this compromises the vascularity of the femoral head (Ferguson and Howarth, 1934). In this connection, Hipp (1962) claimed to have demonstrated vascular insufficiency of the vessels supplying the head by angioradiography.

Experimental investigations have for the most part involved disruption of the epiphyseal blood supply by crude methods and then studying the effects of total avascular necrosis. No contribution has been made by so reproducing in an animal a common and easily observed happening in man – a criticism that applies to many animal experiments.

Kemp (1969) approached the problem in a more sophisticated fashion. Basing his investigations on the fact that some breeds of dog are subject to the naturally occurring disease and some are not, he sought the difference in epiphyseal blood supply. In vulnerable animals the epiphyseal vessels ran an exposed extraperiosteal course and were therefore subject to changes in intra-articular pressure. Immune animals carried their vessels within the bone. furthermore, he was able to reproduce epiphyseal necrosis by raising intra-articular pressure in the first group, but not in the second. This brings us back again to the role of transitory pressure changes in, for example, transient synovitis.

The variability of the vascular arrangements between species of dogs stimulated an interest in the possibility of similar genetic factors operating in man. The disease has been reported in identical twins several times, and surveys of large series have variously estimated familial associations at between 5 and 20%. Studies at The Hospitals for Sick Children (Catterall) and Edinburgh (Wynne-Davies) have shown an association between Perthes' disease and genitourinary abnormality.

Histological reports are scanty. Ferguson and Howarth's observations on the vascular changes have been mentioned. Ponseti (1956) found disorganization of the epiphyseal plate and irregular enchondral ossification. Premature fusion is not uncommon and it may be assumed that this is due to ischaemia of developing cartilage cells.

Specimens from the epiphysis itself are rarely obtained. In his recent monograph, Catterall (1982) has reviewed histological material collected from various centres throughout the world, which shows avascular necrosis undergoing revascularization, with areas of normal bone alternating with areas of necrosis undergoing osteoblastic absorption and replacement by granulation and, later, fibrous tissue. Elsewhere there is active osteoblastic activity with new bone being laid down on the surface of the dead trabeculae. In the single specimen report by McKibbin and Ralis (1974) the microscopic appearances were correlated with microradiography. This showed that increased opacity represents new bone laid down in dead trabeculae, whereas radiolucent areas represent absorption and fibrous replacement. The joint space commonly appears widened; this is due to ischaemia affecting the cells of the epiphysis, such that ossification does not spread from the bony nucleus towards the periphery. At the same time, cartilage proliferation in the surface layers of the femoral head continues, nourished by synovial fluid, and so there is both a relative and an absolute increase in the thickness of cartilage that shows an increase in the joint space. In severe cases premature closure of the growth plate may be seen, with widening and shortening of the femoral neck. There are changes in the acetabulum, with irregularity of the subchondral bone and adaptation of the acetabulum to the shape of the deformed femoral head, producing the so-called state of 'congruous incongruity' of the hip joint.

Radiologically the head changes are sometimes irregular, with areas of apparent translucency and presumably viability in one part, and density suggesting sequestration in others (Goff, 1954; O'Gara, 1959; Catterall, 1971).

The histological and radiological variability suggests that Perthes' disease represents incomplete ischaemic necrosis which does not necessarily occur in one moment in time. Thus sequestration and repair seem to run concurrently in some areas whereas in others, sequestration or normal texture predominate (segmental necrosis). In this way one may explain the clinical differences between avascular necrosis following a fracture or epiphyseal displacement which cause total ischaemia of the head and the articular cartilage, and the more benign course of partial ischaemia seen in Perthes' disease.

Clinical features

Initially the clinical features resemble transient synovitis, with limp predominating over pain. Abduction in flexion is invariably limited. Rotation at the hip is nearly always limited – usually internal rotation but occasionally external rotation. Wasting is related to the duration of the disease at the time of diagnosis, and shortening suggests collapse of the head and, later, premature epiphyseal arrest.

The time taken for evolution from onset to final healing is about 4 years, but following an initial period of hip joint irritability the disease causes little or no discomfort even when it is not treated.

Radiological features

Radiological features are divided traditionally into three phases. These descriptions assume that the whole head is involved, and make no concessions to the variability of the early radiographic appearances and the possibility of partial involvement. The following account refers to the anterior projection only, but it should be emphasized that some early signs and later, more subtle, signs are better seen in the lateral projection.

The initial phase lasts about 6 months and varies from normality to some porosis, with apparent increase in joint space and capsular thickening. This is followed by increasing opacity of the epiphysis, which is reduced in both diameters. There is often a radiolucent zone in the metaphysis and in the subchondral area of the epiphysis. In the patient who has the clinical signs and symptoms of Perthes' disease but the X-ray appears normal, a bone scan can be very useful in confirming the diagnosis, as in Perthes' disease it will show a definite cold segment within the femoral head which corresponds to the area of segmental avascular necrosis.

The fragmentation phase follows and lasts for about 1 year. The homogenous density is broken up by radiolucent areas, suggesting that revascularization is beginning. Further radiolucent areas may spread from the epiphyseal plate into the metaphysis.

The phase of repair lasts for 2 years or more. In the head the radiolucent areas gradually encroach upon the dense, until normal bone density is restored. During this time the head may be seen to flatten, bulging from the cup of the acetabulum, and the neck thickens to support the coincidental widening of the epiphyseal plate. The metaphyseal lesions heal, the growth plate may fuse early and the trochanter lengthen in sympathy. At worst, in the final state the head is as flat as a mushroom, bulging and subluxating laterally, supported on a short neck.

This is a general description of the evolution of the disease when the whole head is involved. We will discuss the variations seen in partial involvement later.

Differential diagnosis

Although femoral capital necrosis complicates several dissimilar conditions such as traumatic or congenital dislocation, sickle cell anaemia and so on, difficulty only arises in practice when bilateral Perthes' disease is mistaken for dysplasia epiphysealis multiplex. This is resolved in favour of the latter when changes are found in the epiphysis of wrist or ankle. It is also extremely uncommon to see identical changes in both femoral heads in bilateral Perthes' disease, whereas in multiple epiphyseal dysplasia the changes are usually very similar in the two femoral heads.

General prognosis

The development of late osteoarthritis is related to residual deformity of the head at maturity (Helbo, 1953; Stulberg *et al*, 1981). In general, the outcome is influenced by age of onset (the earlier the better) and sex (girls are affected worse than boys). The stage at which the diagnosis is made is important in that those who would benefit from treatment are best treated early, for established deformity is irremediable. The extent of head involvement rather than delay in diagnosis is often more important.

Ratliff (1978) followed a group of unselected patients with Perthes' disease into adult life. His conclusions were that, after 30 years, only two in five patients would be radiologically normal, but four out of five would be clinically fully active and free from pain. In a further smaller group followed for 41 years there was little evidence of further deterioration. The appearance of 'congruous incongruity' appears to be compatible with good function up to the age of 50. When the upper femoral epiphysis remains well contained either following no treatment in mild forms of Perthes' disease or following containment treatment in severe forms, the long-term result is likely to be good.

Factors influencing the natural history of the disease

These may be considered under two categories. Firstly the effect of treatment and secondly those factors inherent to the disease.

Treatment

If 'treatment' is taken to mean relief from weight bearing only (bed rest, caliper and so on) and the results obtained are considered, there is an immediate difficulty, for the results of any one method are variable although they do relate to age of onset, sex and, in some, the stage at diagnosis. Unless the results of different methods can be compared in comparable patients their relative contributions remain uncertain.

Evans and Lloyd-Roberts (1958) compared inpatient traction followed by an outpatient caliper regimen with outpatient management alone using a Snyder sling. This was later compared with a series of patients who were given no treatment (Murley, 1962), and it appeared that there was no significant difference between the two series. We now know that this conclusion is fallacious and probably none of these treatments affects the natural history of the disease, so it is not surprising that they produce a similar result.

Further scrutiny, however, revealed that a disproportionate number had only half of the head involved (good prognosis) or total collapse at the time of diagnosis. In both these situations treatment is unlikely to be of great benefit (*see* below).

If protection from weight bearing alone is an advantage, complete, enforced and prolonged bed rest with traction should give the best results. Brotherton and McKibbin (1976) reported a series of 103 hips followed up for an average of 17 years, treated by recumbency and containment in broomstick plasters for an average period of 26 months. This series showed remarkably good results, particularly in those hips with the most severe form of Perthes' disease.

Inherent factors

From that already said, it is clear that there is lack of one or more further parameters by which one can distinguish between one hip and another so that the natural history in each may be anticipated. One could then decide rationally for or against treatment and, if for, which method to use. The most promising development is based on distinguishing between the proportion of the head which is abnormal and possibly necrotic, and that which seems normal. The assessment must be radiological and so suffers from the limitations of visualizing a sphere in only two planes.

Goff (1954) noted that the disease frequently involved only the anterior non-weight-bearing segment and that healing in these was much more rapid and complete. O'Gara (1959) definitely established that the prognosis was very good in those with anterior half involvement. Catterall (1971) studied patients at The Hospitals for Sick Children and concluded that there are four main groups in which the outcome varies.

Group 1

Anterior half only necrotic; no collapse; no sequestration. Restoration of head shape very good. This is similar to O'Gara's variety and the distinction between normal and abnormal is well seen in the lateral view (Figure 13.13).

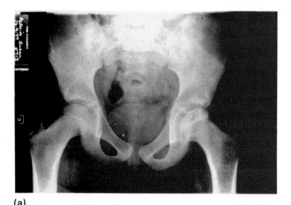

(a)

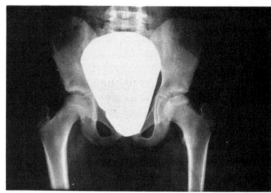

(b)

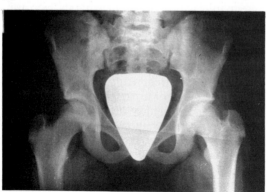

(c)

Figure 13.13 Group 1 Perthes' disease. (a) At diagnosis. (b) Same patient 10 months later, with no treatment. (c) Same patient 3 years later. Treatment was observation only. Note that the head has re-formed well without significant loss of height or deformation

Group 2

More than anterior half necrotic. Sequestration occurs and collapse is unlikely but possible; healing is good. On the radiograph there is often a central dense area with normal radiolucency at both ends.

Group 3

Only the posterior third is viable. Collapse and bulging beyond the rim of the acetabulum is common. There may be a small area of normal density at one pole of the necrotic area.

Group 4

The whole epiphysis is necrotic. Collapse is severe; bulging is lateral and posterior giving the appearance of a mushroom head (Figure 13.14).

There are difficulties in the interpretation of radiographs, particularly early in the disease when it may be necessary to wait until the type becomes recognizable.

In general, groups 1 and 2 have good results, but groups 3 and 4 have fair or poor results with conventional modes of treatment excluding containment (discussed later). The factor of age is still valid because below 4 years of age results are good and uninfluenced by treatment. The factor of sex and the unfavourable course in girls is explained by the predilection of girls for groups 3 and 4 (overall incidence in relation to boys, 4:1; groups 3 and 4, 2:1).

Observations on treatment

It is evident that one must not think of Perthes' disease as a single entity with a constant pattern of behaviour, but rather as a varying manifestation of a common cause.

All conventional methods have disadvantages. Prolonged bed rest in hospital must be unchallengable to justify its social and economic disadvantages. The Snyder sling with crutches is too easily rejected by the patient and is a cause of unnecessary shortening. An ischial bearing caliper often encourages subluxation in poliomyelitis and the same criticism applies in Perthes' disease.

The contemporary concept is one of containment of the head deeply within the acetabulum so that during the phase of softening the

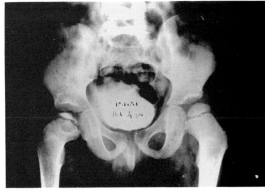

(a)

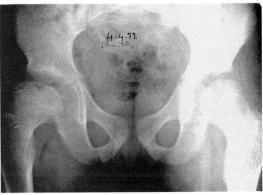

(b)

Figure 13.14 Group 4 Perthes' disease. (a) At age 4 years. Note the involvement of the whole head and the marked metaphyseal changes. (b) Same patient 5.5 years later at 10 years of age. Note the lateral extrusion of the head and significant flattening. The only treatment was weight relief on crutches

anterolateral segment of the head is moulded by the socket and prevented from bulging outwards, thus allowing the hip to subluxate. As usual, this method is not entirely new. W. R. Bristow insisted that the Jones frames, upon which these children were nursed, be abducted widely to contain the head within the acetabular mould. The Brotherton and McKibbin (1976) series, in which bed rest was combined with containment, provides further evidence that such treatment can produce good results.

Abduction and therefore containment may be achieved by broomstick plaster (Petrie and Bitenc, 1967) in which the child walks with some abduction and internal rotation. Harrison, Turner and Nicolson (1969) reported good results using a similar device in moulded leather with crutches. Our preference is for a femoral varus and external rotation osteotomy allowing the child full freedom after union (Axer, 1965).

The selection of patients for operation is based on the concept of the 'head at risk' – that is, a head which can be shown to be progressively subluxing laterally. The other signs associated with the head at risk are speckled calcification lateral to the epiphysis, radiolucency of the lateral margin of the epiphysis, a diffuse metaphyseal reaction and a horizontal growth plate. Lateral extrusion is by far the most important sign, and examination under anaesthetic combined with an arthrogram is the most satisfactory way of demonstrating not only the 'head at risk' but also whether abduction and internal rotation will contain the head satisfactorily within the acetabulum. We now believe that all hips with evidence of the 'head at risk', which can be improved on abduction and internal rotation as shown by examination under anaesthetic and arthrogram, should be treated by containment. We prefer to use an upper femoral adduction external rotation osteotomy to achieve this containment. In his recent monograph, Catterall (1982) makes two important points. The first is that in the patient with group 4 disease who is over the age of 8, it is probably best to do a containment osteotomy before there is evidence of the head at risk because of the rapid deterioration of these hips and the generally poor results obtained if they are left in these older patients. The second point is that, if it is not possible to achieve containment in a subluxed hip, and the hip appears to be hinging into abduction when examined with an arthrogram, then correcting the adduction deformity by abduction osteotomy will sometimes be the treatment of choice (Quain and Catterall, 1986). Despite a great deal of interest in this condition over the past few years, we are still far from understanding it fully. At present it is felt that containment treatment can influence the ultimate end result of the process we call Perthes' disease. Only further long-term studies of the results of this type of treatment will confirm whether or not this is true.

Osteochondritis dissecans

Osteochondritis dissecans (Figure 13.15) has the same appearances in the hip as osteochondritis elsewhere – that is, part of the convex

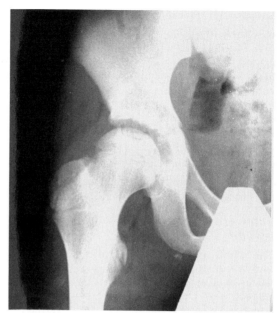

(a)

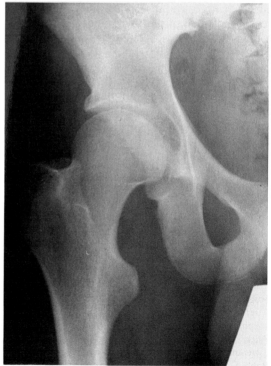

(b)

Figure 13.15 Osteochondritis dissecans of the hip. (a) At diagnosis. (b) Same patient, showing healing, 7 years later. In children it is most likely to be the aftermath of Perthes' disease – a segment that fails to revascularize. In older patients, however, it may arise primarily

surface of the joint becomes dense and separated from its surroundings by a radiolucent line. The lesion in the hip encroaches upon the weight-bearing area but, because of the congruity of the joint in this situation, loose bodies rarely occur.

Fortunately, the symptoms are usually mild and tend to improve despite failure of healing. Ratliff (1976) reported two patients followed for 30 years without healing but with good hips. It is fortunate that an expectant attitude is justified (Guilleminet and Barbier, 1957).

Some other conditions involving the hip and thigh

The hip in myelomeningocele and in cerebral palsy is discussed on pages 66 and 58, respectively. Delay in femoral head ossification occurs in several general disorders, notably mongolism, cretinism, achondroplasia, osteochondrodystrophy and diastrophic dwarfism. Dysplasia epiphysealis multiplex (page 5) resembles bilateral Perthes' disease. Rheumatoid arthritis and arthrogryposis frequently involve the hip. Coxa vara may complicate rickets (page 23) and osteogenesis imperfecta (page 11). The trochanteric area is a favoured site for fibrous dysplasia (page 28) and osteoid osteoma (page 31). Diaphyseal dyostosis, Engelmann's disease (page 13), Gaucher's disease (page 22), dyschondroplasia and osteopetrosis are prone to involve the shaft of the femur.

References

Adams, J. A. (1963) Transient synovitis of the hip joint in children. *J. Bone Jt. Surg.* **45B**, 471

Amstutz, H. C. and Wilson, P. D. Jr (1962) Dysgenesis of the proximal femur (coxa vara) and its surgical management. *J. Bone Jt. Surg.* **44A**, 1

Angel, J. C. and Dunn, D. M. (1975) Open operative replacement for adolescent slipping of the upper femoral epiphysis. *J. Bone Jt. Surg.* **57B**, 112 [report]

Axer, A. (1965) Subtrochanteric osteotomy in the treatment of Perthes' disease. *J. Bone Jt. Surg.* **47B**, 489

Babb, F. S., Ghormley, R. K. and chatterton, C. C. (1949) Congenital coxa vara. *J. Bone Jt. Surg.* **31A**, 115

Barlow, T. G. (1962) Early diagnosis and treatment of congenital dislocation of the hip. *J. Bone Jt. Surg.* **44B**, 292

Blockey, N. J. (1969) Observations on infantile coxa vara. *J. Bone Jt. Surg.* **51B**, 106

Botting, T. D. J. and Scrase, W. H. (1965) Premature epiphyseal fusion at the knee complicating prolonged immobilisation for CDH. *J. Bone Jt. Surg.* **47B**, 280

Boyer, D. W., Mickelson, M. R. and Ponseti, I. V. (1981) Slipped capital femoral epiphysis. *J. Bone Jt. Surg.* **63A**, 85

Brotherton, B. J. (1976) The long-term results of the treatment of Perthes' disease by recumbency and femoral head containment. *J. Bone Jt. Surg.* **58B**, 131 [report]

Carter, C. and Wilkinson, J. (1964) Persistent joint laxity and congenital dislocation of the hip. *J. Bone Jt. Surg.* **46B**, 40

Catterall, A. C. (1970) The natural history of Perthes' disease. *J. Bone Jt. Surg.* **52B**, 186 [report]

Catterall, A. (1982) *Legg–Calve–Perthes' Disease.* Edinburgh: Churchill Livingstone

Chiari, K. (1955) Ergebnisse mit der Beckenosteotomie als Pfannendachplastik. *Z. Orthop.* **87**, 14

Clarke, N. M. P., Harcke, H. T., McHugh, P., Lee, M. S., Borns, P. F. and MacEwen, G. D. (1985) Real-time ultrasound in the diagnosis of congenital dislocation and dysplasia of the hip. *J. Bone Jt. Surg.* **67B**, 406–412

Colonna, P. C. (1932) Congenital dislocation of the hip in older subjects. *J. Bone Jt. Surg.* **14**, 277

Colonna, P. C. (1965) Capsular arthroplasty for congenital dislocation of the hip: indications and technique. *J. Bone Jt. Surg.* **47A**, 437

Cruess, R. L. (1963) Pathology of acute necrosis of cartilage in slipping of the capital femoral epiphysis. *J. Bone Jt. Surg.* **45A**, 1013

de Valderrama, J. A. F. (1963) 'Observation hip' and its late sequelae. *J. Bone Jt. Surg.* **45B**, 462

Dunn, D. M. (1964) Treatment of adolescent slipping of the upper femoral epiphysis. *J. Bone Jt. Surg.* **46B**, 621

Durbin, F. C. (1960) Treatment of slipped upper femoral epiphysis. *J. Bone Jt. Surg.* **42B**, 289

Dwyer, N. St J. P., Bernard, A. A. and O'Hara, J. N. (1986) Congenital dislocation of the hip. Open reduction by the medial approach in infancy. *J. Bone Jt. Surg.* **68B**, 668

Edgren, W. (1965) Coxa plana. *Acta Orthop. Scand.* suppl. 84

Evans, D. L. and Lloyd-Roberts, G. C. (1958) Treatment in Legg–Calve–Perthes' disease: a comparison of in-patient and out-patient methods. *J. Bone Jt. Surg.* **40B**, 182

Eyre-Brook, A. L. (1936) Osteochondritis deformans coxae juvenilis or Perthes' disease: results of treatment by traction in recumbency. *Br. J. Surg.* **24**, 166

Eyre-Brook, A. L. (1966) Treatment of congenital dislocation or subluxation of the hip in children over the age of three years. *J. Bone Jt. Surg.* **48B**, 682

Fahey, J. J. and O'Brien, E. T. (1965) Acute slipped capital femoral epiphysis. *J. Bone Jt. Surg.* **47A**, 1105

Fairbank, T. J. (1969) Manipulative reduction in slipped upper femoral epiphysis. *J. Bone Jt. Surg.* **51B**, 252

Ferguson, A. B. and Howorth, M. B. (1934) Coxa plana and related conditions at the hip. *J. Bone Jt. Surg.* **16**, 781

Ferguson, A. B. Jr (1973) Primary open reduction of CDH using a median adductor approach. *J. Bone Jt. Surg.* **55A**, 671

Finlay, H. V. L., Maudsley, R. H. and Busfield, P. I. (1967) Dislocatable hip and dislocated hip in the newborn infant. *Br. Med. J.* **4**, 377

Fixsen, J. A. and Lloyd-Roberts, G. C. (1974) Natural history and early treatment of proximal femoral dysplasia. *J. Bone Jt. Surg.* **56B**, 86

Fixsen, J. A. (1987) Anterior and posterior displacement of the hip after innominate osteotomy. *J. Bone Jt. Surg.* **69B**, 361–364

Fredensborg, N. (1976) Results of early treatment of typical CDH in Malmo. *J. Bone Jt Surg.* **58B**, 272

Galloway, H. P. H. (1962) The open operation for CDH. *J. Bone Jt. Surg.* **8**, 539

Ghormley, R. K. and Fairchild, R. D. (1940) Diagnosis and treatment of slipped epiphyses. *J. Am. Med. Ass.* **114**, 229

Goff, C. W. (1954) *Legg–Calve–Perthes' Syndrome.* Springfield, Ill.: Charles C. Thomas

Graf, R. (1983) New possibilities for the diagnosis of congenital hip joint dislocation by ultrasonography. *J. Ped. Orthop.* **3**, 354–359

Griffiths, M. J. (1976) Slipping of the capital femoral epiphysis. *Ann. R. Coll. Surg. Engl.* **58**, 34–42

Guilleminet, M. and Barbier, J. M. (1957) Osteochondritis dissecans of the hip. *J. Bone Jt Surg.* **39B**, 268

Hall, J. E. (1957) Results of treatment of slipped femoral epiphysis. *J. Bone Jt. Surg.* **39B**, 659

Hamanishi, C. (1980) Congenital short femur. *J. Bone Jt. Surg.* **62B**, 307

Hardinge, K. (1957) The etiology of transient synovitis of the hip in childhood. *J. Bone Jt. Surg.* **52B**, 100

Harris, N. H. (1965) A method of measurement of femoral neck anteversion and a preliminary report on its practical application. *J. Bone Jt. Surg.* **47B**, 188 [report]

Harris, N. H., Lloyd-Roberts, G. C. and Gallien, R. (1975) Acetabular development of CDH. *J. Bone Jt. Surg.* **57B**, 46

Harris, W. R. (1950) Endocrine basis for slipping of the upper femoral epiphysis. *J. Bone Jt. Surg.* **32B**, 5

Harrison, J. (1951) *Congenital Dislocation of the Hip.* Springfield, Ill.: Charles C. Thomas

Heikkila, E., Ryoppy, S. and Louhimo, I. (1985) Management of primary acetabular dysplasia. *J. Bone Jt. Surg.* **67B**, 25

Helbo, S. (1953) *Morbo Calve Perthes.* Odense: Fyns Tidendes

Herndon, C. H., Heyman, C. D. and Bell, D. M. (1963) Treatment of slipped capital femoral epiphysis by epiphyseodesis and osteoplasty of the femoral neck. *J. Bone Jt. Surg.* **45A**, 999

Hey-Groves, E. W. (1927) Reconstructive surgery of the hip. *Br. J. Surg.* **14**, 486

Hipp, E. (1962) Perthes' disease. *Z. Orthop.* **96**, suppl.

Ireland, J. and Newman, P. H. (1978) Triplane osteotomy for severely slipped upper femoral epiphysis. *J. Bone Jt.*

Surg. **60B**, 390

Jacobs, B. W. (1960) Early recognition of osteochondrosis of capital epiphysis of femur. *J. Am. Med. Ass.* **172**, 527

Kalamchi, A., and MacEwen, G. D. (1980) Avascular necrosis following treatment of congenital dislocation of the hip. *J. Bone Jt. Surg.* **62A**, 876–888

Kemp, H. (1960) *MS thesis.* University of London

King, R. E. (1969) In *Proximal Femoral Focal Deficiency: A Congenital Anomaly,* a symposium held in Washington, 13 June 1968. ed. G. T. Aitken. Washington DC: National Academy of Sciences, pp. 23–49

Kitaoka, H. B., Weiner, D. S., Cook, A. J., Hoyt Jr., W. A. and Askew, M. J. (1989) Relationship between femoral anteversion and osteoarthritis of the hip. *J. Ped. Orthop.* **9**, 396–404

Klein, A., Joplin, R., Reidy, J. and Hamelin, J. (1948) *Slipped Femoral Epiphysis.* Springfield, Ill.: Charles C. Thomas

Kostuik, J. P., Gillespie, R., Hall, J. E. and Hubbard, S. (1975) Van Nes rotational osteotomy for treatment of proximal femoral focal deficiency and congenital short femur. *J. Bone Jt. Surg.* **57A**, 1039

Langenskiold, A. and Salenius, P. (1967) Epiphyseodesis of the greater trochanter. *Acta Orthop. Scand.* **38**, 199

Le Mesurier, A. B. (1948) Developmental coxa vara. *J. Bone Jt. Surg.* **30B**, 595

Lloyd-Roberts, G. C. (1955) Osteoarthritis of the hip. *J. Bone Jt. Surg.* **37B**, 8

Lloyd-Roberts, G. C. and Pilcher, M. F. (1965) Structural idiopathic scoliosis in infancy. *J. Bone Jt. Surg.* **47B**, 520

Lloyd-Roberts, G. C. and Stone, K. H. (1963) Congenital hypoplasia of the upper femur. *J. Bone Jt. Surg.* **45B**, 557

Lloyd-Roberts, G. C. and Swann, M. (1966) Pitfalls in the management of CDH. *J. Bone Jt. Surg.* **48B**, 666

Lowe, H. G. (1970) Necrosis of articular cartilage after slipping of the capital femoral epiphysis. *J. Bone Jt. Surg.* **52B[R]**, 108

Ludloff, K. (1912/13) Open reduction of congenital hip dislocation by an anterior incision. *Am. J. Orthop. Surg.* **10**, 438

MacKenzie, I. G., Seddon, H. J. and Trevor, D. (1960) Congenital dislocation of the hip. *J. Bone Jt. Surg.* **42B**, 689

McKibbin, B. (1970) Anatomical factors in the stability of the hip joint in the newborn. *J. Bone Jt. Surg.* **52B**, 148

McKibbin, B. and Holdsworth, F. W. (1966) Nutrition of immature joint cartilage in the lamb. *J. Bone Jt. Surg.* **48B**, 793

McKibbin, B. and Ralis, Z. (1974) Pathological changes in a case of Perthes' disease. *J. Bone Jt. Surg.* **56B**, 438

McSweeny, A. (1971) a study of femoral torsion in children. *J. Bone Jt. Surg.* **53B**, 90

Morgan, J. D. and somerville, E. W. (1960) Normal and abnormal growth at the upper end of the femur. *J. Bone Jt. Surg.* **42B**, 264

Mubarak, S., Garfin, S., Vance, R., McKinnon, B. and Sutherland, D. (1981) Pitfalls in the use of the Pavlik harness for treatment of congenital dysplasia, subluxation and dislocation of the hip. *J. Bone Jt. Surg.* **63A**, 1239

Murley, A. H. G. (1962) To treat or not to treat in Perthes' disease. Proceedings of the American Orthopedic Association. *J. Bone Jt. Surg.* **44A**, 1705

Nelson, M. A. (1966) Early diagnosis of CDH. *J. Bone Jt. Surg.* **48B**, 388 [report]

Newman, P. H. (1960) Surgical treatment of slipping of the upper femoral epiphysis. *J. Bone Jt. Surg.* **42B**, 280

Ogden, J. A. and Moss, H. L. (1978)Pathologic anatomy of congenital hip disease. In *Progress in Orthopaedic Surgery*, vol. 2. Berlin: Springer-Verlag

O'Garra, J. A. (1959) Radiographic changes in Perthes' disease. *J. Bone Jt. Surg.* **41B**, 465

Panting, A. L. and Williams, P. F. (1978) Proximal femoral focal deficiency. *J. Bone Jt. Surg.* **60B**, 46

Pappas, A. M. (1983) Congenital abnormalities of the femur and related lower extremity malfunction: classification and treatment. *J. Ped. Orthop.* **3**, 45–60

Pearson, J. R. and Riddell, D. M. (1964) Subtrochanteric osteotomy in the treatment of slipped upper femoral epiphysis. *J. Bone Jt. Surg.* **46B**, 155 [report]

Pemberton, P. A. (1958) Osteotomy of the ilium with rotation of the acetabular roof for CDH. *J. Bone Jt. Surg.* **40A**, 724

Pemberton, P. A. (1965) Pericapsular osteotomy of the ilium for treatment of congenital subluxation and dislocation of the hip. *J. Bone Jt. Surg.* **47A**, 65

Petrie, J. G. and Bitenc, I. (1967) Abduction weight-bearing treatment in Legg–Calve–Perthes' disease. *J. Bone Jt. Surg.* **49A**, 1483 [report]

Platt, H. (1953) Congenital dislocation of the hip. *J. Bone Jt. Surg.* **35B**, 339

Platt, H. (1956) Congenital dislocation of the hip. In *Modern Trends in Orthopaedics – 2*. London: Butterworths

Ponseti, I. V. (1956) Legg–Perthes' disease: observations on pathological changes in two cases. *J. Bone Jt. Surg.* **38A**, 739

Powell, E. N., Gerratana, F. J. and Gage, J. R. (1986) Open reduction for congenital hip dislocation: the risk of avascular necrosis with three different approaches. *J. Ped. Orthop.* **6**, 127–132

Quain, S. and Catterall, A. (1986) Hinge abduction of the hip. *J. Bone Jt. Surg.* **68B**, 61

Ratliff, A. H. C. (1967a) Perthes' disease. *J. Bone Jt. Surg.* **49B**, 102

Ratliff, A. H. C. (1967b) Osteochondritis dissecans following Legg–Calve–Perthes' disease. *J. Bone Jt. Surg.* **49B**, 109

Ratliff, A. H. C. (1978) In *Hip Disorders in Children*, eds. G. C. Lloyd-Roberts and A. H. C. Ratliffe. London: Butterworths, p. 150–164

Ring, P. A. (1959) Congenital short femur. *J. Bone Jt. Surg.* **41B**, 73

Ring, P. A. (1961) congenital abnormalities of the femur. *Archs Dis. Childh.* **36**, 410

Sallis, J. G. and Smith, R. G. (1965) A study of the development of the acetabular roof in CDH. *Br. J. Surg.* **52**, 44

Salter, R. B. (1961) Innominate osteotomy in the treatment of congenital dislocation and subluxation of the hip. *J. Bone Jt. Surg.* **43B**, 518

Salter, R. B. (1969) *Recent Advances in Orthopaedics*. London: Churchill

Salter, R. B. and Field, P. (1960) Effects of continuous compression on living articular cartilage. *J. Bone Jt. Surg.* **42A**, 31

Salter, R. B., Simmonds, D. F., Malcolm, B. W., Rumble, E. J., MacMichael, D. and Clements, N. D. (1980) The biological effect of continuous passive motion on the healing of full-thickness defects in articular cartilage. *J. Bone Jt. Surg.* **62A**, 1232–1257

Scaglietti, O. and Calandriello, B. (1962) Open reduction of CDH. *J. Bone Jt. Surg.* **44B**, 257

Scott, J. C. (1953) Frame reduction in CDH. *J. Bone Jt. Surg.* **35B**, 372

Smaill, G. B. (1968) CDH in the newborn. *J. Bone Jt. Surg.* **50B**, 524

Somerville, E. W. (1953) Open reduction in CDH. *J. Bone Jt. Surg.* **35B**, 363

Somerville, E. W. (1957) Persistent foetal alignment of the hip. *J. Bone Jt. Surg.* **39B**, 106

Somerville, E. W. (1967) Results of treatment in 100 congenitally dislocated hips. *J. Bone Jt. Surg.* **49B**, 258

Somerville, E. W. and Scott, J. C. (1957) The direct approach to CDH. *J. Bone Jt. Surg.* **39B**, 623

Staheli, L. T. (1981) Stilted acetabular augmentation. *J. Ped. Orthop.* **1**, 32

Stulberg, S. D., Cooperman, D. R. and Wallenstein, R. (1981) The natural history of Legg–Calve–Perthes' disease. *J. Bone Jt. Surg.* **63A**, 1095–1108

Sugioka, Y. (1984) Trochanteric rotational osteotomy in the treatment of idiopathic and steroid-induced femoral head necrosis, Perthes' disease, slipped capital, femoral epiphysis and osteoarthrosis of the hip. *Clin. Orthop. Rel. Res.*, **184**, 12

Trevor, D. (1960) Treatment of congenital hip dysplasia in older children. *Proc. R. Soc. Med.* **53**, 481

Van Nes, C. P. (1950) Rotation-plasty for congenital defects of the femur. *J. Bone Jt. Surg.* **32B**, 12

Van Nes, C. P. (1964) Transplantation of the tibia and fibula to replace the femur following resection: 'turn-up plasty of the leg'. *J. Bone Jt. Surg.* **46A**, 1353

Vaughan-Jackson, O. J. (1956) Reducibility of slipped femoral capital epiphysis. *Proc. R. Soc. Med.* **49**, 812

Von Rosen, S. (1968) Further experience with CDH in the newborn. *J. Bone Jt. Surg.* **50B**, 538

Wainwright, D. (1976) The shelf operation for hip dysplasia in adolescence. *J. Bone Jt. Surg.* **58B**, 159–163

Waldenstrom, H. (1931) On necrosis of cartilage. *Acta Chir. Scand.* **67**, 936

Wilkinson, J. A. (1963) Prime factors in the aetiology of CDH. *J. Bone Jt. Surg.* **45B**, 268

Wilkinson, J. and Carter, C. (1960) Congenital dislocation of the hip. *J. Bone Jt. Surg.* **42B**, 669

Wynne-Davies, R. (1970) Acetabular dysplasia and joint laxity: two etiological factors in CDH. *J. Bone Jt. Surg.* **52B**, 704

Further reading

Catterall, A. (1982) *Legg–Calve–Perthes' Disease*. Edinburgh, London, New York: Churchill Livingstone

Somerville, E. W. (1982) *Displacement of the Hip in Childhood*. Berlin, Heidelberg, New York: Springer-Verlag

Tachdjian, M. O. (1982) *Congenital Dislocation of the Hip*. New York, Edinburgh, London: Churchill Livingstone

Wilkinson, J. A. (1985) *Congenital Displacement of the Hip Joint*. Berlin, Heidelberg, New York, Tokyo: Springer-Verlag

14

The knee and leg

A. M. Jackson

The knee

Genu recurvatum (back knee, hyperextended knee)

Symmetrical bilateral genu recurvatum of mild degree, especially in the female, may be physiological or a manifestation of one of the ligamentous laxity syndromes. When unilateral or severe the cause is much more likely to be pathological, either primary (congenital) or secondary to some other disorder. Radiologically one should distinguish between congruous hyperextension, anterior subluxation of the tibia and anterior dislocation of the tibia.

Primary congenital genu recurvatum

In primary congenital genu recurvatum the knee is dislocated and seems back to front – an illusion exaggerated by the development of an anterior skin crease, the prominence of the femoral condyles posteriorly, and forward subluxation of the hamstrings which cause increase in deformity if left untreated (Figure 14.1). Laurence (1967) collected cases of 41 knees from various centres and found that they could be divided into two groups. About half the cases achieved a fair outcome after conservative treatment with stretchings, strapping or serial plasters, whilst the other half were recalcitrant to conservative treatment. Undue force should not be applied or fractures may occur. The favourable or responsive group are usually neonates who have been subjected to abnormal moulding *in utero*, but who are otherwise normal. Examination at birth may show that the legs fit the curve of the abdomen

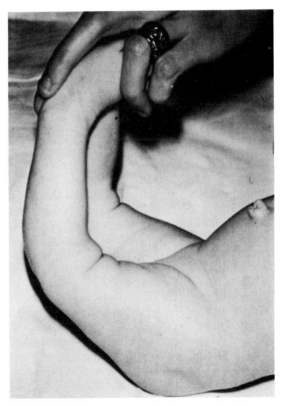

Figure 14.1 Genu recurvatum: the knee seems back to front

and the feet tuck under the chin. Dislocation of the knees in these children is perhaps analogous to the more common phenomenon of neonatal instability of the hip in an otherwise normal child.

In the more severe group, the cause seems to be amyoplasia of the quadriceps which are fibrotic. These patients usually fit somewhere under the broad heading of arthrogryposis. The patella is hypoplastic and may be adherent to the femur and the suprapatellar pouch obliterated, a feature which may be demonstrated on an arthrogram. The recalcitrant group tend to have less passive flexion at birth, averaging 12 degrees compared with 63 degrees in the favourable knees, and they are also commonly associated with other deformities such as club feet and dislocated hips which may make management difficult. In general, the knee should be treated before the hip so as to avoid the complication of quadriceps tension causing redislocation of the hip that has just been reduced.

Vigorous conservative treatment should be undertaken from day one, and the recalcitrant knees should be operated on when this diagnosis has become apparent. Curtis and Fisher (1969) have given a good account of the operative technique in which the quadriceps are lengthened, anterior capsulotomy is performed and the collateral ligaments are mobilized. The menisci usually have a normal appearance. The anterior cruciate ligament, if present, will be elongated and incompetent, in which case a procedure to tighten this structure seems a sensible addition to the operation. The importance of early treatment when there is a greater chance of achieving reduction and before secondary joint changes occur, is clear.

Congenital anterior subluxation of the tibia in extension is a rare condition. On flexion the knee reduces with a snap as the hamstrings and the ileo-tibial band pass posterior to the axis of knee flexion. This may cause symptoms of instability if not corrected by the time the child starts to walk. Early conservative treatment holding the knee at 90 degrees in a cast for 6–8 weeks has not been helpful, but a modification of the MacIntosh procedure has proved useful. A strip of ileo-tibial band still attached distally is passed obliquely behind the knee joint anterior to the vessels and through to the medial side of the knee, where it is attached through the vastus medialis to the margin of the rectus tendon.

Secondary genu recurvatum

Secondary genu recurvatum is a common feature of several neurological conditions and may become more pronounced as the child grows. In cerebral palsy and sometimes after head injury, the knee may be forced into hyperextension by spastic equinus deformity of the foot produced by increased tone in the soleus muscle. If spotted early, significant genu recurvatum may be prevented by timely lengthening of tendo Achillis. Muscle imbalance above the knee, either when spastic quadriceps are opposed by weak hamstrings or sometimes after an overenthusiastic hamstring release, will also produce this deformity. In polio, too, paralysis of the hamstrings in the presence of active quadriceps may produce stretching of the posterior soft tissues of the knee and gross recurvatum. However, in the flail knee it is well to remember that slight hyperextension may be essential for the stability of the knee in walking.

The same muscle imbalance is seen in spina bifida patients with a neurological level of L3/4 but this seldom interferes with the fitting of calipers or poses a clinical problem unless the knee becomes stiff in the extended position. When this happens, problems are encountered in daily living; for example, sitting at a table to work or to eat and getting into a car pose particular difficulties. If above-knee calipers are necessary anyway, quadriceps tenotomy can achieve knee flexion with ease. However, problems with the skin over the front of the knees must be anticipated since this skin may never have been stretched before. Further difficulties arise when there are fixed rotational deformities at the hips so that the knees do not flex in parallel. When this is the case, rotational femoral osteotomies will be required and there are dangers here, too. Correction of a major rotational deformity may compromise the blood supply and therefore the osteotomy is best controlled with a Rush nail so that adjustments can be made after release of the tourniquet should this prove necessary. The stiff hyperextended knee may also be a feature of arthrogryposis, and it is a rare sequel to injection-induced quadriceps contracture.

Damage to the growth plates on either side of the knee from any cause may result in a secondary genu recurvatum. In particular, iatrogenic damage should be avoided (Figure 14.2). For example, tibial tubercle surgery should not be performed before skeletal maturity and care should be taken when performing epiphysiodesis for leg length inequality (Poirier, 1968). When the recurvatum is due to bony deformity the increase in

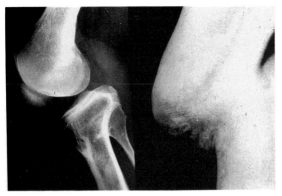

Figure 14.2 Tibial tubercle surgery in early childhood has resulted in tibia recurvatum and unsightly knee deformity

extension is accompanied by a corresponding decrease in flexion.

Knee flexion deformity

Knee flexion deformity is most commonly a secondary phenomenon but it should be recalled that there is invariably a transient physiological flexion deformity at birth. Of the many causes, myelomeningocele and arthrogryposis multiplex in particular may cause flexed knees at birth. In contrast, in cerebral palsy, myopathic and infective conditions, juvenile rheumatoid arthritis and permanent lateral dislocation of the patella the deformity appears later.

In planning treatment, two aspects must always be borne in mind. First, correction by serial plasters is liable to be spurious. The knee hinges open posteriorly without the tibia gliding forwards on the femoral condyles as in normal extension. In effect, the result is posterior subluxation of the tibia. To overcome this problem in haemophilia, a reversed dynamic sling may be used with the aim of producing gentle congruous extension (Stein and Dickson, 1975).

Secondly, when fixed flexion deformity in the younger child is treated by posterior capsulotomy and soft tissue release, restoration of muscle balance is most important if recurrence is to be prevented. The posterior release is best performed through medial and lateral incisions rather than from behind. Once skeletal maturity is approaching and there are established secondary changes in the joint,

supracondylar extension osteotomy is the preferred method of achieving correction. It may prove necessary to shorten the femur a little if the soft tissues will not stretch. A common error is to perform this osteotomy too high. The surgeon is wise to use X-ray control.

Flexion deformities with congenital skin webbing (popliteal web syndrome) are likely to be associated with other and grievous abnormalities. Sometimes an atavistic ischiocalcaneal band is present. Correction is difficult because neurovascular structures tend to lie in the free edge and resent the stretching needed to straighten the knee. Wound closure with Z-plasties and postoperative serial plasters are helpful, but even if good correction is achieved, there is a tendency to recurrence. On occasion, even femoral shortening has been of only temporary benefit in severe cases. As in arthrogryposis, postoperative splintage is of paramount importance.

Rarely, a bony block to extension is seen when an anterior cruciate avulsion of the intercondylar eminence has been inadequately reduced.

Genu valgum (knock knee)

Genu valgum is rarely other than idiopathic but may be secondary or apparent.

Idiopathic knock knee

Idiopathic knock knee is a very common physiological variant. Surveys of unselected children of different ages show a declining incidence with increasing age. For example, Morley (1957) examined 1000 school children and found 22% with a knock knee interval of 5 cm or more between the ages of 3 and 3.5 years, whereas at 7 years of age only 2% were similarly affected.

The appearance of a child with knock knee is well known (Figure 14.3). He stands with knees together and feet apart, with valgus calcaneum and pronated (flat) foot. He is usually active and agile, and in no way troubled by the deformity. To estimate the severity and assess progress, the knock knee interval is measured; that is to say, the distance between the medial malleoli with the child lying supine, the patellae pointing at the ceiling and the knees straight and in contact. Serial photographs are also helpful.

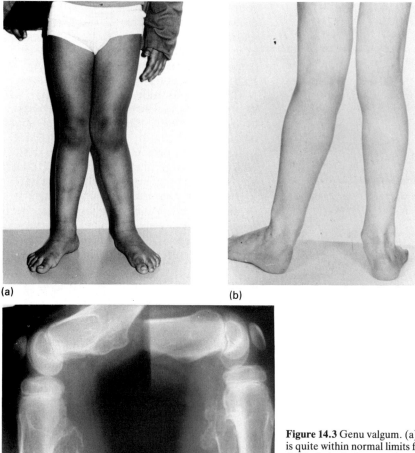

(a)

(b)

(c)

Figure 14.3 Genu valgum. (a) This degree of genu valgum is quite within normal limits for a child of this age (4 years). (b) Pathological genu valgum. The deformity is asymmetric. There are bony lumps visible at the knees and ankles, and the condition runs in the family. (c) The X-ray shows multiple exostoses (diaphyseal aclasis)

This, like some other postural and physiological variations, often engenders a surfeit of both anxiety and treatment, in spite of the probability of spontaneous correction. Furthermore, even if some deformity persists it becomes less conspicuous with growth. Thus a gap of 5 cm at 3 years of age looks quite different in a man of 1.8 metres.

The natural prognosis is so good that it is not possible to assess the effects of the treatments that are so freely prescribed. It is very hard to believe that an inside wedge on the shoe will transmit sufficient force through the ankle and subtalar joints to influence growth of the knee. A bumptious 4-year-old child is hardly likely to co-operate with any form of remedial physiotherapy and night splints are generally more helpful in maintaining a correction after surgery than in achieving it. Lastly, how often does one see an adult presenting in the outpatients' department complaining of knock knees?

Our practice is to teach the mother to measure the knock knee interval and to bring the child back only if the interval exceeds 10 cm. We then observe the child ourselves and resolve that if this deformity persists within 2 years of skeletal maturity, we will staple the lower medial femoral epiphysis. The 10 cm distance is chosen because it is possible that with time the lateral compartment of the knee may suffer or the patella sublux. The time is chosen because Pilcher (1962), in an earlier study of epiphyseal stapling in patients at The

Hospitals for Sick Children who were followed to maturity, found that a gap of 10 cm was corrected during about 1 year's growth. Furthermore, the later the operation, the fewer the candidates. Applying this nihilistic attitude to idiopathic knock knee, with its high rate of spontaneous resolution, has proved most satisfactory. Surgery is very seldom indicated.

Secondary knock knee

Deformity of significant degree (i.e. requiring treatment) is sometimes seen in heavy patients with paralytic conditions (notably meningomyelocele), juvenile rheumatoid arthritis, endocrine imbalance (adiposogenital) and following growth plate damage due to infection, trauma and radiotherapy. The deformity may be seen in syndromes such as homocystinuria and the Ellis–Van Creveld syndrome (Figure 14.4). In this latter condition and in some of the bone dysplasias, delay in ossification may make it difficult to discern the joint line. An arthrogram will help resolve this problem and may influence the decision on whether to perform a femoral or tibial osteotomy.

Patellar tracking should always be checked when valgus deformity is apparent; when correcting severe deformity, an extensive lateral soft tissue release may be necessary, taking care to protect the common peroneal nerve. In patients with polio who walk with the leg in external rotation for stability, the valgus deformity noted clinically and on standing radiographs may be due in part to laxity of the medial ligament. Although this looks impressive, it is seldom painful and does not progress once skeletal maturity has been achieved.

The operations for correction of significant valgus deformities are either osteotomy or inhibition of growth on the medial side of the knee. Rarely, when a discrete bone bridge can be demonstrated crossing the growth plate, the Langenskiold (1975) operation is indicated.

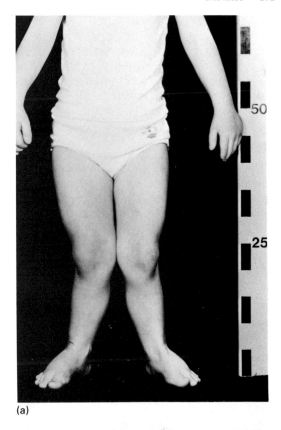

(a)

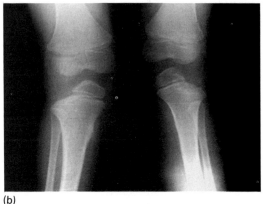

(b)

Figure 14.4 Ellis–Van Creveld syndrome. (a) Age 4 years – delay in ossification of the lateral half of the tibial epiphysis makes the joint line difficult to assess. (b) X-ray appearance

Apparent knock knees

A knock knee gait without a knock knee intermalleolar interval is usually due to one of three causes. First, fat thighs make it difficult to walk with knees and feet aligned. Secondly, joint laxity and hypotonia combine to allow the knee to tilt into valgus on weight bearing only. Thirdly, patients with the triple deformity of anteverted femoral necks, squinting patellae and compensatory external tibial torsion may demonstrate apparent valgus.

Genu varum (bow legs)

The bow leg interval is the distance between the medial femoral condyles when the medial malleoli are in contact and the knees straight. The deformity may be apparent, physiological or pathological.

Apparent bow legs

These children usually present shortly after walking starts, on account of a bow-legged gait. Examination on the couch with the patellae pointing towards the ceiling reveals an absent or negligible bow leg interval. The illusion is due to the broad-based gait of the toddler, the internally rotated posture of the hips and the distribution of subcutaneous fat in the 'chubby' leg. It may be accentuated if the knees go into slight recurvatum.

Physiological bow legs

Salenius and Vankka (1975), studying the normal tibiofemoral angle, have shown that

before the age of 1 year there is a marked varus position which changes to valgus when the child is between 18 months and 3 years old. Children with a marked degree of normal bowing and those correcting late may present with a true bow leg deformity which is termed 'physiological' and which is invariably accompanied by marked internal tibial torsion. The radiographs show medial beaking of both the femoral and the tibial metaphyses, tapering of the medial parts of the ossific nuclei on either side of the joint and thickening of the medial tibial cortex. Whilst most of these knees correct spontaneously, a few will progress to true Blount's disease. The initial radiological appearances may be indistinguishable and therefore these children should be followed up in the short term (Figure 14.5).

Physiological bow legs should be distinguished from prenatal genu varum in which skin dimples are present over the apex of the curvature and the fibula has a slightly S-shaped appearance. This condition also tends to correct spontaneously.

If bowing is asymmetrical or unilateral,

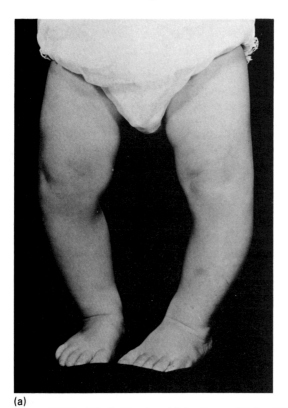

(a)

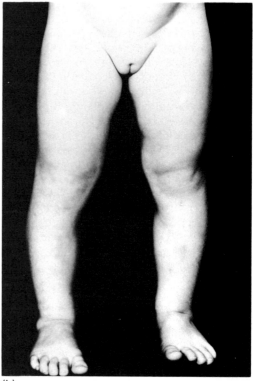

(b)

Figure 14.5 Physiological bow leg. (a) Age 1 year. (b) Age 2.5 years. No treatment has been given

noted to be progressive, or if the child is of short stature, the cause is much more likely to be pathological.

Pathological bow legs

Blount's disease (Blount, 1937)

This title embraces two separate clinical entities distinguishable by the age of onset. Infantile tibia vara is usually bilateral, painless and first noted when walking starts. As well as varus, there is marked internal tibial torsion, slight genu recurvatum and flat foot. In unlateral cases there may be shortening of the order of 1 cm. The aetiology is uncertain, but it is thought that the damage to the posteromedial aspect of the growth plate and the progressive varus follow abnormally high stresses across the physis in some patients with marked physiological bowing. Bateson (1968) noted that Jamaican children were prone to more severe physiological bowing and walked earlier than English children. He thought this accounted for the increased incidence of infantile tibia vara in that population.

Adolescent or juvenile tibia vara arises between 6 and 13 years, and should be regarded as a medial growth plate arrest probably due to trauma. The deformity is less severe and usually unilateral, and the patients may present with pain in the knee. Internal tibial torsion is unusual, and up to 2 cm of shortening may be apparent.

Infantile tibia vara

This is suspected when a physiological bow leg, with internal tibial torsion, is severe enough to cause a true bow leg interval which either does not improve by 2–3 years of age, or deteriorates. Radiologically the first definite sign that a physiological bow leg has progressed to Blount's disease is irregularity and areas of lucency in the medial metaphyseal beak. It is

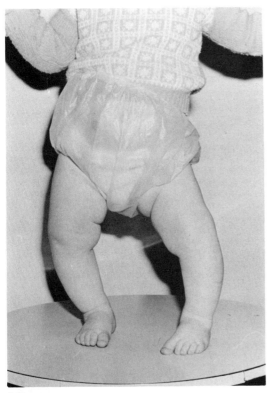

(a)

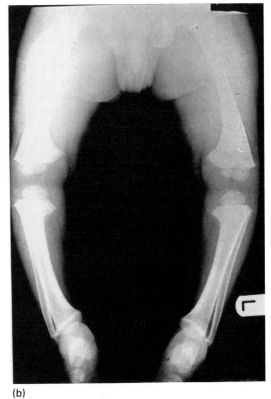

(b)

Figure 14.6 Blount's disease. (a) Clinical appearance in a child 2 years of age. Note the sharp medial angulation and considerable medial torsion. (b) X-ray of the same patient. Note the crumbling appearance of the medial upper tibial epiphysis

possible that the metaphyseal–diaphyseal angle described by Levine and Drennan (1982) may permit earlier differentiation between Blount's disease and physiological bow leg.

This disease is diagnosed too frequently. One should bear in mind that the incidence is estimated to be of the order of 0.05 per 1000 live births (Zayer, 1973), although this may vary a little from population to population. The irregularity of the medial metaphyseal beak may appear at between 18 months and 4 years (Figure 14.6); until it is seen, the diagnosis of Blount's disease should not be made. If in doubt, time is the final arbiter.

Once the features of infantile tibia vara are established, if left untreated, the prognosis is poor. There will be radiological progression from the metaphyseal stage already described to the epiphyseal stage at the age of 5 years onwards, in which the underdeveloped medial part of the epiphysis ossifies and the extent of deformity in the joint becomes apparent. Arthrograms may demonstrate that compensation for the deformity is made to some degree by thickening of the articular cartilage and enlargement of the medial meniscus. If left untreated, at maturity gross varus and damage to the joint will be apparent, and this will be accompanied by ligamentous instability.

Golding and McNeil Smith (1963), in common with Langenskiold (1952), recommended valgus osteotomy of the upper tibia as soon as the diagnosis was certain. They found that early correction when the angle of varus was less than 15 degrees produced a reversal of the changes and a return to normality. More recently, Hoffman, Jones and Herring (1982) have emphasized that early osteotomy must be performed before permanent epiphyseal damage and subsequent incongruity of the joint occur. A study of 12 patients with 19 affected knees followed up at a mean of 12 years revealed symptomatic degenerative changes in 12 knees. Most of their patients were operated on after the age of 6 years. They suggest that varus angulation in excess of 5 degrees in a patient over the age of 3 with proven Blount's disease should be treated by osteotomy. The procedure should be performed below the tibial tuberosity, and rotational deformity as well as varus should be corrected. If performed later, when permanent damage to the growth plate has occurred, repeated osteotomy may be necessary.

Kessel (1970) suggested that a simpler and safer solution should be applied to the younger child in whom a diagnosis of true progressive Blount's disease has recently been made. An upper tibial forage procedure aimed at producing a transient increase in tibial growth may correct the varus deformity due to the lateral tethering effect of the fibula. Also, the vertical offset of the fibula on the tibia acts as a 'cam-shaft', causing unwinding of the internal tibial torsion.

Adolescent or juvenile tibia vara

These patients deteriorate if conservative treatment is attempted, and osteotomy is invariably followed by recurrence of deformity (Figure 14.7). Lateral stapling is probably the best method of treating this difficult deformity, providing the growth plate is intact. If not, osteotomy should be combined with epiphysiodesis.

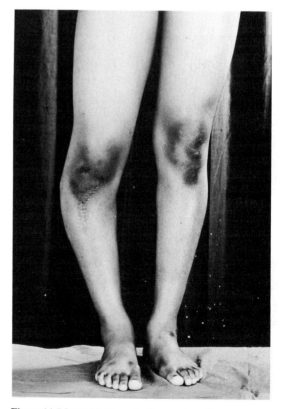

Figure 14.7 Juvenile Blount's disease. Age 10 years – recurrence of deformity after osteotomy

Secondary bow legs

Bow legs are a common feature of achondroplasia and osteogenesis imperfecta. Rickets of any type causes this deformity rather than knock knee. If nutritional, correction of the diet is usually followed by improvement, but in resistant rickets delay in diagnosis may lead to deformity which tends to persist and require operation. Metaphyseal dysplasia may have an appearance similar to rickets and this diagnosis should be suspected if the biochemistry is normal.

Quadriceps contracture

Hnevkovsky (1961) and Fairbank and Barrett (1961) first drew attention to the symptoms of quadriceps contracture, suggesting that the muscular fibrosis was idiopathic. Two years later, Gunn (1964) and Lloyd-Roberts and Thomas (1964) simultaneously noted the association of the great majority of these cases with intramuscular injections and infusions. There is usually a history of premature birth, low birth weight and a very stormy postnatal period in which many injections were given. A precise injection history is often hard to obtain and whilst in the early cases vitamin K appeared prominent, it is now known that almost any intramuscular injection may be incriminated. These are usually antibiotics, analgesics or anticonvulsants.

For reasons that are not clear the quadriceps contracture may not become apparent until the age of 2 or 3 years and may then progress quite rapidly (Figure 14.8). The contracture is invariably bilateral, though not symmetrical, and usually presents as a progressive and painless loss of knee flexion so that in severe cases the child walks with stiff extended knees. The parents will bear witness to difficulties in running, squatting, kneeling and sitting cross-legged, and describe their children as clumsy. Less commonly, knee flexion is maintained at the expense of habitual dislocation of the patella in flexion.

The site of the intramuscular fibrosis in the UK is typically anterolateral, involving the vastus lateralis and sometimes the intermedius

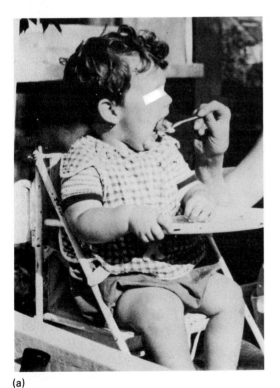

(a)

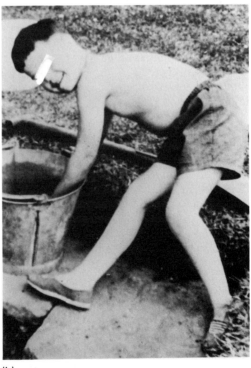

(b)

Figure 14.8 Injection-induced contracture. Note the delayed onset: neonatal injections were given. (a) Mobile knees at 18 months. (b) Stiff knees age 7 years

and rectus femoris as well. Often there is a dimple in the thigh over the affected area and this becomes more prominent as the knee is forced to the extreme of flexion. This dimple is formed by the tethering of scarred muscle to the overlying fascia lata and not, as has been previously suggested, by fat atrophy. Contracture of the rectus femoris muscle should be tested for by flexing the knee with the hip extended.

Once established, this type of contracture does not respond well to conservative treatment. When loss of knee flexion is marked, a proximal operation centred over the site of the pathology is recommended (Jackson and Hutton, 1985). The findings are either a dense island of fibrous tissue within the substance of the muscle or, alternatively, multiple fibrous bands. In either event, a soft tissue release can be performed and knee flexion achieved. Postoperatively the knee is splinted at 90 degrees and mobilized from the flexed position. If the quadriceps contracture is associated with dislocation of the patella then a distal operation realigning the patella and lengthening the rectus tendon is indicated, although this is sometimes followed by a permanent extension lag.

A review of our patients with quadriceps contracture reveals a high incidence of patella alta and fragmentation of the lower pole of the patella. Minor patella/femoral symptoms are common in adolescence and, rarely, patellectomy may be necessary.

Dislocation of the patella

Dislocation of the patella in early childhood differs from that in the second decade in that congenital anomalies are more prominent as a cause than trauma. Below the age of 5 years the condition is difficult to recognize since the patella is small and ossification has not commenced. At this age, careful palpation is the key to diagnosis.

Dislocations of the patella may be classified as acute, recurrent, habitual or permanent, but this classification on its own is not entirely satisfactory. One also needs to distinguish between dislocation and subluxation, to note any deviation from the normal path of patellar tracking and to look for associated abnormalities and syndromes.

Acute and recurrent dislocation

Acute dislocation occurs most commonly during adolescence, when the knee gives way without warning during strenuous activity. Usually a valgus/external rotation force is the precipitating factor. Direct trauma to the kneecap is an uncommon cause. The patella dislocates laterally and there is extensive tearing of the medial structures. Fragments of bone or cartilage may be avulsed from the medial border of the patella and there may also be partial detachment of the patellar tendon insertion. The dislocation almost invariably reduces spontaneously, but, if it does not, all that is required to affect reduction is extension of the knee. In addition to medial structure damage, the possibility of osteochondral fractures with loose body formation should not be overlooked; rarely, associated tears of the medial meniscus may further complicate the picture. The standard treatment of uncomplicated acute dislocation is conservative, splinting the knee in extension for 3 weeks followed by knee mobilization and quadriceps exercises, with special attention to the vastus medialis.

However, following acute dislocation, recurrent dislocation is the rule and there are those who favour immediate repair following acute dislocation. If treated conservatively, the chances of a further dislocation have been estimated by Heywood (1961) to be 85%. After two or three further episodes, some of these knees will satisfactorily stabilize again. The remainder will require surgical treatment. Whilst it should always be possible to stabilize the patella in these knees by operation, in the long term patellofemoral osteoarthritis may mar the result.

Recurrent subluxation of the patella in which the patella deviates momentarily from its normal line of tracking may occur without previous trauma and is responsible for a feeling of instability and giving way. The feeling of instability can be reproduced clinically by a positive apprehension test. Episodes of recurrent subluxation may precede an acute dislocation.

Habitual dislocation

When the patella deviates from the normal line of tracking on every occasion that the knee flexes or extends, this is called habitual dislocation or subluxation. When the dislocation occurs in flexion it is obvious, but habitual lateral subluxation of the patella in extension will be missed if extension of the knee under load is not specifically observed by the clinician. It should be noted that, if the patella is subluxed laterally in full extension, the quadriceps or Q angle (Insall, Falvo and Wise, 1976) will be difficult to interpret, and only at operation when the patella is held in the reduced position can the degree of quadriceps malalignment be fully appreciated. Furthermore, spurious measurements of the Q angle occur because the patella tendon insertion is not always centred over the palpable tibial tuberosity. Marked lateral subluxation in extension exposes the patella to a choice of routes that it may take on flexion (Figure 14.9). Either it can centralize and follow the normal route down the trochlear groove or it can pass down the outside of the lateral condyle and dislocate.

Treatment of recurrent and habitual dislocation

Many different operative procedures have been advised for the treatment of these patellar dislocations, and each case needs to be assessed on its merits. Lateral release alone has no part to play in the treatment of knees in which the patella subluxates laterally in extension, or in knees in which complete dislocation of the patella occurs. Usually a quadriceps realignment is indicated and satisfactory results should regularly be achieved in the presence of good bony anatomy. Tibial tubercle surgery should not be performed until the patient has achieved skeletal maturity. In general we have found the Roux–Goldthwaite procedure to be effective in the younger patient and the Elmslie–Trillat operation to be a suitable alternative once skeletal maturity has been achieved. It is a useful discipline before embarking upon surgery to consider whether there are abnormalities of the passive restrainers, of the active restrainers or of the bones themselves. There may be generalized ligamentous laxity or laxity of the medial retinaculum alone. Alternatively, the lateral structures may be tight and there may be abnormal fibrous bands (Jeffrys, 1963). There may be imbalance between the vastus medialis and the vastus lateralis or malalignment of the whole quadriceps mechanism, producing a

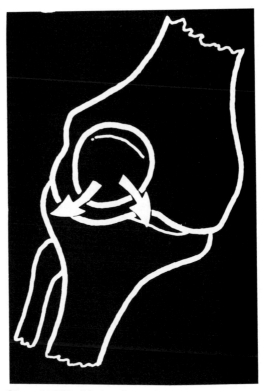

Figure 14.9 The 'choice of routes'

bow-stringing effect on the patella. There may be abnormalities within the substance of the quadriceps muscle itself in the form of fibrous contractures and, lastly, there may be patella alta, a hypoplastic patella as in the nail–patella syndrome, or a Wiberg type III patella which is said to be seen more commonly in patients with dislocation.

Permanent dislocation

Since this diagnosis is seldom made below the age of 3 or 4 years, it is often difficult to know whether the dislocation was indeed present at birth. These knees are very often dysplastic, and the dislocated patella should perhaps be regarded as the obvious feature of a knee whose anatomy is likely to be far from normal. Tight lateral bands are invariably found. The patella is usually hypoplastic and the trochlear groove absent. The condyles are dysmorphic and on occasion the medial condyle is completely obscured by an enlarged and thickened medial plica. The menisci may be absent or discoid. We have seen congenital dislocation of the patella with fixed flexion deformity of the knee combined with congenital absence of the anterior cruciate ligament. The abnormal anteroposterior glide becomes apparent only after the dislocated quadriceps mechanism has been reduced. Suspicion of the diagnosis of permanent dislocation should be aroused when the contour of the knee is abnormal and confirmed by palpation of the dislocated patella.

The treatment of such knees is open to debate since they obviously cannot be made normal. Some have advocated that the most severe cases should be left alone, but increasing fixed flexion and valgus deformity of the knee with posterolateral subluxation of the tibia have been observed in untreated cases, and with increasing weight the disability becomes more severe. Early operation can be rewarded by satisfactory and congruous development of the patellofemoral joint. The operations tend to be 'ad hoc' procedures, depending on the findings. In every case the knee flexion test must be performed and quadriceps lengthening added to the procedure if the knee will flex only at the expense of patellar dislocation.

Permanent dislocation may also be acquired and a rare sequel to injection-induced quadriceps contracture. The author has treated one patient with a dislocated patella in one knee and limited flexion of the other resulting from this condition.

Anterior knee pain

It is now clear that the syndrome of anterior knee pain in adolescence and early adult life may be caused by conditions other than chondromalacia patellae. The patients in this group (who are more often female) present with aching in front of the knees which is aggravated by exercise and especially on coming down stairs. Sometimes the knee gives way and there is an intermittent effusion. Both knees may be similarly affected, and patellar and peripatellar causes of these symptoms should be sought. Pain on patellofemoral compression and crepitus help to incriminate the patellofemoral joint.

The term 'chondromalacia patellae' embraces two definite pathological entities which have been well described by Goodfel-

low, Hungerford and Woods (1976). They distinguish between age-dependent surface degeneration, which is not a cause of pain in the adolescent and young adult, and basal degeneration which commences as softening and swelling of the deep layers of the articular cartilage breaking through to the surface at a later stage. The early softening and even fissuring may not be recognizable on inspection unless the articular surface is examined with a probe. Basal degeneration may be reversible and is not necessarily a precursor of adult osteoarthritis. Other studies have shown microfractures in the subchondral bone, and technetium bone scans have also been hot, so it appears quite possible that the primary pathology is not in the articular cartilage at all. Furthermore, there is often little correlation between the magnitude of the pathological lesion and the severity of symptoms, and even the pain mechanism has yet to be explained.

Faced with such ignorance about the condition, it is fortunate that, in most patients, symptoms which commence spontaneously or after trauma or overuse tend to be self-limiting. There is generally a good response to isometric quadriceps exercises and the avoidance of aggravating activities. The surgeon should be in no hurry to commit his patient to any kind of surgical procedure. If the symptoms remain severe after 6 months and are associated with definite maltracking of the patella, this will need correction. The maltracking may be assessed clinically, radiologically and arthroscopically via a suprapatellar portal. A lateral retinacular release is the smallest realignment procedure and is appropriate for minor degrees of lateral patellar subluxation in flexion, and also for the excessive lateral pressure syndrome described by Ficat and Hungerford (1977). In more marked cases of maltracking, a distal realignment is indicated, as has already been described above (page 176).

Standard radiological views of the knee and patellofemoral joint should always be taken to exclude rarities such as osteochondritis of the patella and osteochondral fractures. These are small localized lesions of the patella and tend to present with a lot of pain consistently within a small part of the arc of knee flexion. Rarely, well localized lateral patellar pain may be associated with a bipartite patella, and excision of the lateral ossicle will relieve the pain.

Of the peripatellar causes of anterior knee pain, traction epiphysitis at the lower pole of the patella is most easily recognized by the characteristic localized point tenderness. Fragmentation of the lower pole of the patella may be seen on the lateral radiograph. Less easy to be sure of is the plica or medial shelf syndrome, but if anteromedial knee pain is relieved by local anaesthetic injection at the tender area and the symptoms are associated with a thickened fibrous plica and erosion of the upper margin of the medial femoral condyle, then the true entity exists. It is a small matter to excise the plica arthroscopically. Rarely, a complete suprapatellar plica is seen at arthroscopy, and excision of this membrane can relieve symptoms.

The discoid meniscus

This abnormality invariably affects the lateral meniscus, and, whilst its origin is open to some debate, it should probably be regarded as a congenital abnormality rather than arrested embryological development. Often both knees are involved and it is interesting that the discoid meniscus has been seen in conjunction with other congenital abnormalities of the knee; for example, congenital absence of the anterior cruciate ligament and congenital dislocation of the patella.

The anatomy of the discoid meniscus is variable. At the extreme there is a meniscal plate extending right across the lateral joint space separating the lateral condyle of the femur from the tibia. The medial free edge is rounded and as thick as the fixed lateral edge, and there is a central dimple. This situation is difficult to appreciate through the standard anterolateral arthroscopic approach. The least severe example is a meniscus which is approaching normal, but is unusually wide in its middle third.

In addition to abnormal meniscal shape, there are other associated abnormalities. The discoid meniscus may have an abnormal posterior attachment, known as the ligament of Wrisberg, which inserts into the back of the femoral condyle rather than the tibia. This arrangement renders the discoid meniscus hypermobile. An impressive clunk can often be demonstrated as the free edge of the meniscus escapes from the trapped position between the femoral condyle and the tibia, or a clunk occurs near the extreme of flexion as the femoral condyle rolls backwards into a trough in the meniscus created by a tear. This abnormal movement may cause progressive meniscal damage, usually of a shearing kind, with a predominantly horizontal component affecting the posterior half of the disc. Degenerate cysts also occur. The normal convexity of the lateral tibial plateau may be exaggerated.

A review of the presenting features of children with discoid menisci has emphasized that pain was the dominant presenting symptom whilst a clunk was only present in half the knees (Glasgow, Aichroth and Baird, 1982). Lateral joint pain is perhaps caused by traction on the synovium of the meniscosynovial junction. Radiological widening of the lateral joint space is a most unreliable sign.

The presence of a discoid meniscus is not an indication for its removal. Provided the symptoms are sufficient, the traditional surgical approach is complete lateral meniscectomy. If the dissection is performed at the vascular meniscosynovial junction, there is evidence that some sort of meniscal regeneration will occur. Whether the regenerated meniscus functions as normal is unlikely. Presumably, it helps to spread the load and lubricate the joint but it cannot fulfil the important restraining function of the 'hoop ligament' if it does not have a strong posterior attachment to the tibia, and it is doubtful if regeneration can occur across the popliteal tendon. Total lateral meniscectomy in a child leads, not surprisingly, to premature osteoarthritis of the lateral compartment.

At the present time, techniques have been described for arthroscopic partial meniscectomy aimed at converting the discoid meniscus into a more normal looking cartilage, but this is difficult and should probably not be applied to the Wrisberg type of meniscus. However, if the discoid abnormality is less severe, this approach is probably justified. The principle of the surgical technique is to resect an anterior flap first, in order to create a working area, and then to excise the posterior part of the meniscus with the punch.

Osteochondritis dissecans

Some care needs to be taken in distinguishing the chronic lesion of osteochondritis dissecans from acute osteochondral fractures as well as anomalies of ossification. A radiological study of 147 children with normal knees aged between 3 and 13 years is of particular interest (Caffey *et al*, 1958). Eighty per cent of the children under 5 years and 20% of children under 12 years had condylar defects, and in 19 patients these lesions were radiologically indistinguishable from osteochondritis dissecans. When there is doubt about the radiographic interpretation, bone scanning and arthroscopy may help to make the distinction.

True osteochondritis dissecans is a disorder of the adolescent and young adult, being characterized by necrosis of an oval area of subchondral bone, usually on the convex surface of the medial femoral condyle adjacent to the intercondylar notch. Radiologically, this area is often best seen in the tunnel view. The overlying cartilage, which gains its nutrition from the joint, remains viable, and in the early stage of the disease the articular surface looks perfectly normal. If the fragment is stable and the weakened area is protected from repeated trauma, it is likely to heal. Indeed, this is the usual outcome in the preadolescent patient. Sometimes the radiological appearance remains unchanged but the symptoms subside. In the older patient the articular cartilage may fissure at the margin of the avascular bone fragment, which then separates completely from its crater as a loose body or may remain partially attached as an unstable trapdoor lesion. The radiological sign of impending or partial separation of the fragment is sclerosis of the crater margins; in such a case arthroscopy and probing should be undertaken to accurately define the situation.

The usual presentation is that of aching in the knee, which may be localized to one side and may be intermittent. Pain may be experienced when doing a full squat, since in this position the medial facet of the patella is compressed against the lesion. There may be a small effusion, and there may be local tenderness over one or other femoral condyles, best sought with the knee in full flexion. The patient may complain of instability or giving way which is understandable in the presence of a loose body or trapdoor lesion, but this is also seen before separation of the fragment and is possibly due to sudden pain inhibition of the quadriceps.

Repeated minor trauma clearly plays some part in the pathogenesis of this condition, which is frequently encountered in sporting individuals. However, reports of familial influences and multiple joint involvement in some patients, in addition to the abnormalities of ossification already referred to, need to be taken into account.

The management of the younger patient is expectant, with restriction of games until pain and swelling have disappeared. In the older patient, if symptoms are persistent and there is sclerosis of the crater, arthroscopy is indicated to assess stability of the lesion. If the lesion is stable and the articular surface is intact, it is probably best to leave the lesion alone although 'in situ' drilling has been recommended in the past. Postoperative protection in a knee brace which limits flexion, together with reduced activities, may then be rewarded by healing. If the fragment then becomes unstable or if an unstable lesion is found at arthroscopy, it should be removed, as should a loose body. The crater is curetted and drilled in order to stimulate healing of the defect with fibrocartilage. The short and medium results of this procedure have been gratifying but, as is so often the case, long-term follow-up is often anecdotal. Reattachment of separated fragments with pins, which may themselves cause problems and need further surgery for removal, is not routinely indicated but there may be a place for reattachment with bone pegs or Herbert screws when large fragments of the weight-bearing surface have been displaced. Articular cartilage grafting is another possibility.

Osteochondritis dissecans of the lateral femoral condyle may be associated with a discoid meniscus. Rarely, the patella is involved and in this case it may be associated with subluxation. Here, too, Edwards and Bentley (1977) have reported good results from excision and drilling. Osteochondritis of the tibial plateau has also been observed.

Instability of the knee

Instability of the knee is a very unusual symptom in children. Recurrent subluxation and dislocation of the patella and osteochondritis dissecans have already been mentioned. Radiolucent cartilaginous loose bodies have been found in the knees of patients with hypophosphataemic rickets and the Stickler syndrome (hereditary arthro-ophthalmopathy). Meniscal tears are uncommon; if peripheral, repair rather than meniscectomy should be the rule. Synovial chondromatosis in childhood is extremely rare. Three other possibilities should, however, be entertained: first, a pedunculated synovial polyp (sometimes haematogenous); secondly, a tendon snapping over an osteochondroma; and, lastly, hypermobility of the superior tibiofibular joint. In the last condition the clicking sensation of the fibula slipping out of place may be felt on the outer side of the knee, usually as the knee approaches full flexion. This joint often stabilizes spontaneously with age and with the slight reduction of childhood ligamentous laxity that occurs during adolescence. If this instability is disabling, it can be eliminated by establishing cross-union between tibia and fibula in preference to excision of the proximal fibula with its important ligamentous attachments.

There is now increasing awareness of rare congenital ligamentous deficiencies of the knee. Some of these children may have wildly unstable knees on the examination couch while, surprisingly, their performance is little impaired. We have on record ten patients with proven congenital absence of the anterior cruciate ligament often in association with tibial or femoral dysplasia or congenital dislocation of the patella (Thomas, Jackson and Aichroth, 1985). The long-term future of these knees is unknown. In some of these children there is habitual anterior subluxation of the tibia as the knee extends. It is particularly important to appreciate this instability in children with significant leg length discrepancy, since its presence is a relative contraindication to femoral lengthening.

Foreign body arthritis

Children are prone to fall on their knees and it is not surprising that pieces of wood, needles and other foreign bodies penetrate into such a superficial joint. In the acute stage the radiological appearance of gas within the joint may provide a clue to the depth of injury, if the foreign body is not radio-opaque. In the chronic case there may be a low grade infective arthritis resembling tuberculosis and synovial biopsy may be contemplated. However, if the possibility of a foreign body is considered before operation, the history, scars and point tenderness may suggest the diagnosis and the surgeon to place his incision over the likely area.

Osgood–Schlatter disease

Pain, tenderness and swelling over the anterior surface of the proximal end of the tibia in childhood cause understandable anxiety. These signs, if localized specifically to the tibial tubercle, are pathognomonic of Osgood–Schlatter disease. The typical case is an active athletic boy over the age of 10 years and commonly both knees are involved. The symptoms are aggravated by games, and, in the clinic, kneeling and getting up from a squatting position are demonstrably painful. The patient points precisely to the tibial tubercle as the site of pain. Short-term advice to avoid those activities which cause more discomfort than he is prepared to tolerate is usually rewarded by a reduction in symptoms and total resolution within a year or so. The parents are reassured that this is a self-limiting condition. In the severe case it is traditional to rest the knee for 6 weeks in a plaster cylinder but this is badly tolerated in the bilateral case, and symptoms tend to return upon removal of the plaster. Infiltration with bupivacaine (Marcaine) and hydrocortisone around the tibial tuberosity may be followed by striking improvement. Surgical drilling and bone pegging have no part to play. In the late unresolving case, if a discrete ossicle is present in the patellar tendon just proximal to the tibial tubercle, symptoms are often relieved by its removal. Late complications are rare but very occasionally premature fusion of the anterior part of the upper tibial growth plate causes mild genu recurvatum or symptoms persist into adult life as local tenderness over a prominent tibial tubercle.

Osgood–Schlatter disease is caused by high stresses placed upon an immature tendon insertion at the time of the adolescent growth spurt. At this stage of development the Sharpey fibres which help anchor the mature ligament to bone are not yet formed and the patellar tendon is attached by fibrocartilage, cartilage and a tongue of epiphysis to the tibial metaphysis. It is not surprising that failure of this insertion occurs from time to time, either as a result of repeated minor traumatic avulsions or due to a traction epiphysitis. The radiological picture is variable, sometimes suggesting avulsion and sometimes fragmentation of the tuberosity.

Popliteal cysts

Popliteal cysts are twice as common in boys and usually present under the age of 10 years as an asymptomatic, fluctuant swelling just to the medial side of the popliteal fossa. If there is doubt about the cystic nature of the lesion, transillumination will settle the issue. The cyst is probably the semimembranosus bursa, and on examination it is better felt in extension than in flexion. The knee is otherwise normal. Dinham (1975) has drawn attention to the very high recurrence rate after surgical removal and the natural tendency of these cysts to disappear

spontaneously. Operation without very good reason is unjustified.

Miscellaneous conditions around the knee

Many conditions which are not primarily disorders of this area present around the knee. Occult fractures such as greenstick buckles of the lower femur or stress fractures of the upper tibia may explain obscure limp or pain. They are also common when movement begins after prolonged immobilization. It was here, too, that premature growth arrest occurred during long-term treatment for tuberculosis elsewhere when the growth plate herniated into surrounding porotic bone.

Acute and subacute osteomyelitis and septic arthritis, rheumatoid arthritis and haemophiliac arthritis favour this area. Tumours and cysts show a similar predilection. Among the

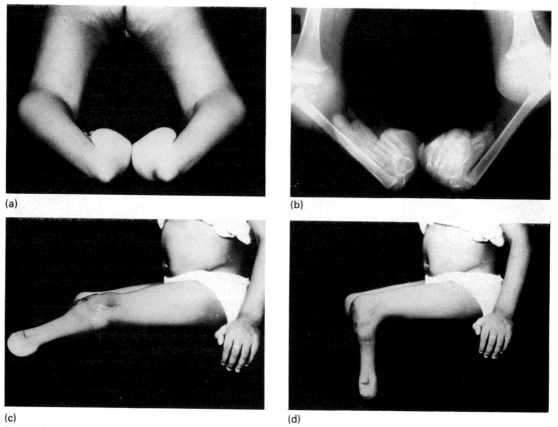

(a) (b) (c) (d)

Figure 14.10 Congenital aplasia of the tibia. (a, b) The presenting deformity. (c) A through-knee amputation has been performed. (d) The fibula has been fused to an upper tibial anlage preserving a useful knee joint

general diseases, nail–patella syndrome, dysplasia epiphysealis multiplex, epiphysealis hemimelica, dyschondroplasia and rickets frequently present here. Bone contour is altered in Gaucher's disease, osteopetrosis and achondroplasia. The epiphyseal appearance is delayed in cretins and there may be a linear metaphyseal translucency in scurvy and leukaemia. The patella is the most common of the potentially bipartite bones.

It should never be forgotten that the child with a limp and pain in the knee may suffer from hip pathology.

The leg

Congenital aplasia and dysplasia of the tibia with intact fibula

The tibia is absent or dysplasic but the fibula is relatively normal and the foot may be augmented, usually on the medial side. The different degrees of the malformation have been well described by Jones, Barnes and Lloyd-Roberts (1978), who stress the difficulty in interpreting the initial radiograph. Delay in ossification of a portion of the tibia may suggest a more severe deformity than that which actually exists, and care must be taken to avoid a needlessly high amputation if, for example, a cartilaginous unossified upper end of the tibia is present. In this case the knee joint can be preserved. If the lower end of the femur looks normal on the initial radiograph, the upper tibia is probably present even though not radiologically visible at this stage. Sometimes it can be palpated.

Treatment should be based on the true morphological deformity. When the upper tibia is not present, disarticulation through the knee poses least problems to the limb-fitters and a satisfactory functional result can be achieved in a short time. If the upper tibia is present, some stability can be achieved by placing the fibula within this upper fragment and performing a Syme's amputation as a second stage (Figure 14.10). When the problem is a short tibia and long fibula with

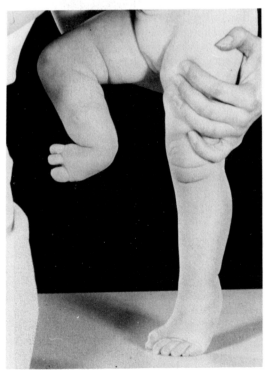
(a)

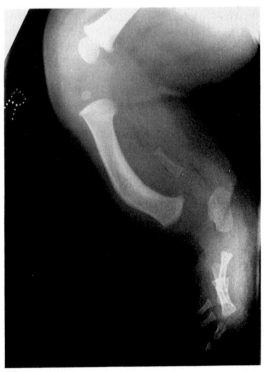
(b)

Figure 14.11 (a) Congenital short tibia and absent fibula. Note the dimple over the tibia and the absence of lateral two rays of the foot. (b) X-ray of congenital short tibia with small fibular remnant distally. Note the tibial bowing and absence of lateral two rays of the foot.

diastasis of the ankle mortice and a varus foot, shortening will dominate the problem and the best solution is a Syme's amputation. In the least severe cases a useful foot should always be preserved. The shortening can be managed with a shoe raise if necessary until the appropriate age for a leg equalization procedure is achieved.

Congenital hypoplasia and absence of the fibula

This is the commonest congenital long bone deformity. The fibula may be totally absent, absent in part, or thin and dysplastic (Figure 14.11). At birth the tibia is bowed anteriorly in most cases, thickened and sclerotic with a dimple at the apex of the kyphosis. Quite major degrees of bowing may correct spontaneously without the need for osteotomy. The foot frequently lacks one or more of the lateral rays and there is often fixed valgus deformity. When the fibula is absent this valgus deformity is associated with a tight fibrocartilaginous band which presumably represents a fibular remnant. With deficiency of the outer rays, the peroneal muscles have abnormal insertions. The feet are often stiff and there may be a tarsal coalition with shortening between the medial malleolus and the sole. In most cases there is some shortening of the ipsilateral femur, and examination of the knee may elicit evidence of congenital cruciate deficiency.

The principal factors that determine the outcome are the expected leg length discrepancy at maturity and the state of the foot. When the fibula is completely absent, foot deformity is usually gross and the expected shortening is likely to be in excess of 10 cm. Disarticulation at the ankle is the logical treatment for both unilateral and bilateral deformity, and we normally advise operation at about the age of 1 year. The technique of Syme's amputation in this anomaly was described by Wood, Zlotsky and Westin (1965). Postoperatively the heel flaps should be set squarely on the tibia and its position maintained by transfixing it with a Kirschner wire. The shortening allows room for an end-bearing prosthesis with an ankle joint. The management of those cases with a less severe anomaly is more difficult because the degree of shortening is less predictable. Primary amputation should be deferred if it looks possible to correct leg length discrepancy by lengthening or epiphysiodesis procedures in the future, and the priority is to obtain a useful weight-bearing foot. Removal of the lateral fibrocartilaginous fibular anlage (Thomas, Straub and Arnold, 1957), posterior release of the ankle and lengthening of the peroneal muscles may all be necessary to correct the equinovalgus deformity. More radical correction with lasting stability may be achieved by the Gruca procedure (Serafin, 1967) in which a bony ankle mortice is fashioned. At a later date the shortening must be corrected, but if this is unattainable a Syme's amputation may still be required (Thomas and Williams, 1987).

Congenital pseudarthrosis of the tibia

Congenital pseudarthrosis is a misnomer for what should better be called pre-pseudarthrosis of the tibia, since only rarely is a fracture or pseudarthrosis present at birth. Most commonly, the fracture occurs within the first two years of life, and it may become manifest at any stage until maturity is reached.

The tibia itself is invariably congenitally abnormal in shape and structure (Figure 14.12a). There is anterolateral bowing, usually combined with some shortening. Two main radiological appearances are seen: first, narrowing of the tibia and sclerosis encroaching upon the medullary cavity at the junction of the middle and lower thirds, and, secondly, a cystic lesion at any level but again commonly in the lower third. Neurofibromatosis is more common than fibrous dysplasia in the aetiology, and one or other of these conditions is often demonstrable in either the bone or the periosteum provided that previous operations and resulting scar tissue have not confused the microscopic appearances. The fibula is either normal or affected, possibly showing a pseudarthrosis which may precede that in the tibia, or there may be segmental sclerosis or cyst formation. Rarely in the absence of neurofibromatosis, a tibia which may have appeared normal in the early years starts to bow at between the ages of 5 and 12 years and may proceed to fracture (Hardinge, 1972).

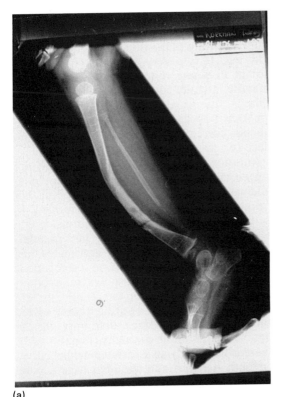
(a)

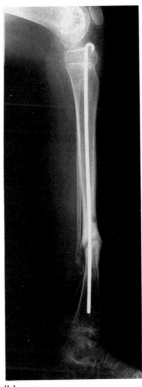
(b)

Figure 14.12 Congenital pseudarthrosis of the tibia. (a) Note the sclerosis and loss of marrow cavity, and the loss of the distal fibula. (b) After intramedullary rodding and grafting

Clearly, pseudarthrosis of the tibia has a considerable variety of clinical presentations and it is a pity that the presenting characteristics of the individual case are not a reliable guide to the prognosis which has, to date, been generally poor. Of the patients reviewed by Hardinge, 29% had undergone amputation.

The treatment of this condition remains one of the most challenging problems in orthopaedic surgery. The aim is to correct the deformity and achieve solid, permanent bone union with the minimum of shortening. The universal problem with the old established procedures is graft resorption and failure to obtain solid and lasting union of the shaft to the small dysplastic distal segment. Sometimes several grafting procedures have been required and even then success is far from guaranteed.

Prophylactic surgery combined with a protective orthosis is worthwhile in patients with bowing or cystic change in the intact tibia because, if left untreated, fracture and pseudarthrosis are almost inevitable. Boyd and

Sage (1958), Eyre-Brook, Baily and Price (1969) and others have recommended grafting dangerous cystic areas. The anterior bowed tibia can be strengthened by grafting the concavity, perhaps on more than one occasion, or by performing a bypass graft (Lloyd-Roberts and Shaw, 1969). A protective orthosis should be worn until maturity and until the tibia demonstrates a normal cortex and medullary canal.

An established pseudarthrosis will not heal with conventional conservative treatment, neither is union easy to achieve in the younger child. By the age of 8 years, one may be more optimistic about the chances of achieving permanent union. With children aged between 1 and 3 years, McFarland's bypass operation (1951) has been popular, largely because neurofibromatosis has been found in the surrounding periosteum and it seems logical therefore to remain outside it. Also, by not excising the pseudarthrosis, shortening is not increased and the graft placed in the concavity runs in a straight line from knee to ankle and is in compression. The deformity in this case is accepted.

In the older child we have undertaken rodding of the tibia, the lower end of the nail gaining stability in the tarsus. Repeated grafting has often been necessary. The problem is far from solved, but three new developments may prove of great significance: free vascular bone grafts, pulsed electromagnetic fields and the technique of bone carrying.

In a review of the long established methods of treatment, Morrisey, Riseborough and Hall (1981) found that the Farmer operation alone showed any superiority. In this procedure a composite skin and bone pedicle graft is taken from the other leg, bringing with it a new blood supply. This biological approach has been refined by recent developments in microvascular surgery. A free vascularized fibular or rib graft is now an established technique (Hagan and Buncke, 1982; Pho *et al.*, 1985).

Paterson and Simonis (1985) published good results using electrical stimulation in conjunction with correction of deformity, intramedullary fixation and cancellous grafting. Twenty out of 27 pseudarthroses united with this technique.

The principle of bone carrying involves excision of the pseudarthrosis and all involved bone. A modified external fixator is applied to the tibia. The proximal fragment is osteotomized and, using leg-lengthening techniques, the lower segment of the shaft is slowly advanced on a sliding carriage until it reaches the distal fragment. Union must then be achieved (Ilizarov, 1971). All these advances require further long-term evaluation.

Pseudarthrosis of the fibula

Although usually associated with tibial disease, pseudarthrosis of the fibula may occur alone. The junction of the middle and lower thirds is the usual site. If untreated, there is progressive valgus deformity of the ankle. Union is difficult to obtain and lower tibial osteotomy of transient effect only. Furthermore, if a lower tibial osteotomy is attempted, it may prove difficult to control the small cancellous lower tibial fragment when the fibula also is unstable. a satisfactory alternative is to establish cross-union between the lower fibula fragment and the tibia.

Bowing of the tibia

Lateral bowing of the tibia is considered under bow leg. It is a very common physiological variant in young children. Persistence of the infantile laterally curved and inwardly rotated tibia is the usual cause of intoe gait and apparent bow legs in the very young. Spontaneous correction is the rule, and there is no place for corrective splintage (see earlier).

Anterior bowing occurs in tibiae that are congenitally short with fibular dysplasia. Spontaneous correction with growth may occur, but if not osteotomy may be safely performed. In contrast, bowing with a fibula of normal length is likely to proceed to fracture and pseudarthrosis, and osteotomy merely anticipates this. Similar bowing is common in osteogenesis imperfecta, when it predisposes to fracture, and often needs operation.

Posterior bowing is associated with severe congenital calcaneovalgus deformity of the foot, which lies in the concavity (Figure 14.13). There is frequently an associated medial curve, but both the foot and the tibia have a good prognosis when the former is treated by stretching. there may, however, be some residual shortening of about 2.5 cm (Heyman, Herndon and Heiple, 1959).

Rotation of the tibia

Excessive medial rotation of the tibia may persist with lateral curvature but is not significant. External rotation develops in uncorrected club feet where the fibula comes to lie posteriorly, and compensates to some extent for the forefoot varus. Similarly, in the triple deformity of anteverted femoral necks, squinting patellae and external tibial rotation, the deformity at the hip is compensated for by the deformity in the tibia. In paralytic disorders, unbalanced muscle action may be responsible.

Growing pains

Growing pains are mentioned here only because they are most commonly felt in front of the shins. In spite of suspicion to the contrary, they bear no relation to either juvenile rheumatoid arthritis or rheumatic fever, but a similar aching may be complained of in leukaemia or subacute osteomyelitis.

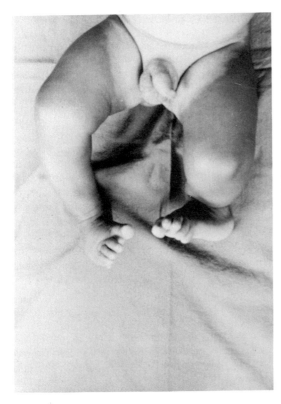

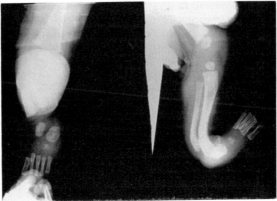

Figure 14.13 Recurvatum of the left tibia. (a) Note the metatarsus varus on the right. (b) X-ray of the same patient

The syndrome is clear cut. A child, usually between 3 and 8 years of age, wakes in the night with pain in the shins. Maternal sympathy, a hot drink and half a paracetamol tablet resolve the problem and he goes back to sleep. He is completely asymptomatic in the morning. This may occur for several consecutive nights and then recover until another episode begins. He finally recovers spontaneously.

The cause is unknown, but pain seems to be related to exercise and barometric pressure. It is not related to sleeping posture. Sometimes the child has cramps rather than bone aching and these are more troublesome, equally mysterious and ultimately self-curing.

References

Bateson, E. M. (1968) The relationship between Blount's disease and bow legs. *Br. J. Radiol.* **41**, 107–114

Blount, W. P. (1937) Tibia vara. *J. Bone Jt. Surg.* **19**, 1–29

Boyd, H. B. and Sage, E. P. (1958) Congenital pseudarthrosis of the tibia. *J. Bone Jt. Surg.* **40A**, 1245–1270

Caffey, J., Madell, S. H., Royer, C. and Morales, P. (1958) Ossification of the distal femoral epiphysis. *J. Bone Jt. Surg.* **40A**, 647–654

Curtis, B. H. and Fisher, R. L. (1969) Congenital hyperextension. *J. Bone Jt. Surg.* **51A**, 255

Dinham, J. M. (1975) Popliteal cysts in children. *J. Bone Jt. Surg.* **57B**, 69–71

Edwards, D. H. and Bentley, G. (1977) Osteochondritis dissecans of the patella. *J. Bone Jt. Surg.* **59B**, 58–63

Eyre-Brook, A. L., Bailey, A. J. and Price, C. H. G. (1969) Infantile pseudarthrosis. *J. Bone Jt. Surg.* **51B**, 604–613

Fairbank, T. J. and Barrett, A. M. (1961) Vastus intermedius contracture. *J. Bone Jt. Surg.* **43B**, 326–334

Ficat, R. P. and Hungerford, D. S. (1977) *Disorders of the Patellofemoral Joint.* Paris, New York: Masson, pp. 123–148

Glasgow, M. M. S., Aichroth, P. M. and Baird, P. R. E. (1982) The discoid lateral meniscus: a clinical review. *J. Bone Jt. Surg.* **64B**, 245

Golding, J. S. R. and McNeil Smith, J. D. G. (1963) Observations on the aetiology of tibia vara. *J. Bone Jt. Surg.* **45B**, 320

Goodfellow, J., Hungerford, D. S. and Woods, C. (1976) Patellofemoral joint mechanics and pathology. 2. Chondromalacia patellae. *J. Bone Jt. Surg.* **58B**, 291–299

Gunn, D. R. (1964) Contracture of quadriceps. *J. Bone Jt. Surg.* **46B**, 492–497

Hagan, K. F. and Buncke, H. J. (1982) Treatment of congenital pseudarthrosis of the tibia with free vascularised bone graft. *Clin. Orthop.* **166**, 34–44

Hardinge, K. (1972) Congenital anterior bowing of the tibia. *Ann. R. Coll. Surg.* **51**, 17

Heyman, C. H., Herndon, C. H. and Heiple, K. G. (1959) Congenital posterior angulation of the tibia with talipes calcaneus. *J. Bone Jt. Surg.* **41A**, 476–488

Heywood, A. W. B. (1961) Recurrent dislocation of the patella. *J. Bone Jt. Surg.* **43B**, 508–517

Hnevkovsky, O. (1961) Progressive fibrosis of vastus intermedius. *J. Bone Jt. Surg.* **43B**, 318–325

Hoffman, A., Jones, R. E. and Herring, J. A. (1982) Blount's disease after skeletal maturity. *J. Bone Jt. Surg.* **64A**, 1004–1009

Ilizarov, G. A. (1971) Basic principles of transosseous compression and distraction osteosynthesis. *Ortop. Traumatol. Protez.* **32**, 7–15

Insall, J., Falvo, K. A. and Wise, D. W. (1976) Chondromalacia patellae; a prospective study. *J. Bone Jt. Surg.* **58A**, 1–8

Jackson, A. M. and Hutton, P. A. N. (1985) Injection induced contractures of the quadriceps in childhood. *J. Bone Jt. Surg.* **67B**, 97–102

Jeffrys, T. E. (1963) Abnormality of tensor fascia femoris in dislocated patellae. *J. Bone Jt. Surg.* **45B**, 740

Jones, D., Barnes, J. and Lloyd-Roberts, G. C. (1978) Congenital aplasia and dysplasia of the tibia with intact fibula. *J. Bone Jt. Surg.* **60B**, 31–39

Kessel, L. (1970) Annotations on the aetiology and treatment of tibia vara. *J. Bone Jt. Surg.* **52B**, 93–99

Langenskiold, A. (1952) Tibia vara. *Acta Chir. Scand.* **103**, 1–22

Langenskiold, A. (1975) An operation for partial closure of an epiphyseal plate in children and its experimental basis. *J. Bone Jt. Surg.* **57B**, 325–330

Laurence, M. (1967) Genu recurvatum. *J. Bone Jt. Surg.* **49B**, 121

Levine, A. M. and Drennan, I. C. (1982) Physiological bowing and tibia vara. *J. Bone Jt. Surg.* **64A**, 1158–1163

Lloyd-Roberts, G. C. and Shaw, N. E. (1969) The prevention of pseudarthrosis. *J. Bone Jt. Surg.* **51B**, 100–105

Lloyd-Roberts, G. C. and Thomas, T. G. (1964) Aetiology of quadriceps contracture. *J. Bone Jt. Surg.* **46B**, 498–582

McFarland, B. (1951) Pseudarthrosis tibia. *J. Bone Jt. Surg.* **33B**, 36–46

Morley, M. (1957) Knock knee in children. *Br. Med. J.* **2**, 976

Morrisey, R. T., Riseborough, E. J. and Hall, J. E. (1981) Congenital pseudarthrosis of the tibia. *J. Bone Jt. Surg.* **63B**, 367–375

Paterson, D. C. and Simonis, R. B. (1985) Electrical stimulation in the treatment of congenital pseudarthrosis of the tibia. *J. Bone Jt. Surg.* **67B**, 454–462

Pho, R. W. H., Levack, B., Satku, K. and Patradul, A. (1985) Free vascularized fibular graft in the treatment of congenital pseudarthrosis of the tibia. *J. Bone Jt. Surg.* **67B**, 64–70

Pilcher, M. F. (1962) Epiphyseal stapling. *J. Bone Jt. Surg.* **44B**, 82

Poirier, H. (1968) Epiphyseal stapling and leg equalisation. *J. Bone Jt. Surg.* **50B**, 61–69

Salenius, P. and Vankka, E. (1975) The development of the tibiofemoral angle in children. *J. Bone Jt. Surg.* **57A**, 259–261

Serafin, J. (1967) Operation for congenital absent fibula. *J. Bone Jt. Surg.* **49B**, 59–65

Stein, H. and Dickson, R. A. (1975) Reversed dynamic slings for knee-flexion contractures in the hemophiliac. *J. Bone Jt. Surg.* **57A**, 282–283

Sutcliffe, M. L. and Goldberg, A. A. J. (1982) The treatment of congenital pseudarthrosis of the tibia with pulsing electromagnetic fields. *Clin. Orthop.* **166**, 45–57

Thomas, I. H. and Williams, P. F. (1987) The Gruca operation for congenital absence of the fibula. *J. Bone Jt. Surg.* **69B**, 587–592

Thomas, N. P., Jackson, A. M. and Aichroth, P. M. (1985) Congenital absence of the anterior cruciate ligament. *J. Bone Jt. Surg.* **67B**, 572–575

Thompson, T. C., Straub, L. R. and Arnold, W. D. (1957) Congenital absent fibula. *J. Bone Jt. Surg.* **39A**, 1229–1237

Wood, W. L., Zlotsky, N. and Westin, G. W. (1965) Congenital absence of the fibula. *J. Bone Jt. Surg.* **47A**, 1159–1169

Zayer, M. (1973) *Natural History of Osteochondroses Tibiae.* C. W. K. Gleerup: Lund, p. 25

Further reading

Macnicol, M. F. (1986) *The Problem Knee: Diagnosis and Management in the Younger Patient.* London: Heinemann Medical

15

The foot

Congenital talipes equinovarus (club foot)

Club foot remains the most difficult of all common congenital anomalies for the surgeon to treat successfully, notwithstanding dedicated care. The problem is fundamentally one of treating a deformity which is in three planes and involves several joints at the same time, in an environment which is constantly changing under the influence of growth.

The incidence is 1–2 per 1000 live births.

Diagnosis

At birth the baby lies with one or both feet inturned from the ankle downwards (Figure 15.1). Boys predominate in the ratio of about 3:1 and there are as many with bilateral as unilateral involvement.

Our first duty is to establish whether this is a fixed structural deformity or a postural attitude

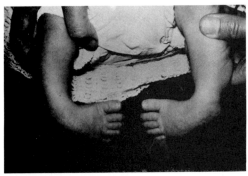

Figure 15.1 Bilateral congenital talipes equinovarus: clinical appearance

possibly accentuated by an intrauterine posture. This is especially likely if one foot is in varus and the other in valgus. The foot of a normal baby may be passively everted and dorsiflexed so that the little toe approximates to, or actually touches, the leg. In a structural club foot this movement is restricted in varying degree.

Mild examples (not always the most amenable to treatment) may dorsiflex to 90 degrees or more, but the heel remains neutral and does not swing into valgus as it should. Severe deformity displays fixed equinus, a fixed varus heel which is small and tucked under the medial malleolus with adduction, supination and cavus of the forefoot. The calf muscles may be lacking in bulk. The degree of rigidity is variable both between feet and between different elements of the deformity in the same foot, and this is of moment in considering prognosis.

Differential diagnosis

The spine is examined to exclude an obvious clue to a neurological determinant. There may be an obvious myelomeningocele or more subtle signs such as a hairy patch or diffuse haemangioma. Sometimes, even in infancy, peroneal or dorsiflexor weakness may be suspected when the spine is superficially normal. Tibial deficiency or constriction rings, if present, indicate a bad prognosis. General examination should not be overlooked because congenital anomalies are frequently multiple or are associated with generalized disorders. In this instance arthrogryposis multiplex congenita and diastrophic dwarfism are considered. In practice the primary treatment is the same in the various varieties, but their early recognition is an aid in prognosis and a precaution against embarrassment later.

The anatomy of the deformity

The anatomy of the deformity varies depending upon age, treatment (and its effects) and growth, so the abnormality may be conveniently divided into the primary changes present *in utero* or at birth, before treatment begins, and those developing without treatment or as a result of treatment (secondary). Radiological changes are described later.

The primary deformity

The primary deformity has received much attention but we remain ignorant of the cause. Wynne-Davies (1964a) investigated genetic factors and found a significant rise in incidence among first degree relations and siblings (2.9 per 1000). This implies that the risk to further children is increased 20 times and that other factors must be concerned as well.

These other factors are unknown, but among the speculations are arrested development when the foot is normally in equinovarus, occult neurological or muscular deficiencies, and abnormal intrauterine compression – but none has factual support. Muscular influences require further discussion because, at operation, tendons sometimes seem abnormal. By this time, however, it is difficult to exclude secondary adaptive changes. These may account for medial prolongation of the tendo Achillis, thickening and surrounding fibrosis of the tendon of tibialis posterior, and a medially displaced tibialis anterior (Wiley, 1959). Deficiency of the calf, however, is an observable primary abnormality.

It would be surprising if the equinus, adduction and inversion deformities of both hindfoot and forefoot were not reflected in the shape of the bones and joints at birth, and indeed this is so. If there is an essential lesion, it is varus deformity of the neck of the talus to 45–65 degrees compared with the normal medial inclination of 25–30 degrees from the body (Irani and Sherman, 1963) and medial displacement of the navicular on the head of the talus (Brockman, 1930). The other bones of the tarsus are relatively normal in shape but

tilted to follow the clinical deformity. Thus the calcaneum is tilted into equinus and the cuneiforms are disposed more vertically. A more recent study by Ippolito and Ponseti (1980) of congenital club feet in infants between the ages of 16 and 19 months, showed extensive changes even at this early age. The tarsal bones are misshapen and smaller than normal. There is a decrease in the size and number of muscle fibres in the distal third of the muscles of the posterior and medial aspects of the leg, with an increase in the fibrous tissue in these muscles, tendons and fasciae. the ligaments on the posterior and medial aspects of the ankle joint are pulled into the joint by severe plantar flexion and varus of the talus, with thickening of the distal tendo Achillis and the posterior capsule of the ankle. Sophisticated three-dimensional computer modelling has added to our understanding of the inter-relationships of the bones (Herzenberg *et al*, 1988).

Secondary bony deformities

Secondary bony deformities follow with growth and adapt themselves at first to the shape of the foot which is imposed by the primary deformity. They later undergo further modifications which seem to alleviate some of the early deformity by indirect means. Thus at first the heel becomes slightly inverted and the subtalar joint inclines upward and medially; the navicular widens medially and becomes vertically longer and narrower. The lateral aspect of the whole foot becomes both convex and longer than the medial. The joints also share in the deformity by alterations in their planes of articulation. The altered alignment of the subtalar joint has been mentioned; the calcaneocuboid is directed more medially, the navicular may so displace at its articulation with the talus that it opposes the medial malleolus, and the metatarsals may adduct on the cuboid and cuneiforms, which in turn adduct and invert at the mid-tarsal joint.

Treatment and walking exert the same force on the deformity. This is towards dorsiflexion and eversion, and in both this represents an attempt to make the equinus and inverted foot plantigrade. If the deformity does not yield where it should – that is, equinus of the ankle and inversion of the subtalar joint – spurious correction may occur in the vertical plane (dorsiflexion) to overcome equinus, and in the horizontal plane to overcome inversion (external rotation). The vertical breach takes place at the mid-tarsal area so that the forefoot dorsiflexes around the fixed plantar flexion of the hindfoot (rocker bottom foot). The horizontal breach occurs at the ankle, the talus externally rotating in the mortice carrying the fibula backwards with it (bean-shaped foot).

The vertical breach causes no other significant changes but the horizontal breach alters the alignment of the foot considerably so its mechanism warrants an explanation. Normal dorsiflexion requires that the posterior structures relax to allow movement at the ankle, and the medial structures relax to allow eversion of the subtalar joint. If either or both are tight (as in club feet) and dorsiflexion is forced, external rotation takes place at the ankle mortice. Recently Scott, Catterall and Hosking (1983) reported an anatomical study of the ankle and subtalar joint in normal and clubbed fetal feet. They showed that in normal feet there is rotatory movement of the talus in the ankle mortice, the lateral surface moving in a greater arc than the medial surface, and the fibula normally moves forward on the os calcis. Prevention of this movement by an inextensible tether placed posterolaterally between the fibula and the os calcis blocks dorsiflexion which, if forced carries the fibula backwards and the talus into external rotation.

The secondary effects include internal rotation of the posterior part of the calcaneum which lies behind the axis of rotation, and external rotation of the rest of the foot. Thus the anterior part of the talus, although adducted, is externally rotated to overlie the anterior calcaneum and the varus of the forefoot is correspondingly reduced. In walking, the effect is reinforced by external rotation of the whole leg seen in the lateral inclination of the patella. The total effect of this adaptation is to reduce the forefoot varus, thus making walking easier (Swann, Lloyd-Roberts and Catterall, 1969). The great complexity of this disorder readily accounts for the generally unsatisfactory results of treatment.

Radiological signs

There is an increasing awareness of the usefulness of radiographs in the management of club feet, provided that they are always made in the same standard positions. Beatson and Pearson (1966) recommended that both the anteroposterior and the lateral projections be taken with the ankle in 30 degrees of plantar flexion. We use this position for the anterior projection but still take the lateral projection with the foot as near 90 degrees to the leg as possible.

Certain normal relationships may be readily seen when all the bones are calcified, but interpretation is more difficult in younger children. In a normal foot in the lateral view the talus, navicular and first metatarsal make a straight line when bisected, and a similar bisection of the calcaneum meets this line in the region of the navicular at an angle of about 30 degrees. In the anteroposterior view the talus and calcaneum diverge at 30 degrees, and again the line bisecting the talus and projected forwards divides the navicular and the centre of the first metatarsal.

In infants under 6–8 weeks of age with club feet, the contour and ossification of the calcaneum and talus are too indefinite for conclusions rather than speculations. At this age the talus and calcaneum are both elongated and bisecting lines may be drawn on the lateral projection. If deformity persists, the talus will be surprisingly anterior and horizontal in the ankle mortice; the calcaneum remains in equinus. These lines may be parallel or meet beyond the foot or within the foot distal to the expected situation at the navicular. Beatson and Pearson regarded 40 degrees as the critical angle beyond which the foot is grossly abnormal. The anteroposterior view is unlikely to be helpful at this age, but later the shadows of calcaneum and talus may overlap, the navicular (when it appears) may be seen to lie too medially on the head of the talus and the line of the talus projected forwards passes through the third or fourth metatarsal. The degree to which all these signs are abnormal depends of course upon the severity of the deformity.

When the foot breaches, further changes are seen in the radiograph. In the vertical breach (rocker bottom) the calcaneum remains in equinus, but its bisecting line no longer continues into the fifth metatarsal because this is now dorsiflexed in relation to the calcaneum, forming an angle centred on the cuboid.

The horizontal breach (Figure 15.2) first declares itself by some posterior displacement of the lower fibula which, if allowed to

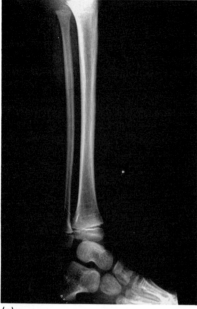

(a)

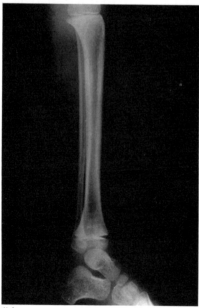

(b)

Figure 15.2 (a) Sagittal breached foot. Note that the fibula appears to be posteriorly displaced, the apparent flat top talus. (b) Same foot internally rotated to place the fibula in the correct position. Note that the hindfoot now looks normal but the forefoot is more deformed

The more the ankle is viewed from the front the more the talus appears 'flat topped' – its normal contour in the anteroposterior radiograph. This is the common cause of this 'deformity' rather than necrosis due to forced manipulation. This external rotation also accounts for the apparent shortening and box-like appearance of the calcaneum and the loss of talocalcaneal divergence in the frontal view. A more normal prospect of the hindfoot is obtained if the lateral radiograph is repeated with the leg internally rotated.

External rotation also modifies the appearance of the posterior calcaneum as seen in the axial view (as for a fracture). Because this is behind the axis of rotation it is seemingly inwardly rotated, but if the radiograph is repeated with internal rotation of the leg the appearance is shown to be largely spurious, for the calcaneum is now longer and straighter. These changes were illustrated and discussed by Swan, Lloyd-Roberts and Catterall (1969).

Management

The growing period may be arbitrarily divided into four age spans, each having an influence upon treatment peculiar to itself. The first is from birth to 1 year, the second from 1–5 years of age, the third 5–12 years of age, and the last the years around skeletal maturity.

The methods that we will now describe are those currently used at The Hospitals for Sick Children, but it must be emphasized that with so much still unknown there are many roads to success (and failure) and we can but try to select the modes which seem most likely to favour success, in varying degree, in the greatest number. Some of these aspects were discussed elsewhere (Lloyd-Roberts, 1964).

To exemplify the variation in attitudes to treatment we may contrast our initial approach with that of Blockey and Smith (1966). We have concentrated on selecting one method of primary treatment which seems the most consistently successful, whereas they used three methods in sequence, with comparable results.

There is in general a continuing trend towards emphasis on early correction of hindfoot equinus rather than postponing this until, in traditional fashion, first the mid tarsal and then the subtalar deformities have been corrected. It is well known that idiopathic congenital calcaneus is associated with valgus,

progress, comes to lie behind the tibia and, as external rotation increases further, an anteroposterior view of the ankle on the same radiograph may be seen as a lateral of the foot.

and equinus with varus, and these patterns are never reversed. Attenborough (1966) made the pertinent observation that a baby's heel cannot be placed in valgus when the foot is in equinus, nor varus when in calcaneus. These, with other observations – clinical, radiological and at operation – support this philosophy.

From birth to 1 year of age

This is the vital period because, if correction is not obtained during this phase, it is unlikely to be achieved at any time in the future.

Treatment cannot begin too early in either the home or the maternity hospital. Should this for some reason not be possible, it should be remembered that healthy newborn babies travel well and may be referred as outpatients to an appropriate hospital department.

When first seen, the diagnosis of structural idiopathic club foot is confirmed by the signs already described. Next attempt to assess the severity. This is no easy matter for we have no reliable criteria. However, the approximate range of movement of ankle, subtalar and mid-tarsal joints are recorded with comments about the size of the foot and calf, the presence of cavus, and so on. Rigidity is described in arbitrary terms, for again we have no sure criteria. Denham (1967) tried to assess the degree of rigidity by using a standard spring-loaded force on the foot and recording photographically the position obtained. Harrold and Walker (1983) have published the results of their series in which the degree of correction that could be obtained by maximum pressure on the foot when it was first examined was recorded photographically. The rigidity of the feet was then classified as mild, moderate or severe, depending on the correction obtained at this initial examination.

After a gentle manipulation, we proceed to strap the foot in the manner attributed to Robert Jones, as described below (Figure 15.3).

Application of Robert Jones' strapping for talipes equinovarus

Materials
Tinc. Benz. Co.
Cotton wool
7 mm thick adhesive surgical felt
2.5 cm wide zinc oxide strapping

Method
Apply Tinc. Benz. Co. liberally over:

1. The dorsal and plantar aspects of the foot.
2. The thigh, above the knee to a depth of 3 cm, or more if a larger child.
3. Both sides of the lower leg.
4. Around the anterior and posterior aspects of the lower leg, between the knee and the malleoli.

Felt
Foot: Take a piece of felt at least 2.5 cm wide and put it round the foot, the distal edge level with the base of the toes, and with the join in the midline on the dorsum of the foot.
Knee: Put a longer piece of felt of the same minimal width over the top of the *fully flexed* knee and down either side of the lower leg, leaving a space of at least 2 cm above each malleolus.

Fixation
Apply the strapping over the felt, starting at the lateral edge, crossing to the medial and round the plantar aspect; then up over the knee, still fully flexed, and down two-thirds of the medial aspect of the lower leg. In doing this, pull the foot with eversion into dorsiflexion as far as possible. If necessary, a second piece of strapping may be applied on top of the first, to increase this correction.

Then put another piece of strapping round the calf, further to tighten and to anchor the vertical pieces. This piece should go round twice, one on top of the other.

Circulation
The peripheral circulation must be checked before the child leaves the department. If after 10 minutes and with the child at rest, the foot, or any part of it, is dusky, check to find the impediment and make the necessary adjustment. If the foot remains dusky after this, take everything off *gently* and start again.

Frequency
Felt and strapping are applied once a week and the correction tightened by strapping on top twice or once during the following 4 days. On the 7th day the mother removes the strapping and felt, leaving the leg free for 24 hours.

The main correcting force is applied around the felt-protected forefoot, so that the free end of the strapping emerges on the lateral side to continue up, above and over the flexed knee to

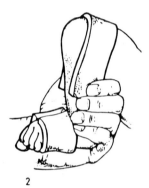

The Hospital For Sick Children
Great Ormond Street, London, W.C.1.

Orthopaedic Dept.
and
Dept. of Physical Medicine

1967

1

Position of operator's hands

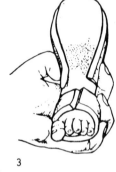 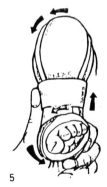

2   3

Application of felt

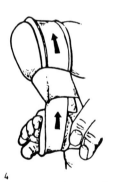

4   5

Application of strapping

Figure 15.3 Robert Jones' strapping for club feet. This
diagram and the explanatory comments in the text
illustrate the method as used at The Hospital for Sick
Children

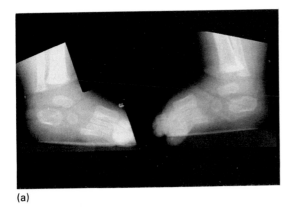

(a)

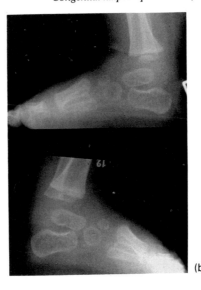

(b)

Figure 15.4 (a) Lateral X-rays of bilateral congenital talipes equinovarus. Note that neither foot is fully corrected. (b) Lateral X-ray of the same patient after posterior release surgery, showing the correction achieved

be fixed to the medial side of the calf. Sometimes a second strip is placed from medial to lateral around the heel and again continued over the knee. The prolongation over the knee is used for added security of fixation and in the belief that, when the child kicks, an added dynamic force is transmitted to the foot.

The mother is taught to manipulate the foot at feeding and nappy changing times, and she returns to the physiotherapist (who manages this stage in treatment) three times each week – twice for overstrapping to take up the slack and once to change the strapping.

The earliest treatment of club feet is by tradition the affair of an outpatient department, but this is somewhat irrational when this is the all-important phase, and results as a whole are far from satisfactory. If beds for mothers were available it would be more rational to admit these babies for constant supervision by the physiotherapist during the first 2 weeks of life.

This method continues for between 6–12 weeks, when the first important decision is taken. If the forefoot corrects on the hindfoot but the hindfoot remains in equinus it should be released by operation. This assessment is based largely on the radiological signs already described (Figure 15.4), but careful inspection of the heel is valuable supporting evidence. If it remains high, there is a sharp convexity at its upper border. At this stage the forefoot is usually corrected but the subtalar joint is likely to lack eversion.

The operation aims to release the hindfoot both posteriorly to prevent a vertical breach (Figure 15.5) and posteromedially to prevent a horizontal breach. It involves lengthening of the tendo Achillis, division of the posterior ankle capsule, posterior talofibular ligament, and tibialis posterior (Perkins' rogue muscle), with flexor hallucis and digitorum longus if their are tight (Attenborough, 1966). We usually add division of abductor hallucis and strip the plantar fascia, with special emphasis on its attachments to the medial face of the calcaneum. Plaster is applied until the wound is healed and thereafter strapping as before. Scott, Catterall and Hosking (1983), following their studies of fetal club feet, have suggested that particular attention should be paid to the

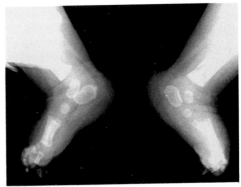

Figure 15.5 Club foot with vertical breach. Note the rocker-bottom contour of soft tissues on the left. The right side has been corrected

posterolateral tether between the fibula and the calcaneum.

This treatment continues until the foot will evert and dorsiflex beyond the neutral position and can be stimulated to do this actively. Although attendances become less frequent, manipulation and strapping may continue for 6 months, and sometimes longer. We next prescribe Denis Browne's bootee splints in which open-ended boots are attached to the hobble splints and joined by a cross-bar. This is a good method of maintaining correction, as opposed to obtaining it. We advise they are used until the child is established in walking.

The results of this method were first analysed by Shaw (1964) and appeared again in Fripp and Shaw's monograph. More recently, Main *et al.* (1972) analysed the results of early operation in the first 6 months of life on 77 club feet which had failed to respond to conservative treatment. They showed that about 50% achieved a satisfactory result following surgery; further surgery improved this to a 70% satisfactory result. In a small group operated on under the age of 6 weeks, 83% were satisfactory. However, the long-term follow-up of these patients (Lloyd Roberts and Green, 1985) showed no significant difference between those operated on early or late. As a result we would now only recommend early surgery and the limited posterior release (Attenborough) operation for those showing correction of the forefoot or the hindfoot at 12 weeks. Patients with severe Harold type III feet not responding to early conservative treatment should be left until 9–12 months of age when the more extensive procedures recommended by Turco can be used.

Fripp and Shaw also analysed the results obtained using Denis Browne splints, which were usually changed, with a manipulation, at 2-week intervals, following an initial month of weekly changes. Out of 105 feet, only 19% were corrected by splinting and manipulation alone, of which very few were lasting. Out of 17 feet treated by serial plasters alone, only two maintained correction at near-maturity. However, this was too small a number to be significant. Kite's method of wedging plasters (1964) is difficult to apply to very small children and unfortunately he gave no details of results in his book. Serial plasters remain the most commonly used conversative treatment. We prefer stretching and strapping but it is probably more difficult to manage in hot climates. Brockman (1930), reporting on the results of stretching and strapping, regarded 50% as corrected without posterior release, a figure which was increased to 70% by later lengthening of the Achilles tendon, manipulation and plaster. These results are the same as ours but are more remarkable because less than half his patients began their treatment within 3 weeks of birth.

Recently, some surgeons have been advocating very early surgery, within the first 1–2 weeks of life. Ryoppy and Sairanen (1983) report remarkably good results in 94 feet treated at a mean age of 12 days. However, they emphasize the necessity for a high standard of neonatal anaesthesia and experience in neonatal orthopaedic surgical techniques and postoperative care as prerequisites for success with this type of surgery. A more radical type of one-stage posteromedial release with internal fixation has been advocated by Turco (1971) in the USA. This can achieve very good results, as given in the same author's report (Turco, 1979), and has also been reported in the UK by Ghali *et al.* (1983). The technique can give very good correction, but sometimes leads to stiffness or overcorrection into valgus. If there is recurrence, requiring reoperation, there is very troublesome scarring to contend with on the medial side. This technique should probably be reserved for very resistant Harold type III feet and operation delayed until 9–12 months. The Cincinnati approach is very helpful for this extensive procedure (Crawford, Marxen and Osterfeld, 1982).

From 1 to 5 years of age

The span of 1–5 years of age is chosen because it begins with the start of walking and ends at the earliest age at which operations on bone (excluding triple arthrodesis and tarsectomy) are feasible. It is also the time when failure of primary correction is most likely to declare itself. There are three common situations.

In the first group are those patients who are apparently corrected on clinical and radiological evidence. These must be watched and the mothers encouraged to continue stretching and exercising. They will have been warned previously that club feet are treacherous. Continued night splintage is commonly advised but in long-term series there is no significant difference between those using splints and those not.

The second group include those with apparent correction who nevertheless walk with their forefeet in varus during the lift off phase. This is not to be confused with fixed forefoot varus with a corrected hindfoot (*see* below). Tendon transfer of tibialis anterior to the lateral side of the foot is indicated. This transfer must be made neither too far laterally nor with tension or a lateral rocker bottom foot, or troublesome forefoot valgus may develop. The tendon should be transplanted to the mid-dorsum or stitched to a detached dorsal tongue of the peroneus brevis tendon which, retaining its distal insertion, increases the effective length of tibialis anterior by about 5 cm. It may seem more logical to transfer tibialis posterior via the interosseous membrane but if tibialis anterior is not moved as well there is a real danger of a secondary medial cavus developing. In practice, transfer of tibialis anterior alone is satisfactory.

Thirdly, there are those cases who are clearly not corrected. If a posteromedial release has not been done already, it should be – or, if inadequate, repeated. This is particularly indicated if the foot is breaching vertically. If there is a fixed forefoot varus, the rest of the foot being apparently satisfactory, correction by serial plasters in combination with a release of abductor hallucis at its origin and insertion usually succeeds in those of moderate severity. In severe fixed deformity, tarsometatarsal release (Heyman, Herndon and Strong, 1958) may be necessary but recent reports are not encouraging (Stark *et al*, 1987). Mild forefoot varus seems to recover spontaneously. Indeed, Wynne-Davies (1964b) noted the tendency of this element of club feet to improve, however unpromising at first.

Lacking these special circumstances we must choose between formal medial soft tissue release operations (Ober, 1920; Brockman, 1930), with their various modifications, and postponing further operation until the patient is 5 years of age. Medial soft tissue operations have limitations and complications, and are difficult to manage afterwards in a rational way. The limitations include failure to influence secondary bony deformity. The complications are a stiff foot and a tendency to recurrence due to contraction of superficial

and deep fibrosis in the scar, which is inevitably placed in an unfavourable position. The exception is recurrent cavus and forefoot pronation which responds well to medial release.

Lastly comes the problem of the duration of postoperative immobilization of a foot in which full correction has been obtained. A short period invites recurrence for the bones are still misshapen; a long period such as 6 months encourages stiffening; and immobility discourages corrective bone growth. Brockman abandoned his operation after a few years because he found no virtue in substituting rigid valgus for mobile varus. Most of these criticisms are overcome if the operation is postponed and combined with calcaneocuboid arthrodesis (*see* below).

Persistence of deformity at this age is rarely associated with a vertical breach (rocker bottom), but very commonly with signs of horizontal breaching (bean shaped). By tradition, manipulations under anaesthesia followed by plaster or wedging plasters (Kite) are the favoured methods. Manipulation with force under anaesthesia is a hazard to mobility and the blood supply of the talus. Serial or wedging plasters applied with gentleness and frequency are innocent of this criticism; however, we very much doubt their value in contributing to true, as opposed to spurious, correction in most feet. Once horizontal breaching (external rotation at the ankle) has begun, this will progress more readily than the responsible fixed deformity which lies further forward in the foot will yield. Pressure, however gentle, towards eversion and dorsiflexion only encourages lateral rotation, whereas lateral pressure on the forefoot may truly correct forefoot varus without affecting the hindfoot. This combination will give an illusion of overall improvement which, however, is largely the result of spurious correction at the ankle joint.

We therefore avoid plaster 'correction' at this age and simply tell the mother to continue to stretch the forefoot into valgus, hoping thereby to reduce the tendency to recurrence of equinus and the amount of forefoot varus that will need correction later.

From 5 to 12 years of age

In the span from 5 to 12 years of age, the degree of deformity and the range of mobility govern our attitude; both factors are not only of great importance, they are also interrelated. It must be emphasized that it is not necessarily desirable to treat every uncorrected club foot at this age. Deformity is variable and function does not always deteriorate with further growth. Deformity is sometimes non-progressive, but more commonly secondary deformity compensates adequately and the foot retains useful function and social acceptance. This is particularly so when good mobility is retained. Laaveg and Ponseti (1980), in their long-term study, have emphasized that a good functional result correlated very well with a good range of motion in the foot and ankle joints, and that an absolute anatomical correction with loss of motion was sometimes worse than accepting some anatomical deformity and retaining mobility. Whatever we do, we must avoid procedures such as forced manipulation and extensive soft tissue release, which prejudice this vital asset. It is better by far to retain movement and accept mild deformity than to correct deformity at the expense of movement.

If treatment seems necessary, any of the operations mentioned in the previous section are applicable for the same indications. We have usually, however, to deal with the bean-shaped foot – that is, varus, cavus and inversion (supination) of the forepart of the foot. Correction may be considered from three aspects. Firstly, we may accept the secondary deformity at the ankle and correct the foot. Secondly, we may realign the ankle by medial rotation of the tibia and correct the forefoot later. Thirdly, we may increase the ankle deformity by rotating the tibia laterally.

The first possibility is the more familiar and certainly the easier. The principle is to externally rotate the forefoot and the heel to align them with the similarly rotated ankle. For the forefoot, Dillwyn Evans' operation (1959, 1961) achieves this admirably (Figure 15.6). The technique involves correction of residual equinus first, a thorough medial release of the talonavicular joint, plantar fasciotomy and stabilization of the correction achieved by calcaneocuboid fusion, having first cut a laterally based wedge from this joint. The virtues are first that the subtalar and peri-cuneiform joints are left intact and a stiff foot is unlikely. Secondly, the convexity of the bean-shaped foot is straightened, shortened and

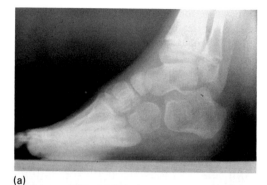

(a)

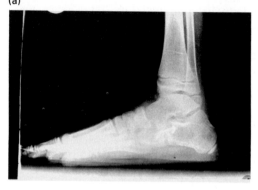

(b)

Figure 15.6 (a) Lateral X-ray of a mid-foot breach before Dillwyn Evans' collateral operation. Note the apparent flat top of the talus, posterior fibula and foreshortened os calcis. (b) Lateral X-ray after the Dillwyn Evans procedure. Note the improvement in the dome of the talus, the position of the fibula and the shape of os calcis

stabilized, thus fixing the correction obtained at the talonavicular joint. Lastly, although the essential improvement is due to external rotation and valgus, both cavus and supination may also be improved by this operation which allows three-dimensional correction. Our results with this procedure (Addison, Fixsen and Lloyd-Roberts, 1983) have shown that the great majority of patients were satisfied with their feet, but inevitably the operation is associated with some stiffening of the hindfoot. If the subtalar joint is mobile, the hindfoot varus will also be corrected. If not calcaneal osteotomy (Dwyer, 1963) preferably from the lateral side will align the weight-bearing posterior plantar surface with the remainder of the foot. Again, no joint is at risk.

Residual equinus with or without deformity of the foot may cause disability during this time. It is unlikely that posterior release will influence this significantly after the age of 8 years or thereabouts. This is because, in rotating laterally, the talus protrudes forwards, and so the medial articular surface extrudes somewhat from the tibial mortice. Attempts to correct equinus at the ankle joint will fail because there is a bony block at this point. Furthermore, the talus is usually horizontal rather than in equinus, the calcaneum providing both clinical deformity and talocalcaneal divergence on the lateral radiograph. Uncorrectable equinus can either be left until nearer maturity or elongation of the tendo Achillis undertaken combined with distal displacement os calcis osteotomy.

The second choice is to medially rotate the tibia, to correct the alignment of the ankle and the heel but increase the deformity of the forefoot. This will need attention later by either Dillwyn Evans' operation or wedge tarsectomy. A secondary advantage of such a tibial osteotomy is that, by angulating it slightly forwards, any residual equinus is improved. We used this for a short period but the size of the wedge tarsectomy required led to severe shortening of the foot and we rarely, if ever, do this now.

The third possibility is to externally rotate the tibia. This is indicated when the foot is severely deformed and stiff, and rigid varus of the forefoot is a handicap in walking. Moderate degrees are naturally compensated for by lateral rotation of the ankle and tibia and reinforced by lateral rotation of the hip on walking. If this mechanism is inadequate, lateral rotation osteotomy of the tibia is helpful.

Skeletal maturity and thereabouts

Provided that some useful movement remains, any of the previously mentioned operations (with the exception of posterior release) may be used to improve the deformity and retain movement. Alternatively, if deformity is moderate, there is no pain and movement is good, it is often best not to interfere.

Triple arthrodesis, regardless of any movement that may remain, has been the final solution for too long. A stiff foot, especially if there is also limitation of ankle movement, is a disability (it is difficult to climb a ladder or cross a ploughed field) and is not entirely blameless as a cause of degenerative arthritis in the ankle later. We are of the opinion that the only absolute indication is unacceptable deformity with rigidity, when this operation converts a stiff deformed foot into a stiff straight foot. this also reduces the risk of pain later. Sometimes, however, wedge tarsectomy with calcaneal osteotomy (preserving the subtalar joint) seems a worthwhile alternative in even severe deformity.

The difficulties encountered in correcting late persistent equinus have been mentioned. Triple arthrodesis is no solution, and, if deformity exceeds that for which a raised heel is compensatory, a solution must be found. If the ankle is stiff, arthrodesis at about 10 degrees of equinus is the natural choice. If not stiff, a low tibial osteotomy is performed. For cosmetic reasons this should be made as low as possible at the level of the growth plate, and is therefore postponed until growth has ceased.

Lastly, a stiff foot and ankle with some equinus and pain are sometimes seen when the talus is deformed due to the effects of forceful manipulation in the past. Astragalectomy should then be considered as an alternative to pan-arthrodesis. This operation is particularly useful even in much younger patients with severely stiff feet associated with arthrogryposis, sacral agenesis and occasionally multiple previous failed surgery where the operation can provide a plantigrade, useful but stiff foot.

Metatarsus varus (hook foot, skew foot)

In metatarsus varus deformity the foot anterior to the navicular is adducted and often supinated. There is usually an associated valgus of the heel which is not appreciated until the child walks. The radiograph shows the main deformity to lie at the metatarsotarsal joints (Figure 15.7).

Three varieties are seen. The first presents in infancy and is usually easily corrected by gentle pressure and sometimes by the baby's active movement. Persistence may be encouraged if the child sleeps prone with knees flexed and his feet tucked up under him. This variety needs no treatment and invariably corrects itself.

The second variety is slightly more severe and will not fully straighten on gentle pressure. The mother should be taught to stretch the forefoot into valgus holding the heel neutral in the meantime. Those with fixed deformity in early infancy may be treated by plasters in

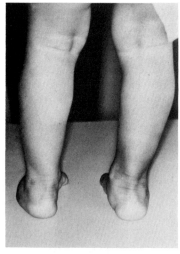

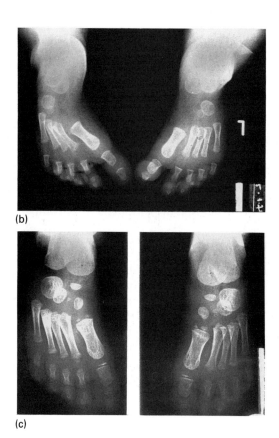

(b)

(c)

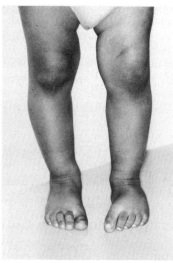

(a)

Figure 15.7 (a) Left metatarsus varus, anterior and posterior views. Note that the head is not in equinus or varus. (b) Right metatarsus varus at age 18 months. (c) X-ray of the patient in (b) at age 3 years after no treatment. Note the spontaneous correction

which care must be taken not to increase the valgus of the hindfoot while correcting the varus forefoot. Alternatively, the condition may be left strictly alone as there is a strong tendency to spontaneous recovery (Ponseti and Becker, 1966; Rushforth, 1978).

Lastly, we infrequently see significant fixed deformity which fails to straighten by 30 degrees or more. In some, release of the abductor hallucis at its origin and insertion followed by corrective serial plasters is effective. In others the radical tarsometatarsal release (Heyman, Herndon and Strong, 1958) seems more appropriate but has recently been criticized (Stark *et al*, 1987). Also, in older children a severe deformity is present at both

fore- and hindfoot so that the whole is distinctly 'S' shaped (Figure 15.8). This seems to represent a different condition in which the foot is serpentine or 'Z' shaped. The navicular lies laterally on the talus. The hindfoot is in fixed valgus. There may be a ball-and-socket ankle present (Lloyd-Roberts and Clark, 1973). This condition is extremely difficult to correct surgically.

Metatarsus varus is almost invariably a benign condition. It is extremely rare to encounter it as a presenting symptom in an adult. Both Ponseti and Becker (1966) and Rushforth (1978) have shown that 85–90% of these patients will correct spontaneously without any treatment by the age of 3–4 years.

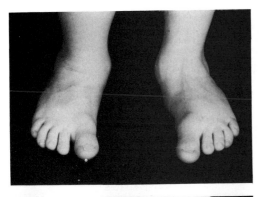

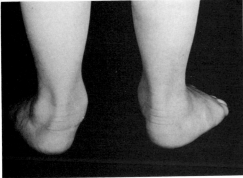

(a)

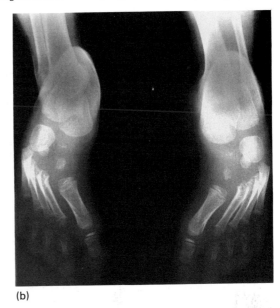

(b)

Figure 15.8 (a) Serpentine or 'Z' foot. (b) Anteroposterior X-ray of true serpentine feet. Note that the navicular is lateral on the talus

Congenital talipes calcaneovalgus

In congenital talipes calcaneovalgus the foot is dorsiflexed and lies everted, so that the dorsum readily touches the anterolateral surface of the leg (Figure 15.9). Plantar flexion ceases at around the mid-position. This is as easy to treat as equinovarus is difficult, and there are no troublesome sequelae – although on first walking there may be a mildly alarming heel valgus. Treatment demands only that the mother stretch the foot into plantar flexion at each feed and nappy change.

The significance relates to other conditions apart from its rare association with posterior angulation of the tibia. Congenital vertical talus (*see* below) is not infrequently overlooked in favour of this diagnosis. If deformity persists after 3–4 months from birth, a neurological cause should be sought. It is also important to look particularly carefully at the hips of neonates with calcaneovalgus because there is an increased incidence of hip instability in association with calcaneovalgus foot and other foot deformities.

Congenital vertical talus (congenital or convex pes valgus)

The rarity of congenital vertical talus does not detract from its interest because it obtrudes into the differential diagnosis of several other abnormalities of the foot. Although it is only seen in relation to club foot in the ratio of about 1:100, it is nevertheless frequently, and therefore incorrectly, diagnosed.

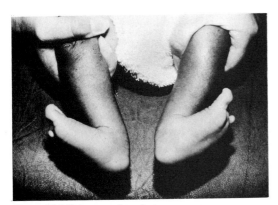

Figure 15.9 Calcaneovalgus feet

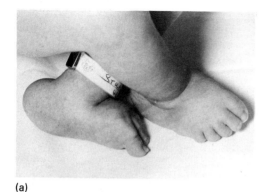

(a)

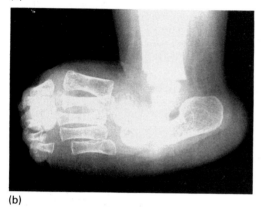

(b)

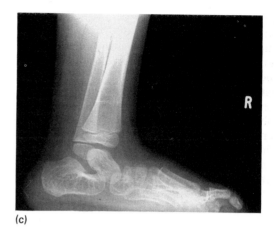

(c)

Figure 15.10 Congenital vertical talus. (a) Bilateral condition. (b) Lateral X-ray. Note the verticality and waisting of the talus. The os calcis is in equinus and the forefoot grossly everted. (c) After corrective surgery

The degree of the deformity varies, but the basic clinical and radiological signs are constant. An older child with marked deformity will walk upon the prominence of the head of the talus which protrudes in the sole. From this point the foot is convex, rising behind to an equinus heel (with slight valgus) and in front to dorsiflexed metatarsals and hallux flexus. There is rigidity, especially at the subtalar joint, which, whatever the severity, is immobile.

The radiograph is characteristic when the tarsal bones are visible, provided (and this is vital) that the foot is placed at 90 degrees to the leg and preferably weight bearing. The calcaneum is in equinus and the talus continues the vertical line of the tibia or departs from this by not more than 20 degrees. The talus is like an hourglass, articulating at the waist, with the navicular in front and the beak of the calcaneum behind (Figure 15.10). This talonavicular dislocation is the essential abnormality, and from this point the cuneiforms and metatarsals rise into dorsiflexion.

In young babies the diagnosis may be difficult, but subtaloid rigidity and the heel in equinus distinguish this from talipes calcaneovalgus. Confusion between these is common, and may wrongly favour one or the other. Interpretation of the radiograph before the navicular appears may be difficult, but the equinus heel and dorsiflexed metatarsals are always visible. Eyre-Brook (1967) emphasized that the position of the navicular may be deduced by observing the movement of the medial cuneiform when the foot is first dorsiflexed and then plantar flexed. Other misdiagnoses include severe paralytic flat foot with collapse of the talus, rigid flat foot with equinus in cerebral palsy, and a vertical breach (rocker bottom) following treatment of club foot. It is rarely an isolated deformity. Commonly it is associated with conditions such as arthrogryposis multiplex congenita, craniocarpotarsal dystrophy (Freeman–Sheldon syndrome) and neurological conditions such as sacral agenesis (Coleman, 1983).

Non-operative treatment is unavailing. In

infancy it is possible that some may be corrected by moulding the foot into full equinus by serial plasters, thereby reducing the talonavicular dislocation, and following this by a posterior release to restore the plantigrade position (Harrold, Silk and Wainwright, 1967). The success of this depends upon relative mobility of the talonavicular joint, and is therefore less likely to succeed when this is rigidly displaced.

In the older child the degree of deformity governs treatment. Moderate or mild deformity is compatible with satisfactory function, and as correction does not improve mobility these are better left. In severe examples an open reduction is necessary. General principles and the details of the standard operation are as described by Herndon and Heyman (1963). Our modification begins as a posterior release followed by mobilization of the talus from the medial side, excision of the navicular to allow room to elevate the talus and fixation by Kirschner wires, with a transplant of tibialis anterior through the neck of the talus. In the more severe case, the forefoot is corrected by dorsal capsulotomies and tendon lengthening at a second stage (Stone and Lloyd-Roberts, 1963). Using Eyre-Brook's (1967) method, one removes only part of the navicular, which is used to block the anterior subtalar joint, and shortens tibialis posterior and the spring ligament. With the Osmond-Clarke (1956) technique, peroneus brevis is transplanted to the talus. This is often a deforming feature on the lateral side. Recently we have performed a full open reduction posteriorly, medially and laterally, stabilizing the correction with K wires and avoiding naviculectomy.

Pes cavus and pes calcaneocavovalgus

In pes cavus and pes calcaneocavovalgus, the medial arch of the foot is abnormally raised in varying degree. Later the heel curls into varus, and the toes claw by extending at the metatarsophalangeal joints and flexing at the interphalangeal joints. Symptoms other than clumsiness are unusual in childhood, but later metatarsalgia, callosities on the toes and disability due to the varus heel are all likely to develop. In calcaneocavovalgus the cavus deformity is much more conspicuous, being accentuated by the calcaneus heel.

Diagnosis is simple but this should be followed by a search for the cause. About 30% must be classified as idiopathic, but because even these are frequently familial, the suspicion remains that a neurological disorder is responsible which will declare itself later. The mechanism by which this deformity develops is uncertain but it is usually thought that intrinsic muscle weakness in the presence of powerful long flexors is responsible. This is difficult to explain other than on a neurological basis, except after injury when local ischaemic contracture may cause it.

Pes cavus is a common presenting symptom in peroneal muscular atrophy (hereditary motor and sensory neuropathy, HMSN types I and II in which familial influences are common) and spina bifida occulta, and less so in spinal dysraphism. In myelomeningocele the paralysis often includes the calf muscles, so a paralytic calcaneocavovalgus is more likely than a simple cavus deformity, as in poliomyelitis. Spasticity in cerebral palsy is sometimes responsible, but although the association with Friedreich's ataxia is well known (especially if this is associated with peroneal muscular atrophy) this is very rarely seen in childhood (Brewerton, Sandifer and Sweetnam, 1963).

Treatment depends upon the degree of deformity, its cause and the rate of deterioration. When first seen there is usually only a minor abnormality which, if truly idiopathic, may not progress, and thus be compatible with normal function. Those with a neurological aetiology, however, are likely to progress because of either neurological deterioration or growth in the presence of muscle imbalance. No form of splinting or physiotherapy has any effect in controlling this deformity.

When the toes remain mobile, growth is still active and there is no significant secondary bony deformity, stripping of the plantar fascia (Steindler's operation), transfer of toe flexors to extensors and extensor hallucis to the neck of the first metatarsal may introduce a dynamic correcting force (Taylor, 1951). When there is fixed clawing of the toes, arthrodesis of the interphalangeal joints and transfer of the long extensors to the necks of the metatarsals is the necessary alternative. The block test described by Coleman (1983) is most useful in assessing the pronation of the forefoot. Plantar and medial release will correct both forefoot pronation and hindfoot varus if it is still mobile. Significant fixed bony deformity may require wedge tarsectomy and calcaneal osteotomy (Dwyer, 1959).

When there is associated calcaneus and valgus, it is tempting to transfer the peronei and one or more dorsiflexors to the Achilles tendon, but this does not seem to delay deterioration significantly. Peroneus longus translocation, however (Makin and Yassipovitch, 1966), in which this tendon is re-routed in continuity via a groove behind the calcaneum, is helpful in poliomyelitis but is rarely applicable in myelomeningocele. Function is relatively good, resembling that after a Syme's amputation, because the child walks on his heel, the forefoot being excluded from weight bearing. Correction may, however, be needed in the interest of appearance and shoe fitting. Elmslie's two-stage triple arthrodesis is a satisfactory method (Cholmeley, 1953).

Equinus deformity

Equinus may occur at the ankle or the mid-tarsal joint (plantaris), and the relative contribution of both is sometimes important in deciding upon treatment. Thus in a cavus foot with metatarsalgia, the abnormal pressure may derive more from calcaneal equinus than the more obvious plantaris associated with the cavus. In practice, however, by equinus we mean that there is fixed plantar flexion of the ankle.

This deformity is usually the result of some obvious primary disorder such as uncorrected club foot, myelomeningocele, conspicuous leg shortening or unequivocal cerebral palsy. However, equinus is sometimes the presenting feature in less florid abnormalities. Thus in a child fresh to walking who tends to tiptoe on one or both sides, the diagnosis of mild spasticity is not always as simple as it may seem. Similarly, minor degrees of shortening of the leg as in infantile coxa vara or contracture of the calf in myopathies may seem equally obscure in origin. If the contracture is so mild that it is obscured by valgus of the heel, as in spastic hemiplegia of trivial degree, or with the hypermobile flat foot (*see* below) with which it is sometimes associated, it is even easier to overlook. Lastly, some children walk temporarily on tiptoe for no apparent reason.

These and other possibilities must be excluded before a diagnosis of idiopathic shortening of the tendo Achillis is considered (Hall, Salter and Bhalla, 1967). In this unusual condition the calcaneal tendon is shortened for unknown reasons, although sometimes there is an abnormally low muscle insertion into the tendon. The contracture is usually mild, and with an effort the child can walk with heels on the ground. There is a tendency to spontaneous improvement, but, if this is not forthcoming in a few months, elongation of the tendon is curative.

Köhler's disease (osteochondritis of navicular)

Variations in the development and pattern of ossification of the tarsal navicular are common, and may exactly simulate this disease. The diagnosis therefore depends upon physical signs rather than radiological changes. The navicular is also variable in the time at which it becomes visible, for this may be from 2.5 to 3.5 years of age. Symptoms arise at between 4 and 5 years of age, and boys predominate.

The child limps and there is pain in the foot. There is tenderness over the navicular and sometimes local swelling, redness and warmth. Movements of the mid-tarsal joint are full. The radiograph discloses either a narrow sclerotic navicular or a bone of normal shape which is dense (Figure 15.11). Within 2–3 years the appearances will return to normal (Waugh,

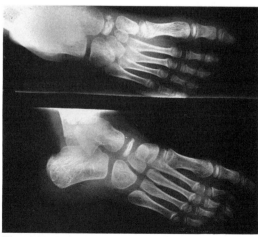

Figure 15.11 Anteroposterior and oblique X-rays showing Köhler's disease of the tarsal navicular

1958). Cox (1958) reviewed 55 patients with Köhler's disease attending The Hospitals for Sick Children and also found no permanent deformity.

Waugh suggested that the changes are due to compression of the navicular (which is the last of the tarsal bones to ossify) between its neighbours. It may then suffer infraction due to insupportable stress. This would certainly account for the symptoms, which are difficult otherwise to explain.

Treatment is obviously symptomatic and in most is unnecessary. Occasionally pain is sufficiently severe to warrant a walking plaster cast but this is seldom needed for more than 6 weeks as symptoms are transitory.

Painful heels in children

Pain in the heel in children is not an uncommon symptom, which may of course be due to some local disorder affecting the calcaneum, such as fibrous dysplasia or osteomyelitis.

The commonest cause is enlargement of the superior and posterior angle of the calcaneum which, compressed by the shoe, causes a tendonitis or bursitis around the tendo Achillis, just above its insertion (os calcis boss). In contrast to this condition in adults, it is very uncommon to have to consider removal of this exostosis in childhood, for the symptoms are transitory and, if not, respond to elevation of the heel of the shoe and removal of the stiffening from the back of that part of the upper which encloses this area.

Sever's disease (osteochondritis of the calcaneal apophysis) is probably a traction lesion of the insertion of the tendo Achillis. It tends to occur in active children, particularly boys between the ages of 7 and 11. The patients present with local tenderness over the insertion of tendo Achillis and find that they are more comfortable in a shoe with a heel than walking barefoot or in tennis shoes. The X-ray shows density and fragmentation, but when an X-ray of the opposite side is taken the same appearances are also present, and this is probably a normal X-ray finding at this age and not a true osteochondritis (Figure 15.12). The symptoms will usually respond to conservative measures such as reducing activity, fitting a small heel pad in the shoe or raising the heel of

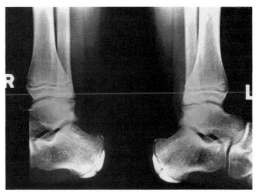

Figure 15.12 X-ray of so-called Sever's disease. The density and fragmentation of the calcaneal apophysis are normal

the shoe to reduce the stretch on the tendo Achillis. Occasionally, in a severe case a short period in a below-knee plaster may be necessary.

Pain in the heels may be due to bruising, and it is easy to miss an os calcis fracture in the normal anteroposterior and lateral views of the foot. If such a fracture is suspected, an axial view of the os calcis should be taken. Plantar fasciitis may develop in juvenile chronic arthritis, sometimes with a heel spur of periosteal new bone. Cushioning the heel with a sorbothane heel pad is useful in this condition.

Flat feet

Physiological and secondary flat feet

Alleged flat feet are a source of disproportionate anxiety among parents and some doctors. Feet are usually declared flat when either the

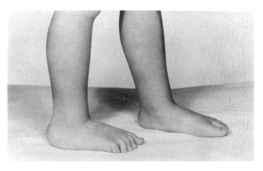

Figure 15.13 Physiological or flexible flat feet in a child with joint laxity

medial side of the foot seems too near the ground or the heel is unduly everted, or there is a combination of both (pronated foot) (Figure 15.13).

Such signs seldom indicate an abnormality provided that there is neither pain or weakness nor loss of movement. Indeed, feet of this type are frequently familial or have a predilection for certain peoples (Jews, West Africans) and are compatible with normal function. Some will remember that great athlete Joe Louis, who would stand in the boxing ring with fully pronated feet, but, rising from this position with astonishing speed and agility when need arose, he was immediately poised for activity. Furthermore, how often are feet of this type seen presenting with symptoms in adult life – other than the occasional young adult with transitory pain on the inner side, or an elderly woman with tenosynovitis of tibialis posterior? This rare happening contrasts with the many children referred for an opinion on their 'flat feet'.

Management is essentially concerned with the exclusion of symptomatic (and therefore abnormal) flat feet, those secondary to some independent condition, and those with abnormalities within the foot itself. Ask about pain, performance at games and the feet of near adult relations, with special reference to their symptoms. On walking, the heel, medial side of the foot, the presence of knock knee and the patellar alignment are noted. Next tell the child to walk in turn on tiptoe, on the point of his heels and in inversion. This establishes that movement and power in these directions are normal. There remain only the range and power of eversion which are tested on the couch. If all is normal, the feet are normal and the mother may be reassured, but if she has been indoctrinated otherwise by shoe shops and friends this may not readily be accepted. On no account should treatment be prescribed to pacify her at the expense of the child. Explanation takes time at the first consultation but saves time in the end, for the child need not return for supervision of treatment. It is often helpful to apply these criteria of normality to the mother's hand and then compare yours with hers, demonstrating the differences and asking which is normal. Rose *et al.* (1985), following a 25-year study, concluded that restoration of the arch on tiptoe or extension of the great toe was the most reliable test of

normality in flat feet.

Secondary flat feet are seen in association with knock knees, when the heels evert to follow the line and thrust of body weight transmitted on their inner sides. A child will often invert his feet (pigeon toeing) to compensate for this. Persistent anteversion of the femoral neck (page 154) produces internal rotation of the thighs (seen at the patellae) and compensatory eversion of the feet. Indeed, this happens so commonly that deliberate external rotation of the thigh in a child not so affected may be used to 'correct the flat foot' in the process of reassuring the mother.

Delay in walking, hypotonia both primary and secondary and joint laxity invariably cause 'flat feet' when walking first starts.

Because painless, mobile and strong 'flat feet' are intrinsically normal or secondary to some other cause, treatment of the feet is by definition unnecessary. Nevertheless, this is frequently prescribed and so merits discussion. Medial wedging of the heel either outside or inside the shoe, plastic heel cups and arch supports are the methods most commonly used. It is difficult to understand exactly what these measures are designed to achieve or the way in which they are supposed to work. We are asked to believe that joints which move in certain directions beyond the average range, but which nevertheless are fully mobile actively and passively in the opposite direction, will in some curious way lose their harmless hypermobility while retaining the other movements. This is attempted nowhere else in the body. Alternative modes are physiotherapeutic and consist of either foot exercises or postural instruction. Foot exercises directed towards strengthening weak intrinsic muscles presuppose that a peculiar paradox exists in flat feet, because paralysis of the intrinsic muscles causes pes cavus and so it is surely more desirable that they should be weak. To correct foot posture the child is taught (and nagged) to walk with his legs laterally rotated at the hips so that the patellae point forwards and counteract eversion of the feet. To develop this habit he must at no time be allowed to walk in any other way. What is to happen when he runs? Is football to be forbidden? How do you 'build up' football boots and should he wear a plastic cup in his gym shoes? Recently Wenger *et al.* (1989) have shown in a carefully controlled trial that corrective shoes and inserts have no effect on the natural history of flexible flat feet in children.

We are of the opinion that there is only one indication for shoe alteration in flat feet and that is to reduce the speed with which the shoes wear out when the heel is in valgus. Sometimes this imposes a strain on the family budget which may be reduced by buying shoes with medial stiffening and asking the cobbler to apply a metal reinforcement to the medial side of the heel.

Symptomatic and pathological flat feet

In symptomatic and pathological flat feet, abnormality may be expressed by pain, by stiffness or by weakness of the foot. These symptoms or signs may occur in isolation or in combination, but for convenience may be discussed separately.

Painful flat feet

In painful flat feet, pain is most commonly transient, felt under the medial border (which is tender) and usually seen in adolescence or early adult life – adolescent foot strain. The mechanism is unknown but pain is assumed to arise from overstretching of plantar ligaments during or after the final growth and weight gain. Whatever the cause, it tends to be a temporary affair with spontaneous remission. If severe, the boy may ask to be taken off games and gym, and then active non-weight-bearing exercises are helpful as an alternative to an arch support to which he may become overattached. This syndrome is usually seen in association with hypermobile flat feet (*see* below). Like many other overuse phenomena in adolescence it is useful to chart the weight and height of the patient who is often over the 90th centile for one or both.

The tarsal scaphoid may be enlarged or duplicated by an accessory bone. There is then a prominence on the medial border of the foot which rubs on the shoe and is painful. If possible, conservative measures should be used to treat this, such as alternative footwear or even wearing a medial arch support to alter the position of the foot in the shoe for a short period. A few will require removal of the prominence or excision of the ossicle. When this is done it is extremely important to remove enough bone to ensure that no prominence is

left following the operation. It is advisable to put the patient in plaster for a short period because the insertion of the tibialis posterior is always disturbed during the operation, and it is important that it heals soundly; otherwise the patient may get a persistent chronic pain at the insertion of this important tendon. Pain is also a feature in peroneal spasmodic flat feet (*see* below).

Weak flat feet

Congenital spinal lesions are the predominant cause of weak flat feet, now that poliomyelitis is a rarity in the developed world. Invertor weakness is followed by valgus displacement of the heel, plantar flexion of the talus into the sole and abduction of the forefoot. This is more likely to be seen with spina bifida occulta or spinal dysraphism than in association with the obvious signs of myelomeningocele. In benign hypotonia with or without joint laxity, the heel sometimes becomes so valgoid that it causes disability and requires stabilization of the subtalar joint before the associated fore-foot pronation becomes a fixed secondary deformity. This may be carried out by subtalar arthrodesis after the child is 5 years of age. The original operation described by Grice requires grafts to be taken from the tibia, and their exact placement is difficult. The Batchelor modification described by Brown (1968), using the fibula as a dowel graft, was very attractive but led to problems with fracture of the fibular graft and disturbance of the growth of the fibula and the ankle mortice. More recently, Dennyson and Fulford (1976) described using a single screw for internal fixation combined with cancellous bone grafting both to obtain accurate fixation of the subtalar joint and to avoid using cortical bone graft from the tibia.

In cerebral palsy there is frequently weakness of the invertors in the sense that there is imbalance between them and the spastic evertors. Indeed, unilateral heel valgus may be a presenting sign in mild hemiplegia. This variety is usually associated with some shortening of tendo Achillis and the peronei so that an element of stiffness is added. Function is generally good and so treatment is rarely indicated for this alone, but a secondary valgus deformity of the big toe is likely to cause symptoms. If treatment seems indicated in the young, subtalar fusion must be combined with tendo Achillis lengthening and division of peroneus brevis, or the deformity will recur with growth. In older children triple arthrodesis is the natural choice, for the foot is both stiff and deformed.

Stiff flat feet

Congenital vertical talus has already been discussed and so has the stiff foot of cerebral palsy. Peroneal spasmodic flat foot is discussed below.

There remains the flat foot associated with shortening of the tendo Achillis and compensatory hypermobility distal to the ankle (Harris and Beath, 1948a). This variety is often painful and seemingly weak, but as restriction of ankle movement is the cause it is discussed under this heading. The calcaneus in equinus provides inadequate support for the talus which plantar flexes and bulges into the sole. There is, however, normal power, and inversion restores the medial concavity of the foot. When the foot is held in this position and dorsiflexed it will be seen that the heel tilts into valgus, and if this is prevented dorsiflexion is limited to about the right angle.

There is considerable variation in severity, many being compatible with good function although prone to foot strain pain in adolescence. If Achillis shortening is conspicuous the child is clumsy, and aching may persist. Stretching in plaster can be helpful, or sometimes slide elongation of the tendo Achillis. In older children subtalar fusion is sometimes indicated. Naviculocuneiform arthrodesis was once a popular remedy but the long-term results were poor, only 30% remaining symptom free (Seymour, 1967).

Peroneal spasmodic flat foot (spastic flat foot)

In spastic flat foot there is fixed valgus deformity of the heel and the forefoot follows, so the foot as a whole is pronated. The peronei stand out when inversion is attempted because they are either shortened or respond by protective muscle spasm. The symptoms are aching pain and clumsiness.

There are two causes – irritative lesions of the tarsus and congenital tarsal anomalies (Harris and Beath, 1948b).

The first group include those acquired

lesions likely to stimulate peroneal muscle spasm, of which the commonest is juvenile chronic arthritis of the subtalar joint. It may, however, develop otherwise with, for example, chronic infection, osteoid osteoma or following injury to the tarsal joints.

The second group (tarsal anomalies) accounts for the deformity more frequently. These are common and may involve any part of the foot (O'Rahilly, 1953) but two varieties are specially important in this context. Fusion between the talus and calcaneum in the region of the sustentaculum tali can be identified only by a special radiographic technique or CT scan, but is responsible in two-thirds of the feet affected. The remainder show a connection between the calcaneum and the navicular which is easily seen in the lateral radiograph (Figure 15.14). Union may be complete or partial, and both are often associated with lipping on the dorsum of the talonavicular joint. The peronei may be structurally shortened.

There are two common clinical problems. Firstly, the condition may be seen but the cause cannot be demonstrated. In these cases there is often a partial talocalcaneal lesion large enough to block inversion and demonstrable at operation, although not visible on the radiograph (Harris and Beath, 1954). Secondly, some with obvious lesions develop symptoms later than others. One can only assume that a strain has precipitated pain and so disclosed the underlying fault.

The prognosis in the first group is that of the cause. In the second, fixed valgus remains but symptoms may disappear. Braddock (1961) followed 12 patients for an average of 20 years and found that 7 were pain free, but in most of these symptoms had continued for many years.

Mitchell and Gibson (1967) and Macnicol *et al.* (1986), reviewing the same patients recently, reported the results of excision of calcaneonavicular bars in children and obtained symptomatic relief in two-thirds of their patients. One patient whose foot we explored in infancy on suspicion of an inflammatory lesion and found and excised a cartilaginous bar, has retained full movement without pain. Talocalcaneal bars lend themselves less to direct attack. Those with persisting and disabling pain are best treated by triple rather than subtalar arthrodesis because of the frequency of talonavicular abnormalities.

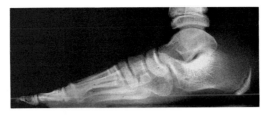
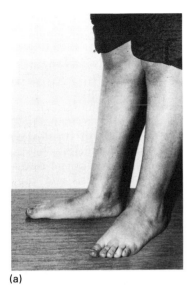
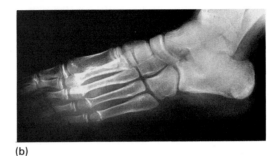

(a)   (b)

Figure 15.14 (a) Bilateral painful peroneal spastic flat feet. (b) Lateral and oblique X-rays showing the partial calcaneonavicular bar in peroneal spastic flat foot

The metatarsals and phalanges

Stress fractures and Freiberg's disease

Stress fractures rarely occur in normal feet below 12 years of age (Figure 15.15). Freiberg's infraction, which involves the head of the second metatarsal, is probably due to stress or an osteochondral fracture rather than to osteochondritis. The second metatarsal is the commonest site, but the condition can develop in other metatarsal heads. It may also develop well beyond skeletal maturity. The head is flattened and dense and the metatarsal thickened below it. There is pain and there are

signs of arthritis in the metatarsophalangeal joint. Symptoms usually resolve if the joint is protected by a metatarsal bar, but are likely to recur later and require excision of the metatarsal head. This may be seen before the age of 12 years, but is unusual.

Hallux valgus

The onset of troublesome adult hallux valgus is frequently traced to childhood. Hardy and Chapman (1951) obtained a history of the deformity before the age of 20 years in half the patients they reviewed, and, if the fickleness of memory is allowed for, the proportion is probably considerably higher.

This immediately introduces the possibility of correction in childhood as a precaution against pain and disability later. Although the results of surgery in adults are on the whole moderately satisfactory, it is preferable if possible to anticipate the need for this.

When a child presents with a valgus deformity at the first metatarsophalangeal joint it is difficult to decide whether to advise correction. On general principles one would expect the younger children to deteriorate as there is more growth ahead of them, but this is not invariably true. It is best, therefore, to take a radiograph with the child standing and compare the angle of deformity by repeating this in

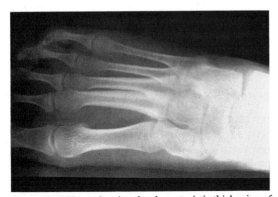

Figure 15.15 X-ray showing the characteristic thickening of the cortex of the second metatarsal following a stress fracture

a year or two. An alternative is an outline drawing in the notes. Piggott (1960) investigated this problem and found that the joint may be congruous, deviated or subluxated. If the joint is congruous it tends to remain so and not deteriorate, but a deviated joint may progress to subluxation. He regarded the normal metatarsophalangeal angle as below 20 degrees, and all his congruous joints were within this range.

The family history may be helpful, particularly if the mother is present and has significant deformity. Symptoms are unusual at this age but, if there is pain on activity or on applying stress to the joint, this would seem an additional reason for interfering. The influence of a varus metatarsal (metatarsus primus varus) is difficult to assess, for it may certainly develop as a result of, rather than as a cause of, hallux valgus.

Treatment is directed towards realignment of the joint rather than arthroplasty. The target is the metatarsal and we may attempt to realign it by tendon transplantation or osteotomy, or both. The adductor hallucis may be transferred from the phalanx to the metatarsal (McBride's operation) and this may be combined with osteotomy at its base (Simmonds and Menelaus, 1960). In Homans' and Mitchell's operations the osteotomy is at the neck (Gibson and Piggott, 1962). For simplicity and reliability and to avoid any risk of stiffness at the metatarsophalangeal joint, Wilson's short oblique osteotomy (1963) is difficult to fault. In general, it is better to delay metatarsal osteotomy until or approaching maturity; otherwise, despite good correction, deformity may recur with growth.

Hallux valgus is sometimes associated with interphalangeal valgus (*see* below), in cerebral palsy and in myelomeningocele, when the forefoot is pronated and abducted. Pain and trophic ulceration are indications for operation.

Hallux rigidus

In hallux rigidus in children the signs indicate that there is arthritis of the first metatarsophalangeal joint without deformity and without degenerative changes. There is painful limitation of plantar flexion and dorsiflexion – the latter causing the pain on walking. This may be a traumatic arthritis due to stubbing the big toe; if this is so, protection of the joint in roomy shoes fitted with a rocker often relieves the symptoms and few recur. In some cases, however, symptoms persist, or, having subsided, recur later in adult life.

Persistent or recurrent symptoms may be associated with abnormal dorsiflexion of the first metatarsal but, as in the varus metatarsal, this may be primary or secondary to the loss of phalangeal dorsiflexion. Nevertheless, hallux rigidus certainly complicates metatarsal elevation following a triple arthrodesis and congenital vertical talus. Kessel and Bonney (1958) noted a lesion resembling osteochondritis on the metatarsal head and certainly this sometimes occurs. Whether it is a truly ischaemic lesion or an osteochondral fracture is, however, uncertain. We have seen a similar lesion at the base of the phalanx.

If operation is needed and the child is mature, arthrodesis in a position of compromise (about 20 degrees of dorsiflexion) is entirely satisfactory in men, but less certain in women unless they are prepared to accept a constant height of heel (Harrison and Harvey, 1963). If the epiphysis at the base of the phalanx has not fused, this is clearly undesirable; for these cases Kessel and Bonney suggested that the toe be dorsiflexed by an osteotomy at the phalanx, which appears to give good results.

Interphalangeal valgus of the big toe

Interphalangeal valgus of the big toe is not uncommon in children, and may at first be painful due to shoe pressure. Later, however, callus forms and the pain is usually relieved. The relative rarity in adults suggests that this corrects itself in many patients, but some persist and need treatment in late childhood. This is specially so in cerebral palsy. Corrective osteotomy before and arthrodesis after maturity are both satisfactory solutions.

Hammer toe

In hammer toe, one toe (usually the second) is longer than the others and becomes flexed at the proximal interphalangeal joint and extended at the metatarsophalangeal and distal interphalangeal. This deformity therefore differs from that of claw toes in pes cavus which are correspondingly flexed, extended and flexed. Painful corns on the apex sometimes indicate the need for operation, even in childhood. Excision of the proximal phalanx is simpler and more reliable than arthrodesis with shortening of the flexed joint. Mallet toes (extension, extension, flexion) do not seem to develop in childhood.

Curly toe

In curly toes, the third and fourth toes are usually involved, being rotated medially and flexed and adducted at the distal interphalangeal joint. These are very common and are sometimes associated with partial syndactyly between the second and third toes. By tradition these are strapped in early childhood with the aim of correcting deformity but Sweetnam (1958), after reviewing patients at The Hospitals for Sick Children, found that treatment had no influence on the correction of the deformity and that about one in three straightened spontaneously during the period of observation. The high incidence in children and rarity in adults suggests that most of the others correct later, or, if they persist, do not commonly cause symptoms.

Treatment in childhood is unnecessary unless the toe is giving rise to persistent symptoms. Simple flexor tenotomy will usually alleviate the condition and is less complex than a flexor to extensor transfer, as described for clawing of the toes in association with cavus feet (Menelaus and Ross, 1984).

Congenital elevation of the little toe

In congenital elevation of the little toe, the toe is elevated and rotated medially (Figure 15.16). Being extended at the metatarsophalangeal joint and flexed at the interphalangeal joints it overlies its neighbour. This deformity almost invariably causes pain, because of either a dorsal corn or contact corns between the fourth and fifth toes. When seen in infancy and stretched and strapped assiduously the deformity can sometimes be corrected, but most cases present later with symptoms. Several ingenious operations are described which involve tendon transfer, joint capsulotomies and rearrangement of the skin. Butler's operation described by Cockin (1968) gives good results if carefully performed. A simpler approach is simply to excise the proximal phalanx of the toe.

Miscellaneous conditions seen in the foot

Metatarsal fusions and duplications with dysplastic nails are seen in Ellis–Van Creveld syndrome (page 7) and a short first metatarsal in myositis ossificans (page 85). The nails are also dysplastic in nail–patella syndrome (page 83). Arachnodactyly (Marfan's disease) is characterized by long, thin, hypermobile feet (page 6), and foot deformity is usual in diastrophic dwarfism (page 6). The subtalar joint is very commonly affected in juvenile chronic arthritis (page 80), and, of the neurological disorders, signs in the foot are most frequently the first in spinal dysraphism (page 70) and peroneal muscular atrophy. Congenital lymphoedema (page 21) is commonest here. Duplication of toes and accessory toes are common, especially of the big and little toes. If the little toe is duplicated with its metatarsal, it may be better to remove the fifth ray rather than the accessory sixth. Accessory digits must be excised to the parent metatarsal. Local gigantism of a toe occurs with neurofibromatosis (page 83) and haemangiomatous malformations (page 15). Congenital amputations are usually at the mid-tarsal level and can be readily fitted with blocked shoes. Eosinophilic granulomas (page 77) occur in the calcaneum, and dysplasia epiphysealis hemimelica (page 4) and osteochondritis dissecans affect the dome of the talus.

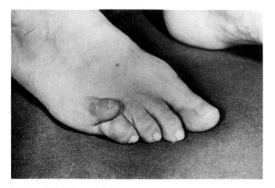

Figure 15.16 Congenital elevation or overlapping of the fifth toe

References

Addison, A., Fixsen, J. A. and Lloyd-Roberts, G. C. (1983) A review of the Dillwyn Evans type collateral operation in severe club feet. *J. Bone Jt. Surg.* **65B**, 12

Attenborough, C. G. (1966) Severe congenital talipes equinovarus. *J. Bone Jt. Surg.* **48B**, 31

Beatson, T. R. and Pearson, J. R. (1966) Method of assessing correction in club feet. *J. Bone Jt. Surg.* **48B**, 40

Blockey, N. J. and Smith, M. G. H. (1966) Treatment of congenital club foot. *J. Bone Jt. Surg.* **48B**, 660

Braddock, G. T. F. (1961) A prolonged follow-up of peroneal spastic flat foot. *J. Bone Jt. Surg.* 43B, 734

Brewerton, D. A., Sandifer, P. H. and Sweetnam, D. R. (1963) 'Idiopathic' pes cavus: an investigation into its aetiology. *Br. Med. J.* **2**, 659

Brockman, E. P. (1930) *Congenital Clubfoot.* Bristol: John Wright

Brown, A. (1968) A simple method of fusion of the subtalar joint in children. *J. Bone Jt. Surg.* **50B**, 369

Cholmeley, J. A. (1953) Elmslie's operation for the calcaneus foot. *J. Bone Jt. Surg.* **35B**, 46

Cockin, J. (1968) Butler's operation for an over-riding fifth toe. *J. Bone Jt. Surg.* **50B**, 78

Coleman, S. S. (1983) *Complex Foot Deformities in Children.* Philadelphia: Lea and Febiger

Cox, M. J. (1958) Kohler's disease. *Postgrad. Med. J.* **34**, 588

Crawford, A. H., Marxen, J. L. and Osterfeld, D. L. (1982) The Cincinnati incision: a comprehensive approach for surgical procedures on the foot and ankle in childhood. *J. Bone Jt. Surg.* **64A**, 1355–1358

Denham, R. A. (1967) Congenital talipes equinovarus. *J. Bone Jt. Surg.* **49B**, 582 [report of demonstration]

Dennyson, W. G. and Fulford, G. E. (1976) Subtalar arthrodesis by cancellous grafts and metallic internal fixation. *J. Bone Jt. Surg.* **58B**, 507

Dwyer, F. C. (1959) Osteotomy of the calcaneum for pes cavus. *J. Bone Jt. Surg.* **41B**, 80

Dwyer, F. C. (1963) Treatment of relapsed club foot by the insertion of a wedge into the calcaneum. *J. Bone Jt. Surg.* **45B**, 67

Evans, D. (1950) Treatment of relapsed club foot. *J. Bone Jt. Surg.* **41B**, 618 [report]

Evans, D. (1961) Relapsed club foot. *J. Bone Jt. Surg.* **43B**, 722

Eyre-Brook, A. L. (1967) Congenital vertical talus. *J. Bone Jt. Surg.* **49B**, 618

Fripp, A. T. and Shaw, N. R. (1967) *Clubfoot.* Edinburgh: Livingstone

Ghali, N. N., Smith, R. B., Clayden, A. D. and Silk, F. F. (1983) Results of pantalar reduction in the management of congenital talipes equinovarus. *J. Bone Jt. Surg.* **65B**, 1

Gibson, J. and Piggott, H. (1962) Osteotomy of the neck of the first metatarsal in the treatment of hallux valgus. *J. Bone Jt. Surg.* **44B**, 349

Hall, J. E., Salter, R. B. and Bhalla, S. K. (1967)

Congenital short tendo calcaneus. *J. Bone Jt. Surg.* **49B**, 695

Hardy, R. H. and Clapham, J. C.R. (1951) Observations on hallux valgus. *J. Bone Jt. Surg.* **33B**, 376

Harris, R. I. (1955) Talo-calcaneal fusion. *J. Bone Jt. Surg.* **37A**, 169

Harris, R. I. and Beath, T. (1948a) Hypermobile flat foot with short tendo Achillis. *J. Bone Jt. Surg.* **30A**, 116

Harris, R. I. and Beath, T. (1948b) Etiology of peroneal spastic flat foot. *J. Bone Jt. Surg.* **30B**, 624

Harrison, M. H. M. and Harvey, F. J. (1963) Arthrodesis of the first metatarsal joint for hallux valgus and rigidus. *J. Bone Jt. Surg.* **45A**, 471

Harrold, A. J. (1967) Congenital vertical talus in infancy. *J. Bone Jt. Surg.* **49B**, 634

Harrold, A. J. and Walker, C. J. (1983) Treatment and prognosis in congenital club foot. *J. Bone Jt. Surg.* **65B**, 8

Helfet, A. J. (1956) A new way of treating flat feet in children. *Lancet* **1**, 262

Herndon, C. H. and Heyman, C. H. (1963) Problems in the recognition and treatment of congenital convex pes valgus. *J. Bone Jt. Surg.* **45A**, 413

Herzenberg, J. E., Carroll, N. C., Christofersen, M. R., Lee, E. H., White, S. and Munroe, R. (1988) Club foot analysis with three-dimensional computer modelling. *J. Ped. Orthop.* **8**, 257–262

Heyman, C. H., Herndon, C. H. and Strong, J. M. (1958) Mobilization of the tarsometatarsal and intermetatarsal joints for the correction of resistant adduction of the fore part of the foot in congenital club foot or congenital metatarsus varus. *J. Bone Jt. Surg.* **40A**, 299

Ippolito, E. and Ponseti, I. V. (1980) Congenital club foot in the human fetus. *J. Bone Jt. Surg.* **62A**, 8

Irani, R. N. and Sherman, M. S. (1963) Pathological anatomy of club foot. *J. Bone Jt. Surg.* **45A**, 45

Kessel, L. and Bonney, G. (1958) Hallux rigidus in the adolescent. *J. Bone Jt. Surg.* **40B**, 668

Kite, J. H. (1964) *The Clubfoot.* New York: Grune & Stratton

Laaveg S. J. and Ponseti, I. V. (1980) Long-term results of treatment of congenital club foot. *J. Bone Jt. Surg.* **62A**, 23

Lloyd-Roberts, G. C. (1964) Congenital club foot. *J. Bone Jt. Surg.* **46B**, 369 [editorial]

Lloyd-Roberts, G. C. and Clark, R. C. (1973) Ball and socket ankle joint in metatarsus adductus varus. *J. Bone Jt. Surg.* **55B**, 193

Lloyd-Roberts, G. C. and Spence, A. J. (1958) Congenital vertical talus. *J. Bone Jt. Surg.* **40B**, 33

Lloyd Roberts, G. C., Swan, M. and Catterall, A. (1974) Medial rotational osteotomy for severe residual deformity in club foot. *J. Bone Jt. Surg.* **56B**, 37–43

Main, B. J., Crider, R. J., Polk, M., Lloyd-Roberts, G. C., Swann, M. and Kamdar, B. A. (1972) Results of early operation in talipes equino-varus. *J. Bone Jt. Surg.* **54B**, 337

MacNicol, M. F., Inglis, G. and Buxton, R. A. (1986)

Symptomatic calcaneonavicular bars. *J. Bone Jt. Surg.* **68B**, 128–131

Makin, M. and Yossipovitch, Z. (1966) Translocation of the peroneus longus in the treatment of paralytic pes calcaneus. *J. Bone Jt. Surg.* **48A**, 1541

Menelaus, M. B. and Ross, E. R. S. (1984) Open flexor tenotomy for hammer toes and curly toes in childhood. *J. Bone Jt. Surg.* **66B**, 770–771

Mitchell, G. P. and Gibson, J. M. C. (1967) Excision of calcaneo-navicular bar for painful spasmodic flat foot. *J. Bone Jt. Surg.* **49B**, 281

Ober, F. R. (1920) An operation for the relief of congenital equino-varus deformity. *J. Orthop. Surg.* **2**, 558

O'Rahilly, R. (1953) Survey of carpal and tarsal anomalies. *J. Bone Jt. Surg.* **35A**, 626

Osmond-Clarke, H. (1956) Congenital vertical talus. *J. Bone Jt. Surg.* **38B**, 334

Piggott, H. (1960) The natural history of hallux valgus in adolescence and early adult life. *J. Bone Jt. Surg.* **42B**, 749

Ponseti, I. V. and Becker, J. R. (1966) Congenital metatarsus adductus: the results of treatment. *J. Bone Jt. Surg.* **48A**, 702

Rose, G. K. (1958) Correction of the pronated foot. *J. Bone Jt. Surg.* **40B**, 674

Rose, G. K. (1962) Correction of the pronated foot. *J. Bone Jt. Surg.* **44B**, 642

Rose, G. K. (1982) Pes planus. In *Disorders of the Foot,* ed. M. H. Jahss. Philadelphia, Eastbourne, Toronto: W. B. Saunders, p. 486

Rose, G. K., Welton, E. A. and Marshall, T. (1985) The diagnosis of flat foot in the child. *J. Bone Jt. Surg.* **67B**, 71–78

Rushforth, G. F. (1978) Natural history of hook forefoot. *J. Bone Jt. Surg.* **60B**, 530

Ryoppy, S. and Sairanen, H. (1983) Neonatal operative treatment of club foot. *J. Bone Jt. Surg.* **65B**, 320

Scott, W. A., Catterall, A. and Hosking, S. W. (1963) Talipes equinovarus: is the tether medial or lateral? *J. Bone Jt. Surg.* **65B**, 221

Seymour, N. (1967) Late results of naviculo-cuneiform fusion. *J. Bone Jt. Surg.* **49B**, 558

Shaw, N. E. and Fripp, A. T. (1966) Comparison of three methods for treatment of congenital clubfoot. *Br. Med. J.* **1**, 1084

Silk, F. F. and Wainwright, D. (1967) Recognition and treatment of congenital flat foot in infancy. *J. Bone Jt. Surg.* **49B**, 628

Simmonds, F. A. and Menelaus, M. B. (1960) Hallux valgus in adolescents. *J. Bone Jt. Surg.* **42B**, 761

Stark, J. G., Johanson, J. E. and Winter, R. B. (1987) The Heyman Herndon tarsometatarsal capsulotomy for metalum adduction. Results in 48 feet. *J. Ped. Orthop.* **7**, 305–310

Stone, K. H. and Lloyd-Roberts, G. C. (1963) Congenital vertical talus: a new operation. *Proc. R. Soc. Med.* **56**, 12

Swann, M., Lloyd-Roberts, G. C. and Catterall, A. (1969) The anatomy of uncorrected club feet. *J. Bone Jt. Surg.* **51B**, 263

Sweetnam, R. (1958) Congenital curly toes. *Lancet.* **2**, 398

Taylor, R. G. (1951) The treatment of claw toes by multiple transfers of flexor into extensor tendons. *J. Bone Jt. Surg.* **33B**, 539

Turco, V. J. (1971) Surgical correction for resistant club foot: one-stage posteromedial release with internal fixation. A preliminary report. *J. Bone Jt. Surg.* **53A**, 477

Turco, V. J. (1979) Resistant congenital club foot – one-stage posteromedial release with internal fixation. *J. Bone Jt. Surg.* **61A**, 805

Waugh, W. (1958) Ossification and vascularisation of the tarsal navicular and their relation to Kohler's disease. *J. Bone Jt. Surg.* **40B**, 765

Wenger, D. R., Mauldin, D., Speck, G., Morgan, D. and Lieber, R. L. (1989) Corrective shoes and inserts as treatment for flexible flatfoot in infants and children. *J. Bone Jt. Surg.* **71A**, 800–810

Wiley, A. M. (1959) Club foot: an anatomical and experimental study of muscle growth. *J. Bone Jt. Surg.* **41B**, 821

Wilson, J. N. (1963) Oblique displacement osteotomy for hallux valgus. *J. Bone Jt. Surg.* **45B**, 552

Wynne-Davies, R. (1964a) Family studies and the causes of congenital club foot. *J. Bone Jt. Surg.* **46B**, 445

Wynne-Davies, R. (1964b) Talipes equinovarus. *J. Bone Jt. Surg.* **46B**, 464

Further reading

Coleman, S. S. (1983) *Complex Foot Deformities in Children.* Philadelphia: Lea and Febiger

Fixsen, J. A. and Lloyd-Roberts, G. C. (1988) *The Foot in Childhood.* New York, Edinburgh, London, Melbourne: Churchill Livingstone

Klenerman, L. (1982) *The Foot and its Disorders,* 2nd edn. Oxford, London, Edinburgh: Blackwell Scientific

Tachdjian, M. O. (1985) *The Child's Foot.* Philadelphia, London, Toronto: W. B. Saunders

Turco, V. J. (1981) *Clubfoot.* New York, Edinburgh, London: Churchill Livingstone

16

General topics

Delay in walking

Most children walk independently at some time between 11 and 15 months of age. Delay until 18 months is not abnormal, provided that the child is standing with the support of his cot side or he is taking a few steps holding on to the furniture. From this point progress to independence is usually rapid, and may often be stimulated in the outpatient department if the child is separated from his mother.

Children of 18 months of age or more who possess neither of these skills are suspected of being delayed by some physical, neurological, emotional or intellectual cause. Nevertheless many are still found to be normal in all respects and develop their independence later.

Physical disabilities are wrongly believed to be a common aetiological factor. In fact, unless the abnormality is obvious, as in severe examples of osteogenesis imperfecta, these are rarely the cause. For example, congenital dislocation of the hip is seldom responsible unless associated with some other feature such as joint laxity.

Hypotonia with joint laxity from whatever cause is the commonest determinant. The child will frequently be brought up with the observation that when put to stand up, the feet lapse into valgus and pronation, and this is the clue which directs attention to joint mobility and muscle tone. Deep reflexes are usually present, but, if absent, a myopathy of early onset is suspected, especially if no progress (however slight) is being made.

Expert crawlers may find walking a comparatively unsatisfactory method of getting

about, especially if they have developed the technique of bottom shuffling.

The possibility of a neurological disorder, especially unsuspected cerebral palsy (page 54), or peripheral flaccid paralysis in association with congenital lesions of the spine must next be considered. If cerebral palsy is responsible, it may well be associated with some degree of intellectual deficit which is likely to be the more important component if the peripheral lesion is so inconspicuous that it has hitherto been overlooked.

Mentally handicapped children are of course generally retarded, including the development of motor skills. Lastly, there are the overprotected and overindulged. This is often justified by serious illness in infancy such as a congenital cardiac lesion which itself contributes to the delay. Sometimes this symptom draws attention to such a situation.

All who are truly delayed display marked valgus of the heels when they begin. This is sometimes confused with the cause. They also have valgus femoral necks on the hip radiograph.

Intoe gait

This is perhaps the single most common reason for referral to a children's orthopaedic clinic. It is a familiar cause for maternal alarm but is seldom due to a significant abnormality. The diagnosis may usually be made by watching the child as he walks towards the examiner (Figure 16.1).

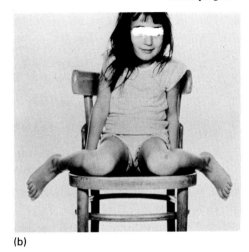

(b)

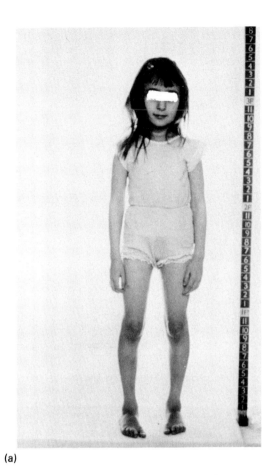

(a)

Figure 16.1 (a) Intoe gait due to persistent femoral anteversion or medial femoral torsion. (b) Same patient sitting in the characteristic 'W' or 'television' position

There are three basic causes for an intoe gait. The first, in the feet, is metatarsus varus with marked adduction of the big toe. This has been discussed in Chapter 15; it corrects spontaneously in the vast majority of cases by the age of 3–3.5 years. The second cause is in the lower leg and is due to so-called physiological bowing of the tibiae, which is always associated with some degree of medial tibial torsion (Chapter 14). Finally, the whole leg may be rotated inwards due to persistent femoral anteversion (Figure 16.1). This frequently runs in families. It occurs in about 10% of the population. These patients characteristically sit between their legs in the so-called 'W' position which is pathognomonic of femoral anteversion (see Figure 16.1b). On the couch with the hips extended they have a far greater range of internal rotation in extension of the hip than external rotation. The great majority correct by the age of 8 – many by increasing the external torsion of the tibia rather than correcting the anteversion (Figure 16.2). It is helpful to suggest that the children sit cross-legged rather than in the 'W' position. There is no evidence of any value in so-called 'twisters' or torsion calipers to correct this condition, nor does any other form of splintage or special shoes affect it. Although it has been suggested, there is no firm evidence that severe anteversion may predispose to osteoarthritis of the hip in later life and also to instability of the patella. In the occasional patient at the age of 10–11 years there may be significant functional and cosmetic disability. In these patients it is occasionally worth considering external rotation osteotomy of the femur to correct the persistent anteversion.

The limping child

There are three common patterns of gait. When there is pain the child moves rapidly off the foot and the stride is shortened on the

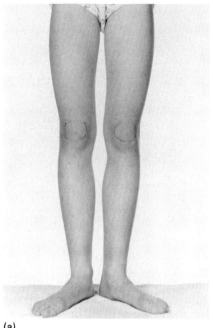 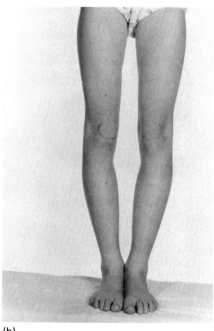

(a)   (b)

Figure 16.2 (a) An older patient with persistent femoral anteversion who has developed compensatory external torsion below the knee, starting with the knees forwards and the feet out. (b) Same patient standing with the feet together, showing characteristic 'squinting' patellae

painful side. If the hip is unstable he lurches towards the affected side (Trendelenburg's sign). Shortening is compensated by equinus on the short side unless, in the very young, it is associated with instability of the hip joint when the foot remains plantigrade but the opposite knee is bent.

A history of pain as given by the child is frequently misleading, for localization is poor, referred pain common and even the sides are confused. However, most arise in the hip and this should be examined first. Next comes the foot where Köhler's disease (page 204) or local painful lesions may be found – such as verruca, calcaneal boss (page 205) and so on. The possibility of injury should not be overlooked, especially if it occurred indulging the pleasures of some forbidden activity. The supracondylar area and the central tibia are favoured sites for these slightly displaced greenstick fractures. Referred pain from the back is very unusual, but pain in the back may be reflected in a cautious and abnormal gait.

Instability is virtually confined to the hip, although foot drop and the extended knee of quadriceps weakness are possibilities. Gluteal weakness, subluxation and dislocation, or infantile coxa vara are all capable of causing hip instability.

Shortening may be apparent or real. Apparent shortening is not exclusively due to pelvic obliquity but may also be the presenting feature in hip flexion deformity. This may arise for reasons within the abdomen such as psoas spasm with acute appendicitis. True shortening should present no difficulty.

Limp in cerebral palsy is most likely to be seen in hemiplegia when the heel reaches the ground by hyperextending the knee, but it may of course be a feature of any variety. Spinocerebellar ataxia may at first be difficult to recognize, as may the limp of slowly progressing acquired spasticity.

Other less common causes include pain from subacute osteomyelitis (page 44), crack fractures in cystic lesions (page 28) and osteoid osteoma (page 31).

Lastly, it should be emphasized that normally painful conditions may declare themselves by limp alone, as in, for example, Perthes' disease and adolescent coxa vara.

Hysterical limp is considered below.

Hysteria

Children are in general unsophisticated people who, if they wish to draw attention to themselves, go about it in a pleasantly straight-forward manner. Thus limp is favoured more than the backache of disgruntled adults.

There are two common varieties: firstly, the imitative limp and, secondly, the grotesque. The imitative limp is the more difficult, for, being borrowed from a member of the family or a neighbour and carefully reproduced, it has a certain verisimilitude. The grotesque limp is easier to recognize for it resembles nothing that one has seen before. One of the advantages of becoming older in medicine is that experience grows with time, so that something entirely outside this at once raises the suspicion of an emotional component.

Most hysterical symptoms in childhood are superficial, when they are reflected in obvious musculoskeletal derangements. Usually a parent, teacher or companion has hit them and they are determined that they will 'show them up' for the brutes they are. The situation is somewhat analogous to the half-hearted suicide attempts of unrequited love. Once they have reached hospital their objective is almost achieved. 'Treatment' is arranged in collusion with the physiotherapist and the child is promised a cure thereby. Most have fully recovered at the next attendance. If not, it is most important to eliminate, as far as possible, any physical cause for the limp, and a bone scan can be a very useful investigation in this situation. If no physical cause can be found for the child's persistent limp, psychiatric opinion should be sought.

Backache

Backache is unusual in young children (Chapter 12) but becomes commoner in adolescence, and is of course commonplace in adults.

In examining the child it is important to realize that abnormalities of contour and rhythm of movement are more prominent signs than loss of movement. Thus in spondylolisthesis there is often a tilt of the whole spine from the lumbosacral junction as the child bends and touches his toes. Similarly, in low grade osteomyelitis (page 44) there may be a short angular kyphoscoliosis apparent only on full flexion. Local tenderness is an important sign and so is pain exacerbated by jumping. Straight leg raising is restricted in low lesions but seldom by pain. Neurological signs in the legs are commonly found as befits the probable serious nature of the underlying cause.

Backache in a young child must therefore be assumed to be of great significance until it is proved otherwise, or disappears spontaneously.

The initial radiographs will disclose many of the causes, including spondylolisthesis and established discitis. As in days gone by when tuberculosis was the feared diagnosis, low grade inflammatory lesions may appear on the radiograph long after they are suspected on clinical grounds. Vertebral collapse in leukaemia and secondary neuroblastoma are other examples of this.

Spinal tumours are usually developmental (spinal dysraphism) so that tell-tale lesions in the overlying skin are sought. In this connection neurofibromatosis is also considered. Dysraphism is supported if there are other radiological signs such as spina bifida, a central spur or a local area of vertebral confusion. Signs of an expanding lesion are best seen as widening of the interpeduncular distance over several segments, for vertebral scalloping may be difficult to distinguish from the normal, especially in the lumbar spine. Enuresis, frequency and urgency are equally important. In all these circumstances myelography, CT scan and sometimes MRI may be indicated.

Children sometimes present with the signs of intervertebral disc prolapse. Recovery is usual on bed rest and the prognosis is therefore more favourable than in adolescence. Miscellaneous painful conditions with obscure vertebral body, appendage or disc lesions are better explored, usually by needle biopsy, and the diagnosis established than treated expectantly.

Inequality of leg length

The disappearance of poliomyelitis in the western world has considerably reduced the patients for whom leg equalization operations are necessary. There remain, however, the discrepancies due to congenital anomalies, the effects of growth plate injury (traumatic or infective) and some with neurological disorders.

The neurological causes are cerebral palsy and myelomeningocele. The discrepancy in the former has rarely been considered to warrant correction for it seldom exceeds 2.5 cm but in myelomeningocele one is confronted by the problem of disabling discrepancy in two ways. Firstly, the neurological deficit may be largely unilateral so that one small paralysed limb is seen, its fellow being relatively normal. Leg lengthening when there is a sensory deficit does not appeal and it seems irrational to shorten the normal side, so amputation and prosthetic correction is preferred. Secondly, when one hip is dislocated and there is an adduction deformity due to pelvic obliquity, the apparent lengthening on the opposite side may be a handicap and leg shortening will be of benefit.

Discrepancy due to lengthening in neurofibromatosis (page 83) and congenital arteriovenous communications (page 18) is treated by shortening of the longer abnormal side either by epiphyseal arrest at an appropriate time or by deliberate shortening which may need to be repeated before the end of growth. When diffuse disease causes unilateral shortening, as in dyschondroplasia (page 7), leg lengthening may now be considered. There is no certain means of calculating the final discrepancy in such conditions, so the extent and timing of correction must be carefully considered.

Shortening due to injury or disease of the growth plate is also somewhat unpredictable, for the lesions are frequently incomplete, such that some growth continues which may, however, be asymmetrical. Furthermore, some compensatory growth may occur from elsewhere such as from the trochanteric epiphysis when the capital epiphysis is lost. In general, therefore, it is best to wait until maturity is approaching and the likely extent of the final disproportion evident. Complete growth plate destruction at, for example, the lower femoral epiphysis, causes a predictable discrepancy and this may be calculated by referring to the lower limb growth tables for boys and girls (Anderson, Green and Messner, 1963). In these circumstances the programme of treatment may be decided upon from the beginning.

Shortening due to congenital dysplasia of the limb, such as short tibia and femur (pp. 182 and 153) tend to remain proportional to the length of the normal side throughout growth. Thus it is possible to reach a reasonable estimate of the likely eventual shortening by determining the proportion by which the limb is short in the young child and then estimating the probable length of the normal femur at maturity by comparing the child with his parents.

We are largely concerned with differences between 3 and 15 cm. If less than 3 cm is involved, leg equalization is not indicated unless the patient is very short. Above 15 cm it is usually necessary to lengthen both bones or to perform repeated lengthenings by the methods described by Wagner (1978) and De Bastiani *et al.* (1986). These are exacting techniques which are sometimes associated with serious complications. Other factors to be considered are the expected final height of the patient calculated from the size of the parents and the usefulness or otherwise of the affected limb. Extreme discrepancy and distal abnormality favour the choice of amputation.

The methods employed are leg lengthening, leg shortening and growth plate inhibition or arrest (epiphysiodesis). There have been major advances in leg-lengthening techniques in the last 10 to 20 years. An excellent review was published recently by Paley (1988). Wagner and De Bastiani (orthofix) use a unilateral lengthening device whereas Ilizarov in Russia and Montecelli in Rome have evolved the circumferential device. The pace of lengthening is approximately 1 mm per day achieved by 4 quarter turns of 0.25 mm. The technique of Callotasi or callus stretching allows the callus to form before lengthening starts and then stretches the callus as the bone is lengthening avoiding the need for plating and grafting as in the original Wagner method. As a result of these advances it is much easier to advise leg lengthening to patients. However it remains a sophisticated and demanding technique, particularly when applied to congenital shortening where all the tissues and not only the bones are short and length is particularly difficult to gain without complications. The overall time taken from the start of lengthening to final consolidation reported by De Bastiani is 30–40 days per centimetre gained. Therefore to gain 5 cm in one bone will take approximately 150–200 days of treatment. This is much quicker than with the old method. The patient remains mobile in the device and is treated largely as an outpatient so that there is much less disruption of normal life for the child.

Deliberate leg shortening is usually performed at or near skeletal maturity. The femur is best shortened at the level of the lesser trochanter but retaining the lesser trochanter. Many surgeons do not like tibial shortening but it can be performed by a step cut in its middle third. Fixation is by nail plate or plate.

Epiphyseal arrest by obliterating the epiphyseal plate is a reliable and predictable operation, but epiphyseal stapling at an earlier age is, in our opinion, too prone to complications and secondary effects to use as a standard method. Pilcher (1962) emphasized this in reporting the results in some of our patients followed to maturity.

Amputation for congenital abnormalities

Amputation may be indicated in neurofibromatosis (page 83) when the limb is painful, deformed and long, and in dyschondroplasia (page 7) for deformity and shortening. Vascular malformations – such as arteriovenous fistula with heart failure or peripheral ulceration – may be an indication for amputation, as are diffuse angiomatous malformations associated with gigantism and uncontrolled anaemia. The choice between disarticulation through the joint and conventional level amputation will depend upon the state of the limb and its joints. It is an interesting observation that, in children, amputation through the bone commonly gives rise to overgrowth of the bone and the necessity for stump revision, whereas amputation through joints rarely does so.

Myelomeningocele with unilateral predominance or intractable ulceration has been mentioned. Disarticulation will be preferred in the presence of diminished sensibility, unless local excisions of part of the foot seem feasible. In arthrogryposis (page 85) or severe stiffness with skin webbing, through-knee amputation should not be unduly withheld if the knee is stiff and flexed and the limb is short. Sometimes this is necessary on both sides.

Congenital amputations rarely require revision except to trim excrescences such as finger buds with nails. Severe dysplasia of one or more bones of the leg is the main indication, when shortening is irremediable and deformity considerable. In these cases disarticulation is preferred, such as Syme's amputation for absent fibula and short tibia (page 182) or through-knee for absent tibia, but less common anomalies will dictate their own levels. Curious, there is a relative lack of skin in these children and flaps should be cut longer than seems necessary (Fulford and Hall, 1968).

Chronology of diseases

During growth, modifications of form and structure are more rapid than at any other time. As a result, we observe a certain age specificity in the presentation of disease which reflects the changing internal environment and the degree of maturity. It is often helpful, therefore, to pay attention to the age of the child when there is uncertainty about diagnosis. Some illustrative situations may be mentioned.

When a baby of less than 3 months of age presents with a swollen limb and the radiograph discloses periostitis, scurvy is most unlikely to be the cause, for by this time the child will not have exhausted the vitamin C with which he is provided at birth. Thus we will suspect the alternatives of injury, osteomyelitis or even congenital syphilis. Even later, when scurvy may be present, it is fruitless to search for bleeding from the gums before the teeth have erupted.

Whereas scurvy is a striking example of time-limited natural immunity, most age-linked conditions are related to the degree of maturation of the system affected – be it osseous, nervous, vascular or some other. Thus it may be impossible to recognize osteochondrodystrophy on the radiograph during the first 2 years of life because ossification is not sufficiently advanced. For the same reason we may fail to recognize the early stages of a disease whose final form is well known. Dyschondroplasia, for example, is at first represented by streaks of translucency spreading from the growth plate towards the metaphysis – a radiological sign which bears little relationship to the deformed and expanded bones so easily recognizable in the adolescent. Similarly, neurofibromatosis sometimes declares itself as tibial kyphosis without pigmentation or superficial tumours. These may not appear for many years whereas pigmentation in fibrous dysplasia frequently anticipates the bone lesions.

The age of onset will often serve as a guide towards an accurate prognosis. Delay in presentation of some general congenital disorders usually suggests a relatively benign variant. Osteogenesis imperfecta, if obvious at birth, usually has a grave outlook whereas when fractures occur for the first time after walking begins, a happier future may be expected. The prognosis in idiopathic scoliosis is closely related to the age of onset for, in general, delay is favourable.

Disorders of the central nervous system frequently cause peripheral deformities to develop at an age related to the onset of the neurlogical deficit. Pes cavus first presenting at 3 years of age is likely to be secondary to myelodysplasia; at 7 years of age to peroneal muscular atrophy or spinal dysraphism; and at 14 years of age to Friedreich's ataxia.

Diseases of joints also have their proper and favoured seasons. Osteochondritis of the capitulum and navicular may occur at 5 years of age; at the knee it is rare before 10 years of age; and the carpal lunate is affected towards maturity. Similarly, signs of arthritis of the hip, if below 5 years of age are likely to be due to juvenile chronic arthritis; from 5 to 10 years of age to Perthes' disease; and from 10 to 15 years of age to displaced femoral epiphysis – if in each case this is not a rapidly resolving synovitis.

A few examples have been given to emphasize the value of a knowledge of the age incidence of disease as an aid to diagnosis and prognosis in many childhood affections.

Genetic considerations

Congenital skeletal abnormalities represent the quotient of genetic and environmental influences (Carter, 1966).

Genetic factors are of three types. Firstly, there are chromosome abnormalities which rarely display skeletal abnormalities as the major fault but in whom these are frequently present. Examples are mongolism with a dislocated hip and Turner's syndrome with Madelung's deformity. Chromosome investigation is specially indicated when skeletal deformity is associated with dysplasia of the sex organs.

Secondly, there is the multifactorial group. In these cases there is an inherited predisposition to some condition but its severity may not exceed the limit of normal variation. When, however, some other marginally abnormal feature is also inherited they may combine to cause a true congenital malformation. For example, congenital but very mild acetabular dysplasia may pass unrecognized, but if in addition there is joint laxity, dislocation is likely.

Lastly, there are mutant genes, the commonest and therefore the most important factors. The fertilized primitive germ cells contain two autosomes (the chromosome complement less the X or Y sex chromosomes) and the abnormal gene may be linked with one or both autosomes or the X chromosome. If genes of one autosome are abnormal the influence is said to be 'dominant'; if of both, 'recessive'. If the abnormal genes are attached to the X chromosome it is 'sex linked'. The genes are attached in large numbers to the many phosphate, sugar and base chains of the chromosome which are in groups of three.

These terms are difficult to orientate because one may not unreasonably think that 'dominant' means dominating and so the effect is likely to be present in every child of affected parents in perpetuity, and that 'recessive' means receding and so less likely to penetrate into all the offspring, and, if so, with less severity than the dominant types. 'Dominant' also suggests that the anatomical abnormality in the cell is worse but in fact only one, rather than two autosomes, is involved. This concept is in part misleading for it applies the term to the child rather than the parents to whom inherited 'dominant' and 'recessive' refer.

Thus in dominant autosomal inheritance the parent is always affected and half the children inherit the obvious abnormality in varying degree. The others escape obvious abnormality and do not carry the abnormal gene as a danger to their children. In dominant mutation some accident occurred at conception, for the parents are normal but one child is abnormal and will pass on his defect to half his children, but further siblings may all be normal and their children are not at risk.

In recessive inheritance the parents are normal clinically, but have by mischance mated not knowing that they both carry this unobtrusive abnormality. Not all the children are affected, for about three out of four escape clinical effect, but, of these, one out of two will carry the same hazard to their children as each of their parents did to them.

'Sex-linked' abnormalities are easier to understand, for, being linked with the X chromosome, they are unlikely to produce a clinical effect in females who have two X chromosomes but will be transmitted by the mother to affect the male who has only one X chromosome (XY). Haemophilia is the outstanding example. When the female has only one X chromosome (Turner's syndrome, XO), she may be affected, and also when she inherits two mutant genes and both X chromosomes are at fault.

Abnormalities of the genes produce their effects by disturbing normal enzyme reactions or stimulating the synthesis of an abnormal biological protein, which in most cases is not yet identifiable. Important though they are, genetic factors seldom account wholly for abnormal development. Thus in identical twins both are likely to be affected, but in dizygotic (ordinary) twins one may be spared. Affected identical twins are seldom equally abnormal, an observation which implies that other factors are of some importance.

Environmental factors are probably equally significant. Experimentally, the developing fetus is influenced by a wide variety of substances, many of which are physiological but in higher than normal concentration, such as insulin and oxygen. In man, however, only a few drugs (thalidomide), some infections (rubella) and ionizing radiation are known to have a direct adverse influence on normal intrauterine development when the genes are normal. Clearly there is still a great deal to be learned about the part played by the environ-ment, and it is from an increasing knowledge of this that we may hope to see a reduction in the incidence of serious congenital abnormalities. With the advent of ultrasound scanning, amniocentesis, fetoscopy and other tests on the fetus, we are able to diagnose certain conditions while the child is still *in utero*. This surely is the growing age of medicine.

References

Anderson, M., Green, W. T. and Messner, M. B. (1963) Growth and predictions of growth in the lower extremities. *J. Bone Jt. Surg.* **45A**, 1

Carter, C. O. (1966) The general aetiology of disorders of the skelton. In *Clinical Surgery*, vol. 13, *Orthopaedics*. London: Butterworths

De Bastiani, G., Aldegheri, R., Brivio, L. R. and Trivella, G. (1986) Chondrodiatasis – controlled symmetrical distraction of the epiphyseal plate. *J. Bone Jt. Surg.* **68B**, 550

Fulford, G. E. and Hall, M. J. (1968) *Amputation and Prosthesis*. Bristol: John Wright

Paley, D. (1988) Current techniques of limb lengthening. *J. Ped. Orthop.* **8**, 73–92

Pilcher, M. F. (1962) Epiphyseal stapling. *J. Bone Jt. Surg.* **44B**, 82

Wagner, H. (1978) Operative lengthening of the femur. *Clin. Orthop. Related Res.* **136**, 125

Further reading

Smith, D. W. (1982) *Major Problems in Clinical Pediatrics,*, vol. 7, *Recognizable Patterns of Human Malformation,* 3rd edn. Philadelphia, London, Toronto: W. B. Saunders

Wynne-Davies, R. (1973) *Heritable Disorders in Orthopaedic Practice*. Oxford, Edinburgh, London: Blackwell Scientific

Index